IMAGES OF WAR

THE ROYAL ARMY MEDICAL CORPS IN THE GREAT WAR

RARE PHOTOGRAPHS FROM WARTIME ARCHIVES

Timothy McCracken

Pen & Sword
MILITARY

First published in Great Britain in 2017 by
PEN & SWORD MILITARY
An imprint of
Pen & Sword Books Ltd
47 Church Street
Barnsley
South Yorkshire
S70 2AS

Copyright © Timothy McCracken, 2017

ISBN 978-1-47389-232-3

The right of Timothy McCracken to be identified as author of this work has been asserted by him in accordance with the Copyright, Designs and Patents Act 1988.

A CIP catalogue record for this book is available from the British Library.

All rights reserved. No part of this book may be reproduced or transmitted in any form or by any means, electronic or mechanical including photocopying, recording or by any information storage and retrieval system, without permission from the Publisher in writing.

Typeset by Concept, Huddersfield, West Yorkshire HD4 5JL.
Printed and bound in England by CPI Group (UK) Ltd, Croydon CR0 4YY.

Pen & Sword Books Limited incorporates the imprints of Atlas, Archaeology, Aviation, Discovery, Family History, Fiction, History, Maritime, Military, Military Classics, Politics, Select, Transport, True Crime, Air World, Frontline Publishing, Leo Cooper, Remember When, Seaforth Publishing, The Praetorian Press, Wharncliffe Local History, Wharncliffe Transport, Wharncliffe True Crime and White Owl.

For a complete list of Pen & Sword titles please contact
PEN & SWORD BOOKS LIMITED
47 Church Street, Barnsley, South Yorkshire S70 2AS, England
E-mail: enquiries@pen-and-sword.co.uk
Website: www.pen-and-sword.co.uk

Contents

Acknowledgements 4

Introduction 5

Chapter One
   Faces of the RAMC 15

Chapter Two
   The United Kingdom 28

Chapter Three
   France and Belgium 85

Chapter Four
   A Global War 147

Chapter Five
   After the Conflict 174

Bibliography 189

Acknowledgements

Mr Bryan Armstrong and Mr William Laidlaw, Dumfriesshire Newspaper Group, Annan, for access to the newspaper group archives.

Dr Sarah Barber and Dr Timothy Hickman, who both provided specialist insight into the use of photographs as historical sources in seminars at Lancaster University.

Mr Chris Buswell for research advice.

Mr Glen Carr who provided an excellent foundation for further study through inspiring school history teaching.

Professor Karl-Erik Frandsen who provided exceptional guidance in developing research skills through seminars at the University of Copenhagen.

Ms Barbara Janman for research advice and willingness to share her extensive knowledge of the RAMC in the First World War.

Mr Peter John for research advice.

Mr Alexander McCracken and Mrs Ruth Latimer McCracken for research advice and assistance in locating photographic sources.

Mr Andrew Read for research advice.

Dr Thomas Rohkrämer and Dr Alan Warburton, who both provided detailed insight into the consequences of the First World War for individuals and societies, in seminars at Lancaster University.

Ms Gail Anderson and the Army Medical Services Museum, Aldershot, for research advice.

Ms Emily Oldfield and the British Red Cross Museum and Archives, London, for research advice.

The late Mr Reginald Leonard Barrett-Cross for research advice and willingness to share his extensive knowledge of the RAMC in the First World War.

* * *

This book is dedicated to all who served with
military and voluntary medical services
during the First World War.

Introduction

The Royal Army Medical Corps (RAMC) was formed on 23 June 1898; the Medical Staff merged with the Medical Staff Corps, uniting senior officers with lower ranks, to form the RAMC. Later in that year the RAMC provided medical support at the Battle of Omdurman in September 1898, during the Sudan campaign. Until October 1899 the RAMC provided support to the army around the globe in conflicts of relatively small scale. The South African War of 1899–1902 would prove a challenge for the RAMC. Around 500,000 British troops were involved in the conflict, with approximately 6,000 killed in combat, 21,000 wounded and 16,000 dying of disease.

The experiences of the South African War made it necessary to review preparations for treating large numbers of battle casualties and the importance of preventing disease, including enteric fever. After the war, Royal Commissions and War Office Committees examined the arrangements for the treatment of sick and wounded. The Russo-Japanese War of 1904–5 also provided important areas of learning. The 1906 Geneva Convention provided a basis for the development of further voluntary aid and enhanced consideration was given to the Army Nursing Service.

In the period between the South African War and the outbreak of war in 1914, many other changes to the administration of the medical services took place. These included the creation of field ambulance medical units; the organisation of zones of work, including casualty clearing hospitals; consideration of transportation systems, including motor ambulances; recognition of the role of specialist RAMC sanitary units; the organisation of hospital accommodation for convalescents and the expansion of temporary hospital provision in a time of war.

In 1902 Queen Alexandra's Imperial Military Nursing Service (QAIMNS) was formed; by 1914 it had more than 290 members. Previously there was an Army Nursing Service, supported by an Army Nursing Service Reserve, founded by HRH Princess Christian in 1896 and officially recognised and established in Army Orders in 1897. The Reserve played an important role in the South African War, with 805 members serving in South Africa, 33 at other locations overseas and 538 in the UK. In 1910 the Queen Alexandra's Imperial Military Nursing Service Reserve (QAIMNSR) was formed which gradually absorbed the members of the Army Nursing Service Reserve.

In 1911 a Civil Hospital Reserve was formed to supplement the nursing services of military hospitals in the event of war; in 1914 there were 800 members of this reserve force. The number of trained nursing staff was further increased by the special training of a number of RAMC personnel by QAIMNS matrons and nursing sisters. Personnel of the RAMC were also eligible for special training as masseurs, as operating room attendants and in electro-therapeutics.

The Territorial and Reserve Forces Act of 1907 created the Territorial Force (TF), abolishing the previous militia and volunteer forces, which formed new RAMC units. Territorial Force field ambulance units were formed throughout the UK, together with plans for twenty-three Territorial Force general hospitals staffed by local medical professionals. Contracts were also arranged to take over the necessary buildings as hospitals and to equip them upon mobilisation. A Territorial Force Nursing Service (TFNS) was also created for the purpose of staffing the RAMC Territorial Force general hospitals. At the outbreak of war the TFNS had 2,576 nurses ready for mobilisation.

A reserve of medical officers with military training was facilitated by the formation of medical companies of the Officers' Training Corps (OTC). This organisation was intended to standardise military training for medical students interested in taking a commission in the Regular Army, Special Reserve or the Territorial Force. Medical units of the OTC were formed at large universities where there were medical schools: at Edinburgh, Oxford and Cambridge Universities in 1908, London University in 1909, Dublin and Belfast Universities in 1910 and Aberdeen University in 1912. London University formed four units, Edinburgh two and the other universities one unit each. The approximate total number of cadets in training at any one time was 500 and the average length of training two-and-a-half to three years. In total around 1,900 medical students passed through the Officers' Training Corps from the time the medical units were formed and the outbreak of war in 1914. This training was very important in ensuring there were a number of medical officers with military training on mobilisation and throughout the conflict.

The formation of the Home Hospital Reserve was authorised from 1 April 1908. On the outbreak of war the St John Ambulance Brigade agreed to provide personnel for the military hospitals in England and Ireland and the St Andrew's Ambulance Association for military hospitals in Scotland. By 1911, there were 2,200 personnel enrolled in the reserve from the St John Ambulance Brigade and 82 from the St Andrew's Ambulance Association. A training schedule was organised for quartermasters and non-commissioned officers of the Home Hospital Reserve of eight days, every two years, in military hospitals. It was estimated 392 medical officers and 2,632 other ranks would be required from the St John Ambulance Brigade and 19 medical officers and 95 other ranks from the St Andrew's Ambulance Association. On mobilisation all personnel would receive equivalent rank in the RAMC, officers being commissioned and other ranks enlisted with permission to wear the uniforms of their voluntary aid organisation. This reserve was felt adequate for the replacement of regular army RAMC personnel in UK hospitals on mobilisation for war.

Following the South African War advances were also made in the training of officers and men of the RAMC in their administrative and military responsibilities in the field. The Army Medical School was moved from Netley, Hampshire to a new Medical Staff College in London. It was felt that this would aid progress through development. By 1907 Queen Alexandra's Military Hospital at Millbank and the Royal Army Medical College were united under the administrative control of the commandant of the college. Courses of instruction were organised for RAMC officers. A senior course, for captains prior to promotion to the rank of major, extended to nine months in 1912 and was one of the most thorough post-graduate medical courses in the United Kingdom.

By the outbreak of war in 1914 the RAMC and other military medical services were better prepared than they had ever been. Summary statistics associated with the UK medical services and the RAMC demonstrate the great challenges and accomplishments made during the First World War. A total maximum of 637,746 hospital beds were equipped and maintained in the UK and in theatres of war around the world. Around 770 medical units of all types were mobilised in the UK and sent overseas in support of military campaigns.

The challenges faced by the RAMC were shared by the medical services of all combatants in the First World War. These included modern weaponry, climatic conditions and the rapidly increasing size of armed forces. From August 1914 – August 1920, a total of 2,655,025 sick and wounded were brought to the UK for further treatment. By the Armistice in November 1918 there were 144,514 officers and other ranks serving in the military medical services, most of whom joined the RAMC and were trained in the United Kingdom.

The official general medical history of the British forces during the First World War is the *Medical Services General History – Official Medical History of the War* by Major General Sir W.G. Macpherson. This work, together with RAMC unit war diaries, provides great detail of, and insight into, the work of the medical services during the First World War. As this study is limited in length, these sources can be consulted for further in-depth information about the many units, campaigns and topics noted in this study. They also provide information about the numerous RAMC units not detailed in this volume.

Whilst the collections of the Imperial War Museum include a range of images illustrating the service of the RAMC in conflict areas, the focus of this study is on those who served with medical units, using images to illustrate some of their experiences.

In a corps as large as the RAMC, carrying out such a diverse range of duties, there was no common personal experience of the conflict. An individual, perhaps amongst many events and feelings, may have been wounded, injured or become ill; could have been taken prisoner of war; may have been decorated for bravery or distinguished service; could have experienced the loss of comrades and a feeling of sadness following the end of the conflict. It is hoped the aspects explored in this study will help to illustrate some of the experiences, shaped by the First World War, of those serving with RAMC units.

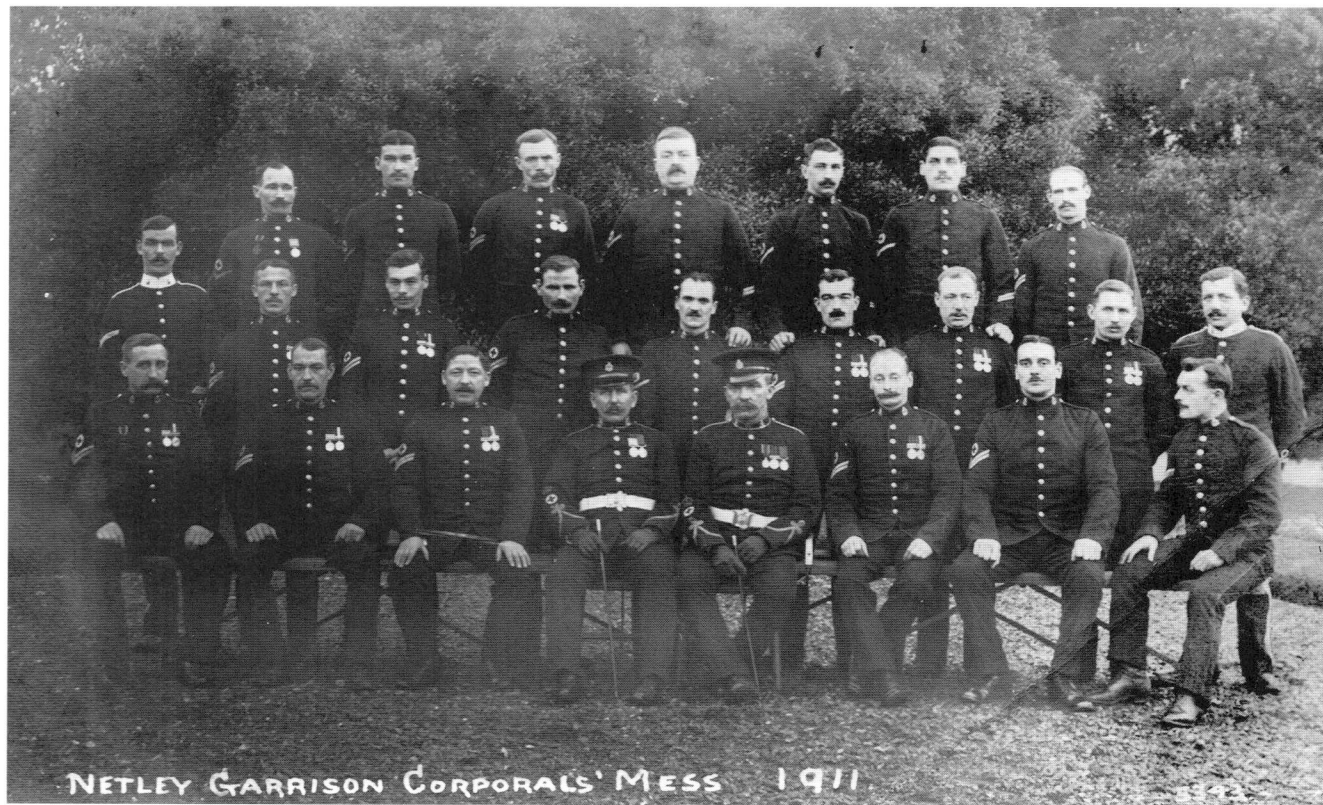

(**Above**) RAMC personnel of the Corporals' Mess, Netley Hospital. Several corporals wear Queen's South Africa and King's South Africa campaign medals, denoting their service in the South African War of 1899–1902. Several Long Service and Good Conduct medals are also worn. The photograph was sent to Lance Corporal Stoneham RAMC, Freetown, Sierra Leone, from London on 30 December 1911.

(**Opposite, above**) Officers and warrant officers at a RAMC Territorial Force unit camp, prior to the First World War. The warrant officer (back left) wears campaign medals from the Sudan campaign of 1898–1899. The warrant officer (back right) wears a Queen's South Africa campaign medal. Sitting front left is a chaplain.

(**Opposite, below left**) A private serving with a RAMC Territorial Force unit wearing dress uniform.

(**Opposite, below right**) A staff sergeant serving with a Territorial Force unit of the RAMC. He wears a Volunteer Long Service Good Conduct Medal and has five proficiency stars on his right sleeve.

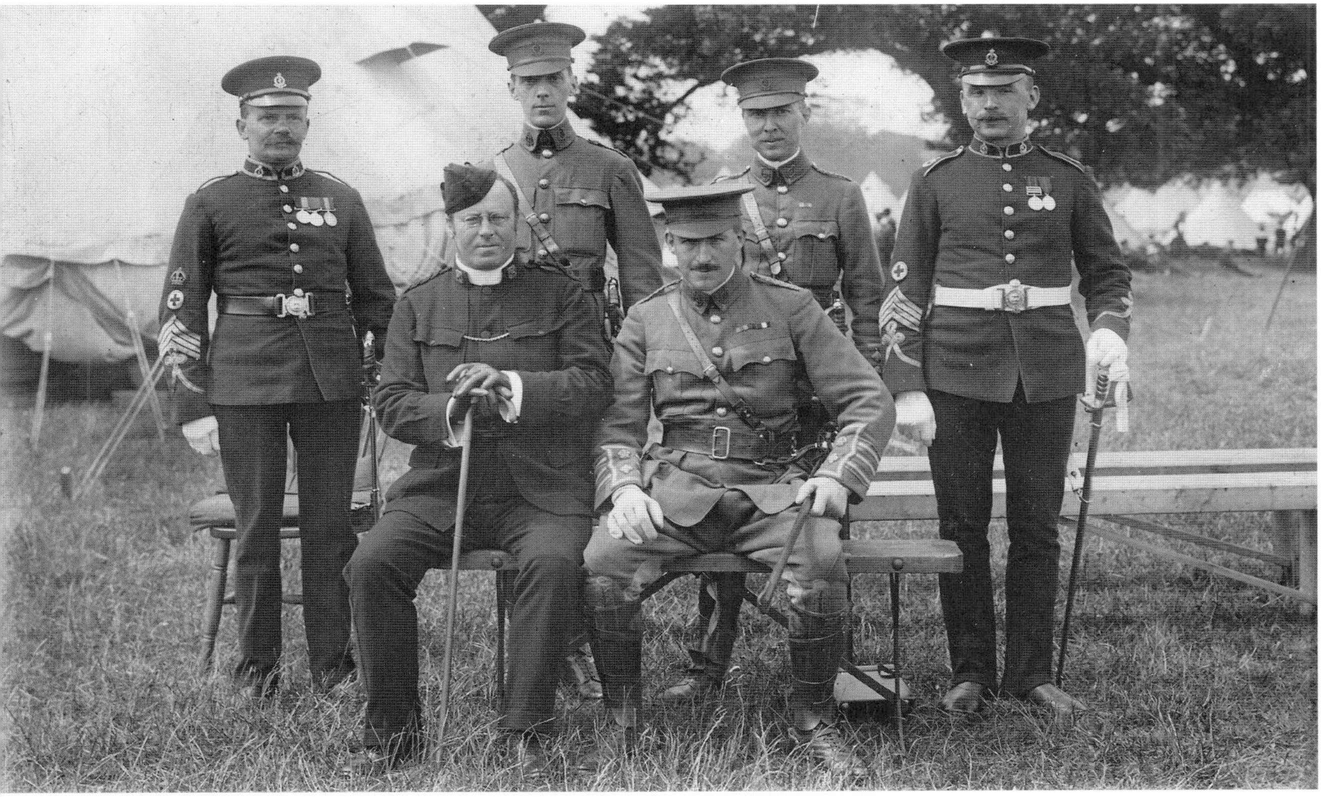

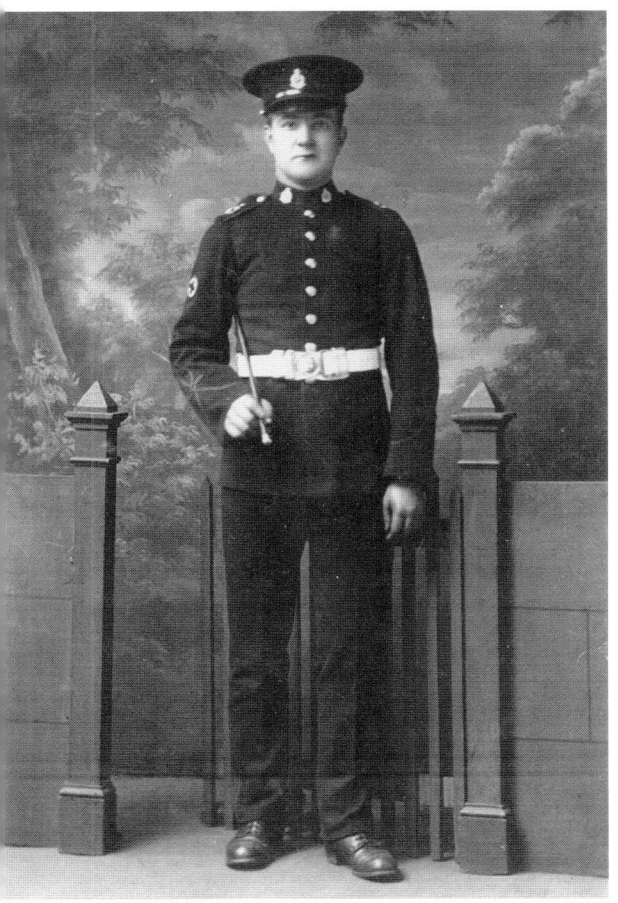
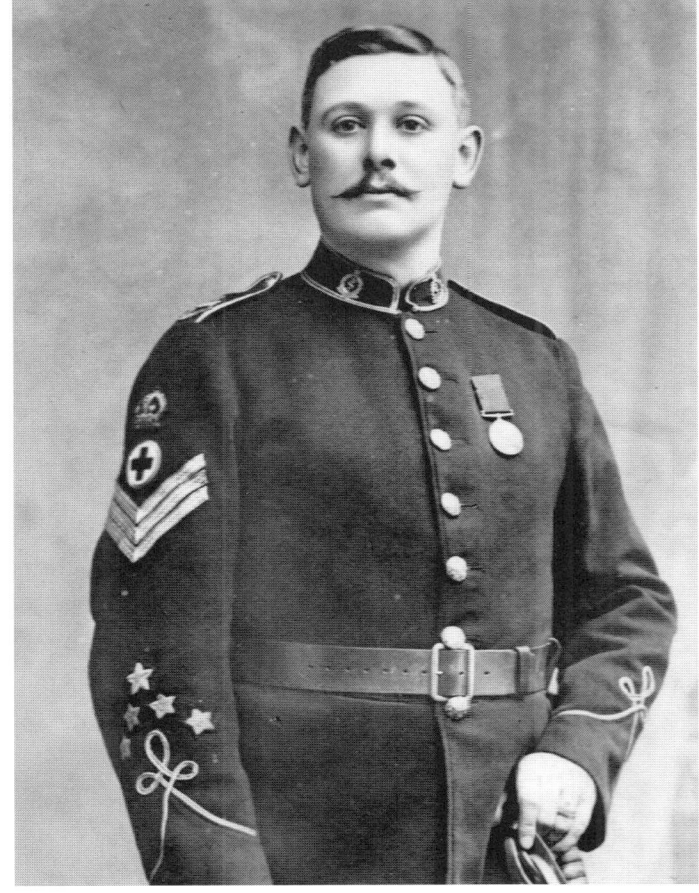

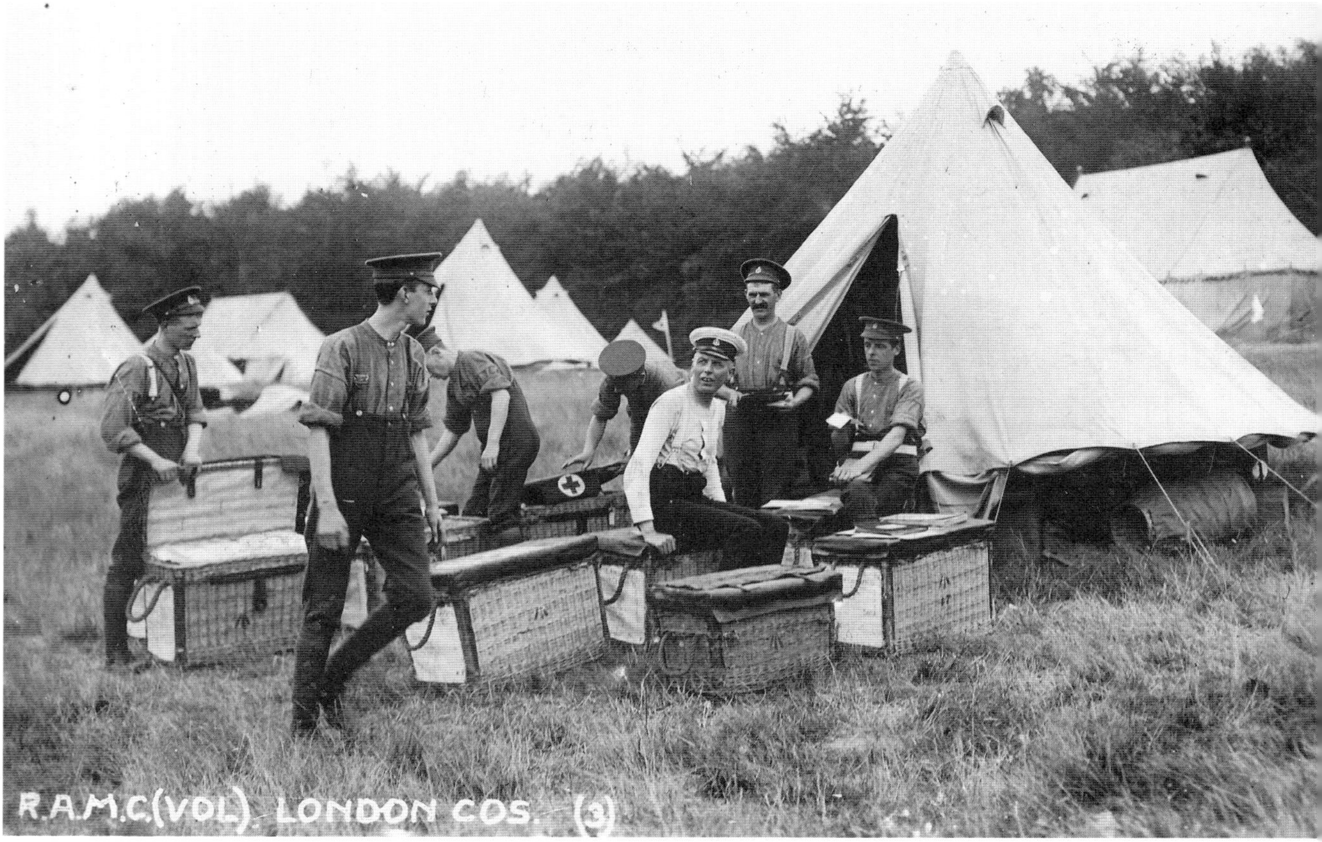

R.A.M.C.(VOL). LONDON COS. (3)

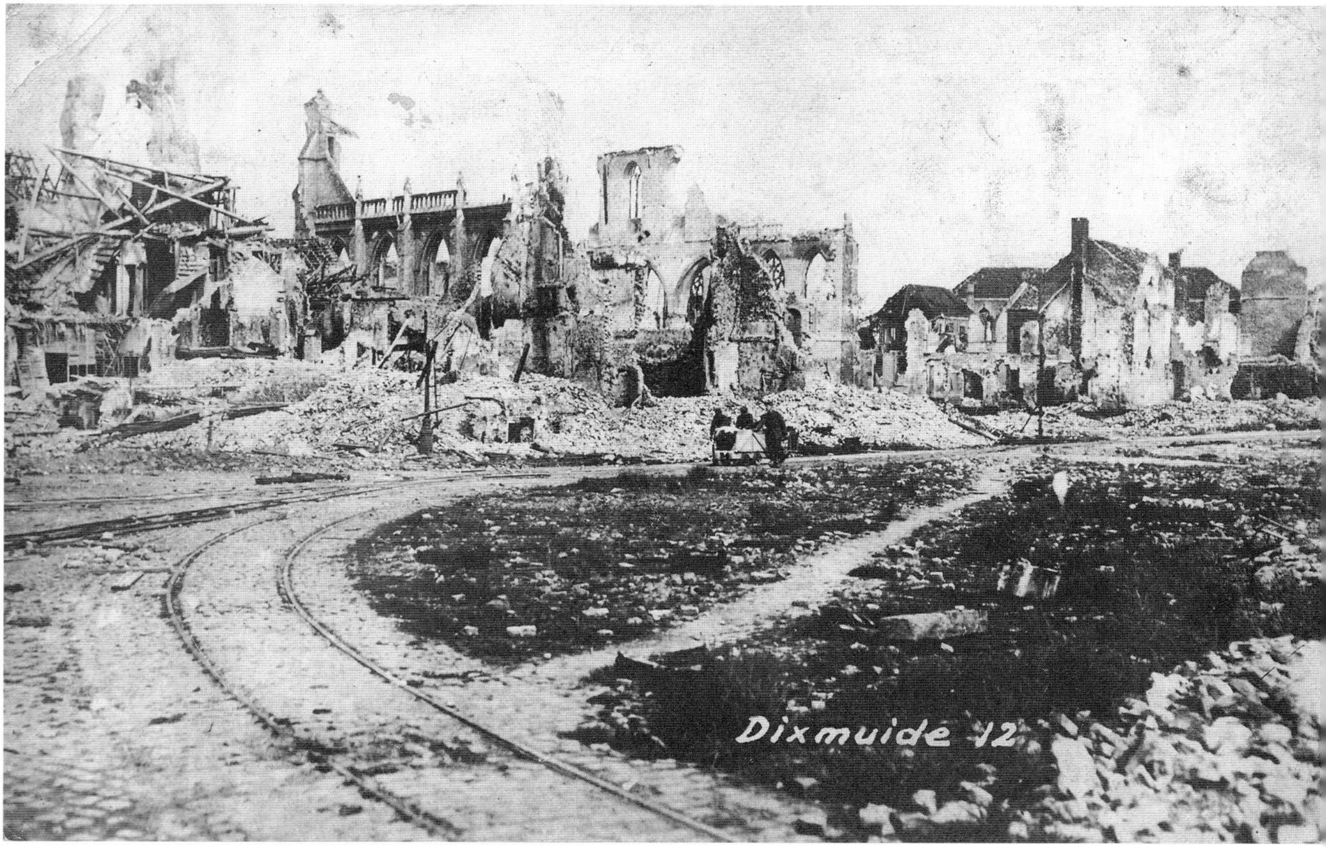

Dixmuide 12

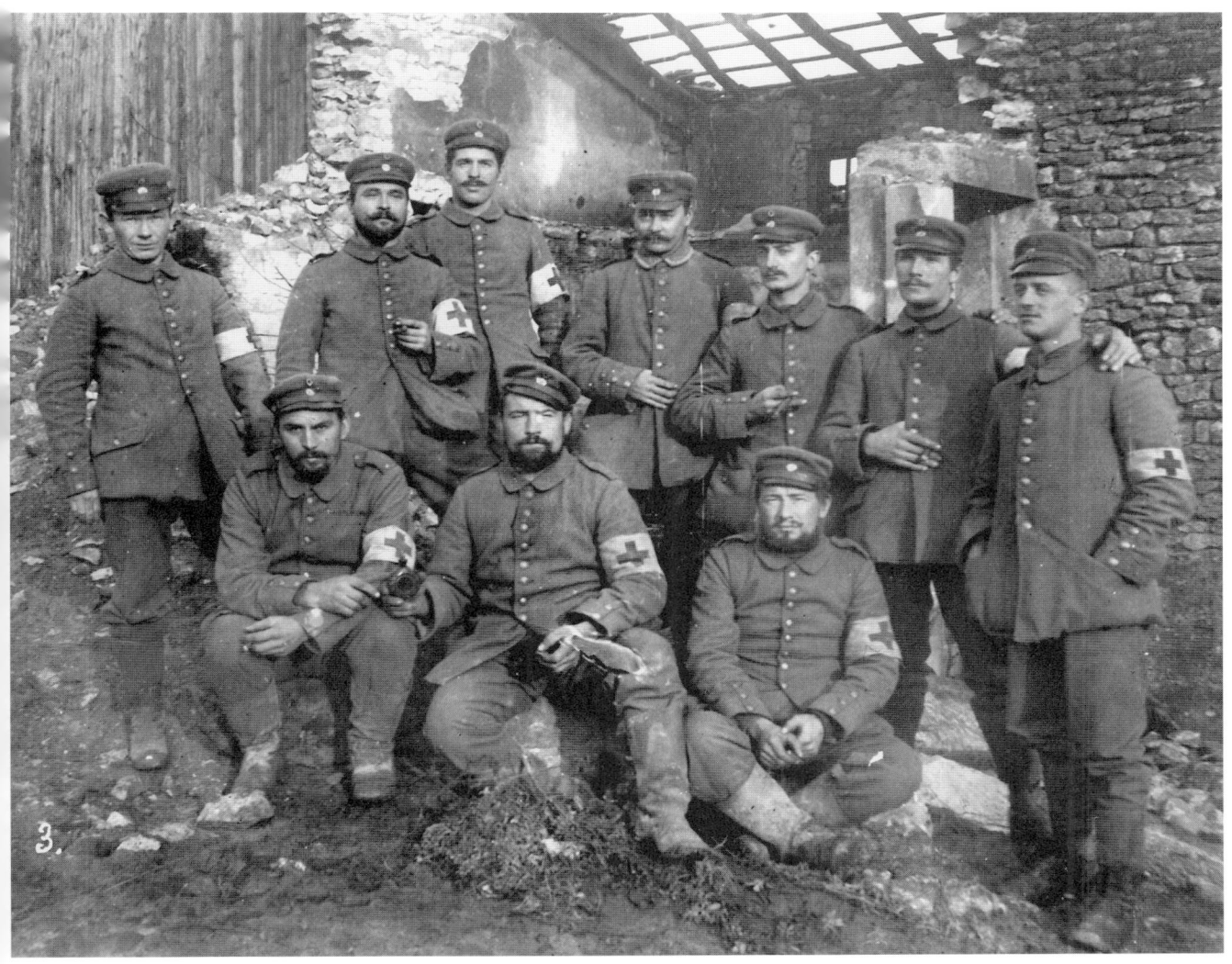

(**Opposite, above**) London Company RAMC (Volunteers), photographed at a training camp.

(**Opposite, below**) A casualty on light railway stretcher, Diksmuide, Belgium. The challenges of casualty evacuation meant combatants needed to develop, and use, a range of transportation methods.

(**Above**) German medical personnel serving with a stretcher-bearer company.

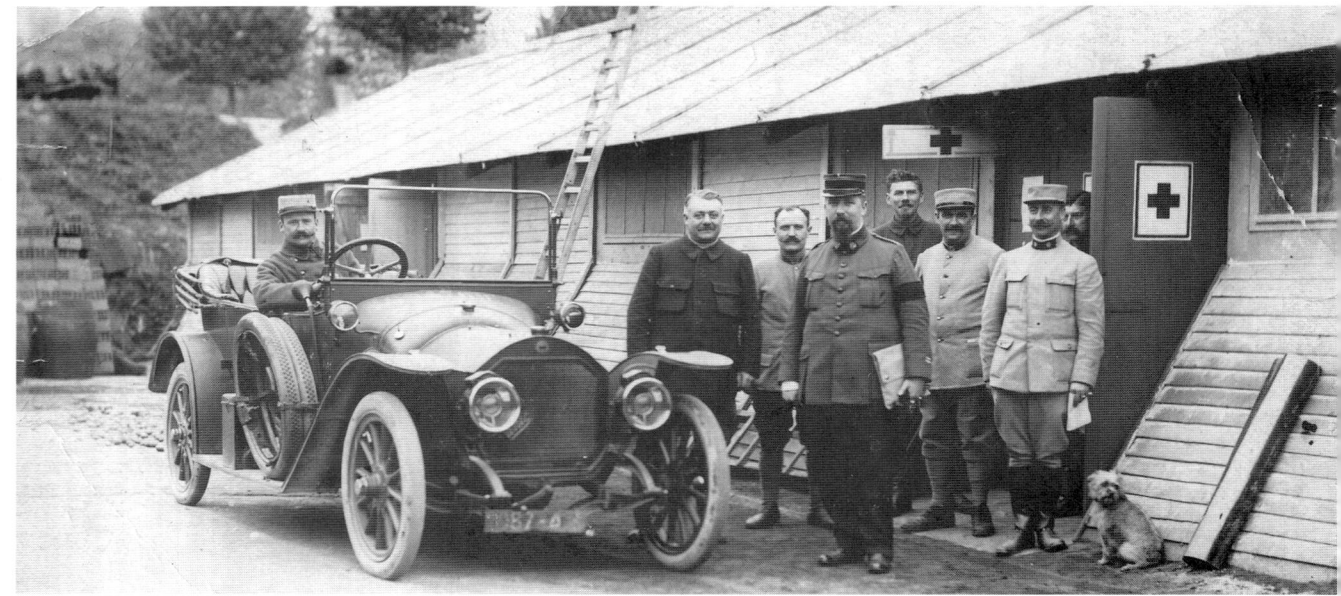

(**Above**) French military personnel outside a medical facility. The high numbers of casualties meant hutted and tented medical facilities were constructed to treat the sick and injured.

(**Opposite**) A French Army medic photographed on the Western Front. In addition to a Red Cross brassard he wears Rod of Asclepius collar badges. The Rod of Asclepius also forms part of the RAMC badge.

(**Below**) Patients and a nurse of Room 21, German Military Reserve Hospital Two, 1917. As the numbers of casualties increased, additional medical accommodation was created in reserve and auxiliary hospitals by all nations involved in the conflict.

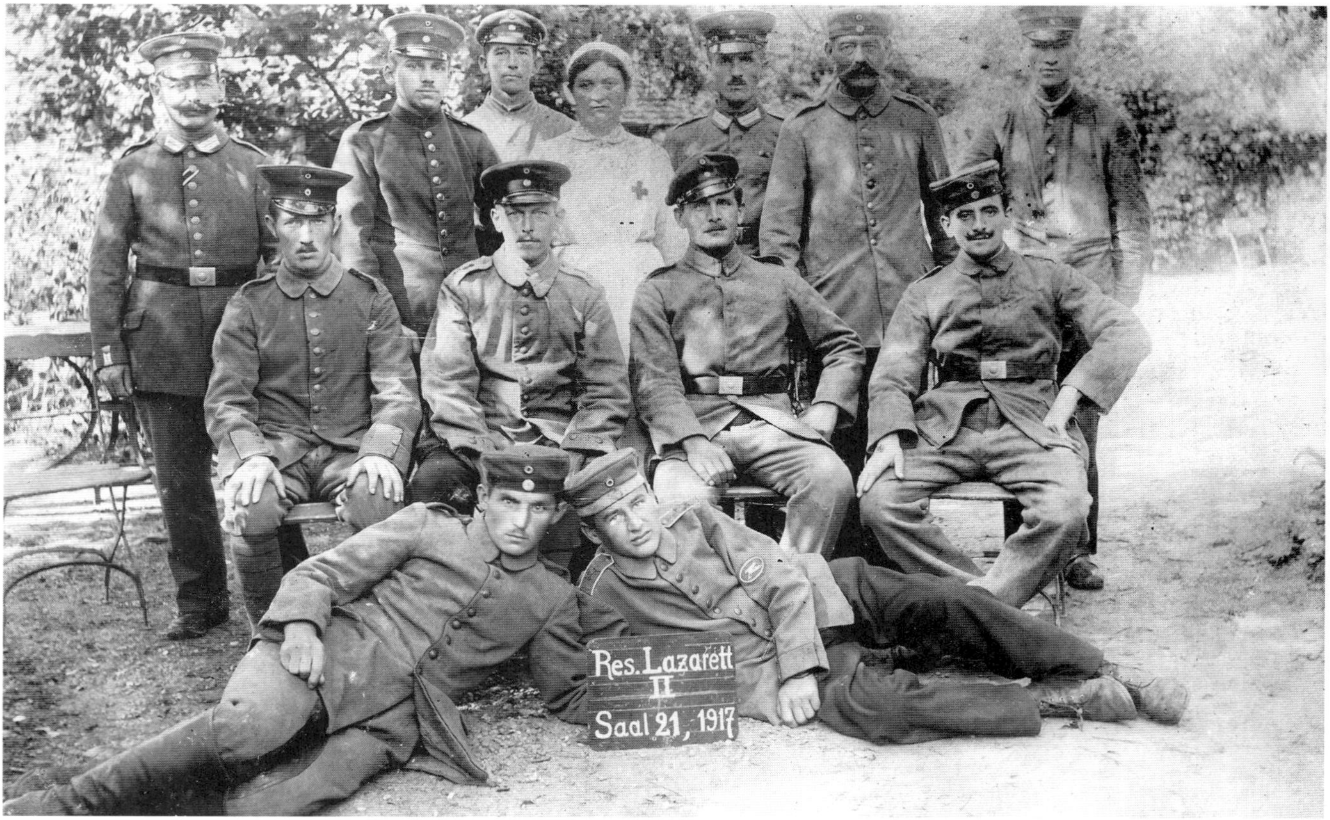

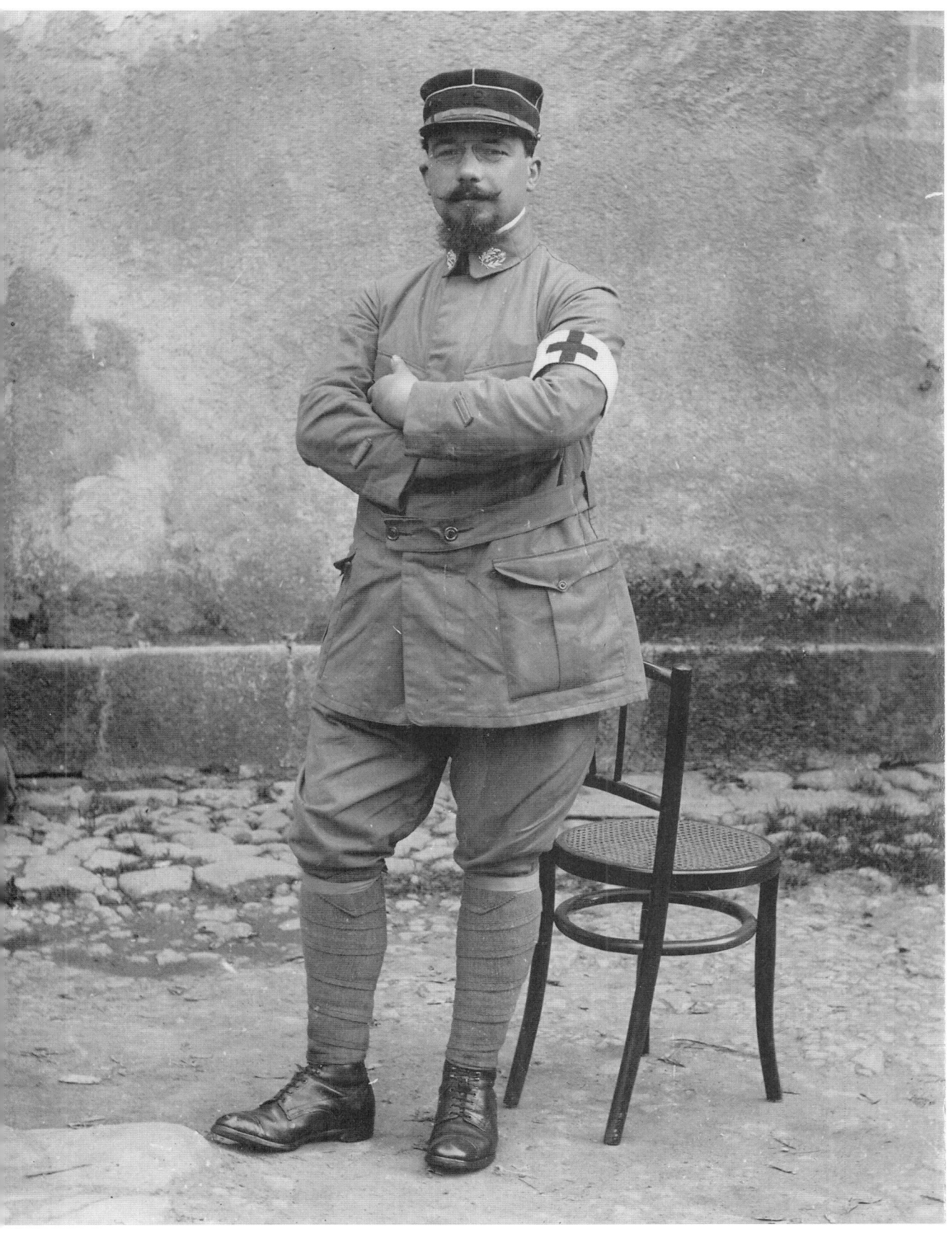

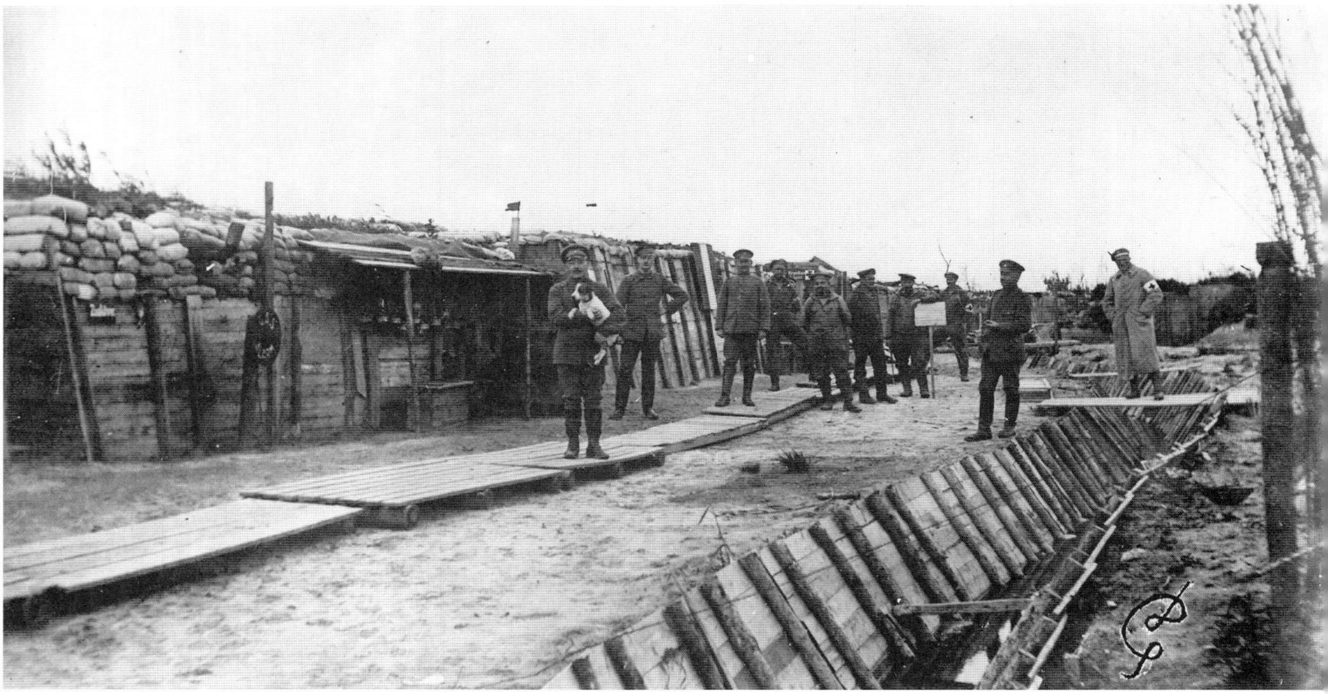

A German medical aid post in the Lombartzyde sector, Belgium.

Wounded French soldiers with an American voluntary nurse. The photo was taken in the American Ambulance Hospital, at Neuilly-sur-Seine, Paris, France, in September 1915. The photo was sent by Corporal Louis Corras, one of the patients in the photograph, to his sister-in-law, on 24 September 1915. Corporal Corras served with the 145th Territorial Regiment.

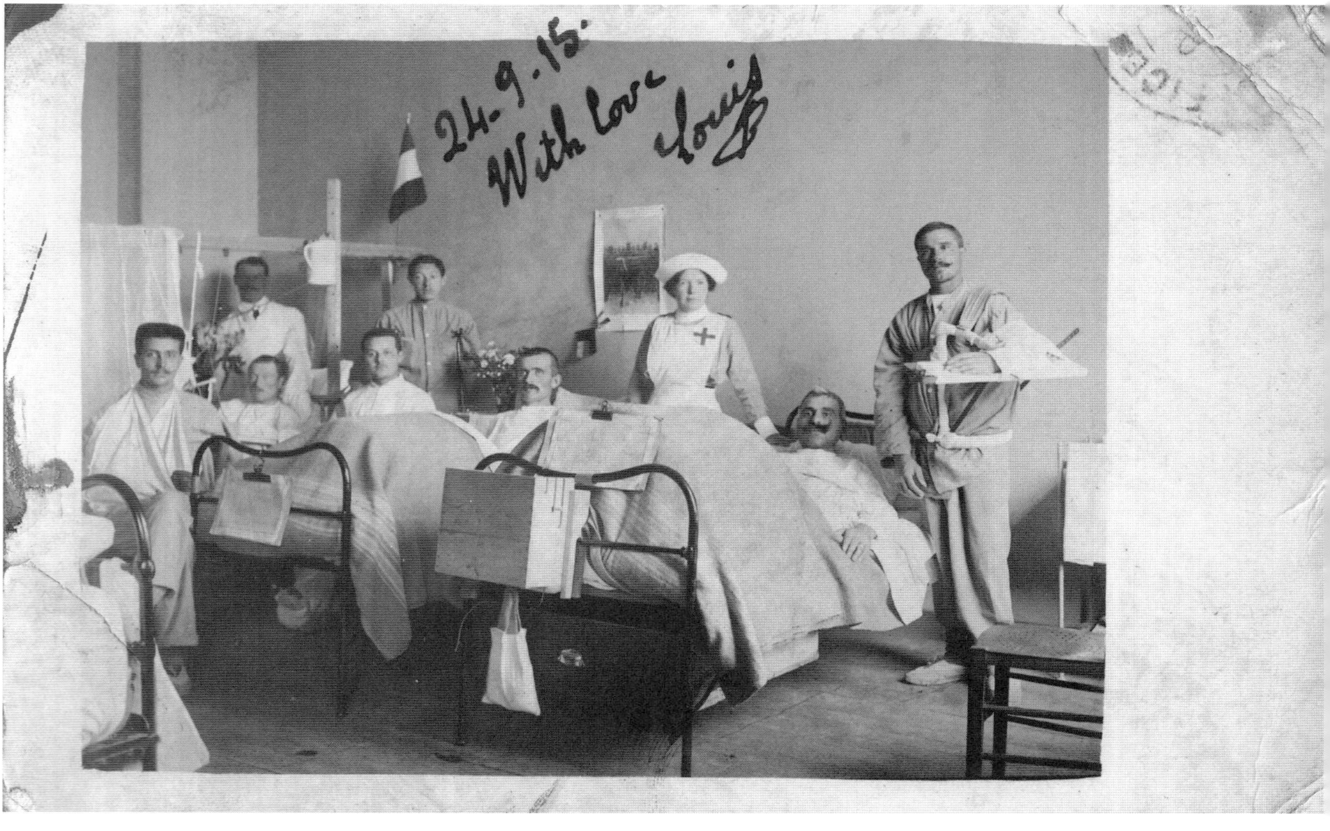

Chapter One

Faces of the RAMC

Throughout the First World War RAMC personnel served in many different units in the UK and overseas. The wide range of specialisms of RAMC personnel reflected the demands of modern warfare and the increasing challenges of providing medical care in a global conflict.

Following the outbreak of war in 1914, recruiting for the RAMC commenced in a similar way as for the rest of the army, except for officers and specialist medical professionals. As the conflict continued, demands for reinforcements for combatant regiments meant that recruiting for the RAMC was limited in numbers as well as military medical categories. Consequently the RAMC had to be assisted in providing hospital services, to a large extent by women. By 31 December 1915 there had been 66,139 voluntary enlistments into the RAMC, including the Home Hospital Reserve, but exclusive of the Territorial Force. After 1915 enlistment into the RAMC was governed by the Military Service Acts and service personnel assigned to the corps were generally of a lower category of physical fitness than that required for combatant units. This meant servicemen of the highest category of physical fitness already in the RAMC were gradually drafted into field medical units, with their positions in medical units on the lines of communication and in the UK filled by women, new recruits of lower physical fitness or service personnel discharged from hospital as unfit for general service. From 1915, Voluntary Aid Detachment (VAD) members were employed in military hospitals to replace RAMC personnel transferred to other medical units.

A brief overview of key aspects of medical service provision helps to illustrate the range of environments in which RAMC personnel served. Medical treatment was started as near to the front line as possible and a medical officer was attached to each infantry battalion (or other combat unit). The RAMC regimental medical officer had a RAMC sergeant or corporal attached to him and several RAMC other ranks. A field ambulance was the most forward of the RAMC units and there was one field ambulance attached to every brigade; each field ambulance also had a number of Army Service Corps (ASC) personnel attached, driving and managing the unit's ambulances. When out of the forward areas, the field ambulances were allocated special tasks such as running a divisional rest centre or a bath unit.

Located behind advanced dressing stations and main dressing stations staffed by field ambulances were casualty clearing stations (CCS). Transportation to a CCS could be via horse-drawn or motor ambulances, each with an ASC driver and RAMC attendant. The casualty clearing stations were intended to facilitate movement of casualties from the battlefield to hospitals and there was one CCS per division. Casualty clearing stations were usually situated mid-way between the front line and the base areas, in close proximity to a main railway line allowing ambulance train transportation. They provided surgical facilities and nursing staff worked with RAMC personnel. Nursing staff from a range of units including the QAIMNS, QAIMNSR and TFNS served at casualty clearing stations; this was the closest to the front line they served. Casualties could then be moved to stationary hospitals or general hospitals for further treatment.

General hospitals were located near railway lines to facilitate movement of casualties from the CCS. In the original mobilisation plans, two stationary and two general hospitals were to mobilise with each division. However, as these units expanded in size to 400 beds for stationary hospitals and 1,040 beds for general hospitals, they eventually mobilised in accordance with the requirements of hospital accommodation in each theatre of war, rather than with each division. As with casualty clearing stations, RAMC personnel worked with staff from a range of military nursing units and also nurses from Voluntary Aid Detachments and the Red Cross.

Casualties could also be transported via hospital ship to the UK for further expert treatment in military hospitals operated by RAMC personnel. RAMC staff also served in a number of specialist areas including sanitary sections and medical store units.

This overview of a range of RAMC units, which is not exhaustive, helps to illustrate their wide experience in the First World War and the many specialist roles they fulfilled.

In the years prior to the First World War photography had grown in popularity and photographers were located in towns and cities throughout Britain. This meant there was a range of opportunities for recruits to be photographed in the UK, both as individuals and with their RAMC unit comrades. When serving overseas, photographers in the rear of battle zones provided personnel with photographs of themselves, reproduced as postcards, as a souvenir of their overseas service.

The many and varied locations where medical staff served provided a range of opportunities for photographs to be taken, sometimes in a studio setting, at training camps, within medical facilities or in the field. Many of these surviving photos do not include any way to identify those photographed or the unit with which they were serving. However they can often provide information about those photographed through either uniform detail, the background in the photo or the location the photograph was taken. The following images help to demonstrate how much can be deduced from photographs of unidentified medical personnel.

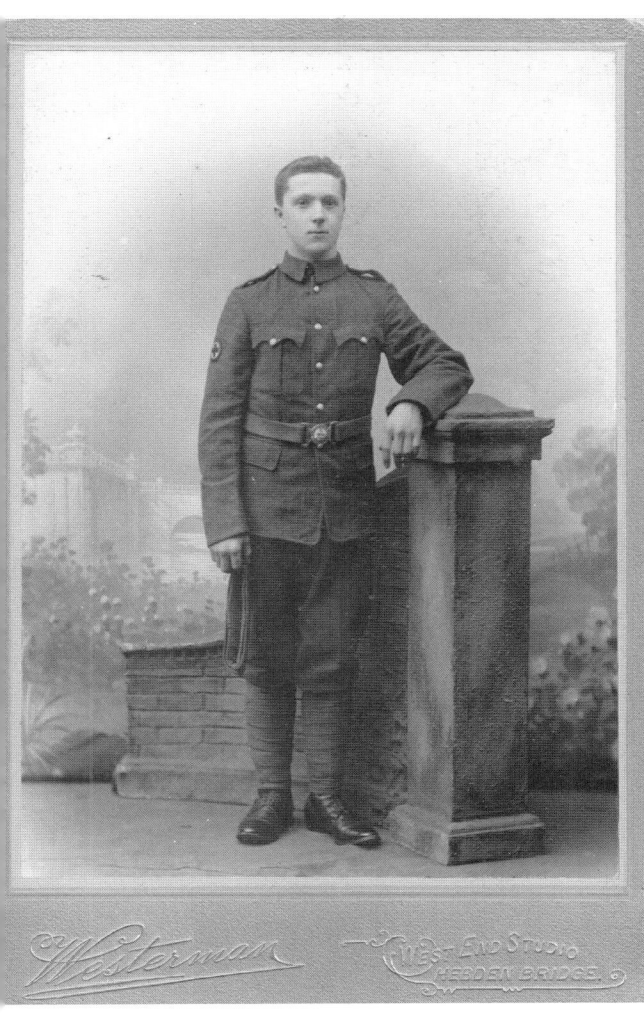

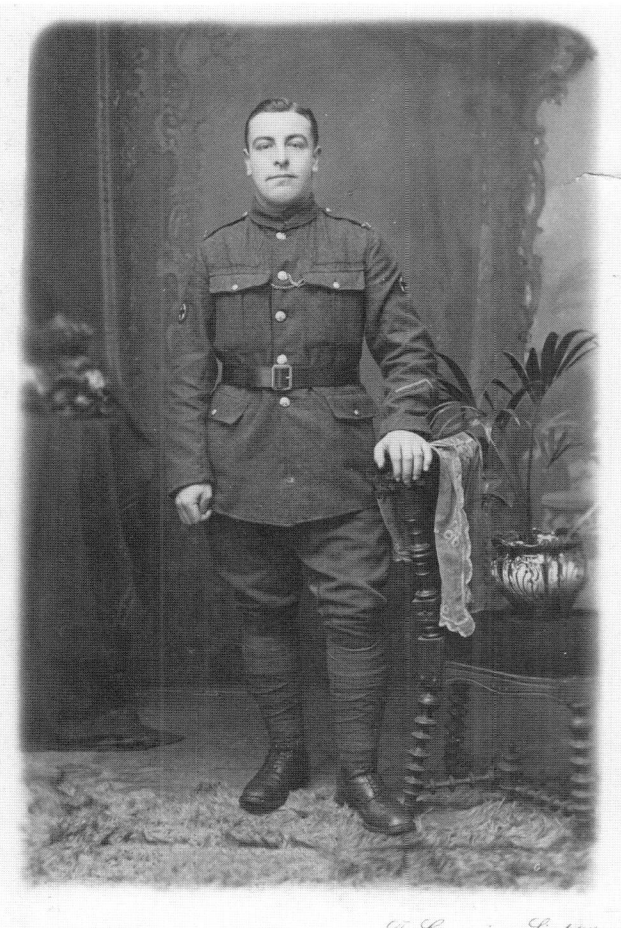

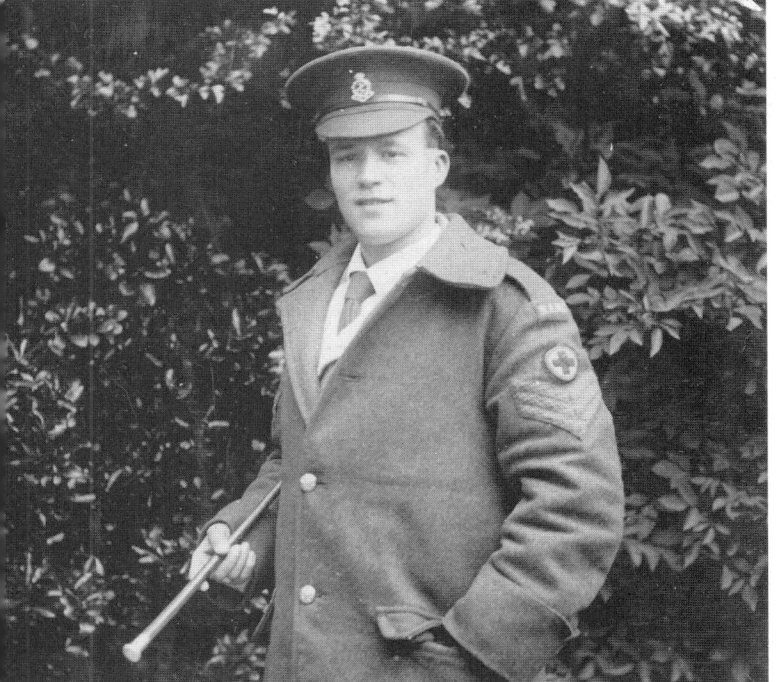

Studio photos were sometimes mounted on card, and can include information about where a photograph was taken. Photographs taken during the First World War were often printed on blank postcards. These can also include information which provides an indication of where they were taken.

The uniforms worn by RAMC personnel can assist with understanding. In this photograph 'hospital blues' uniform is worn by the sergeant under his greatcoat, showing he was a patient at a military hospital.

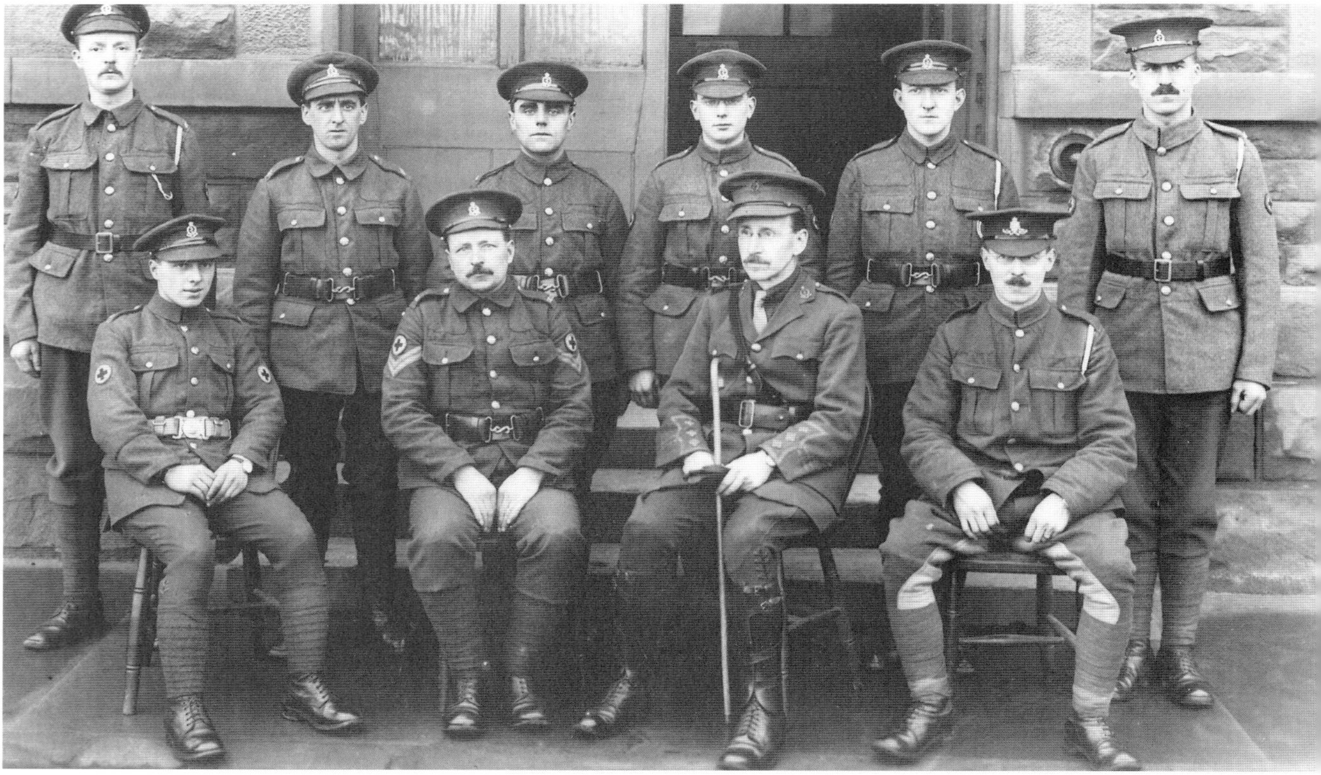

Cap badges can help to identify the unit in which they served. In this photo a RAMC captain is photographed with a corporal and privates. A Royal Artillery gunner is sitting front right.

A group of RAMC non-commissioned officers, photographed on 12 August 1915; sometimes photos were taken in formal style.

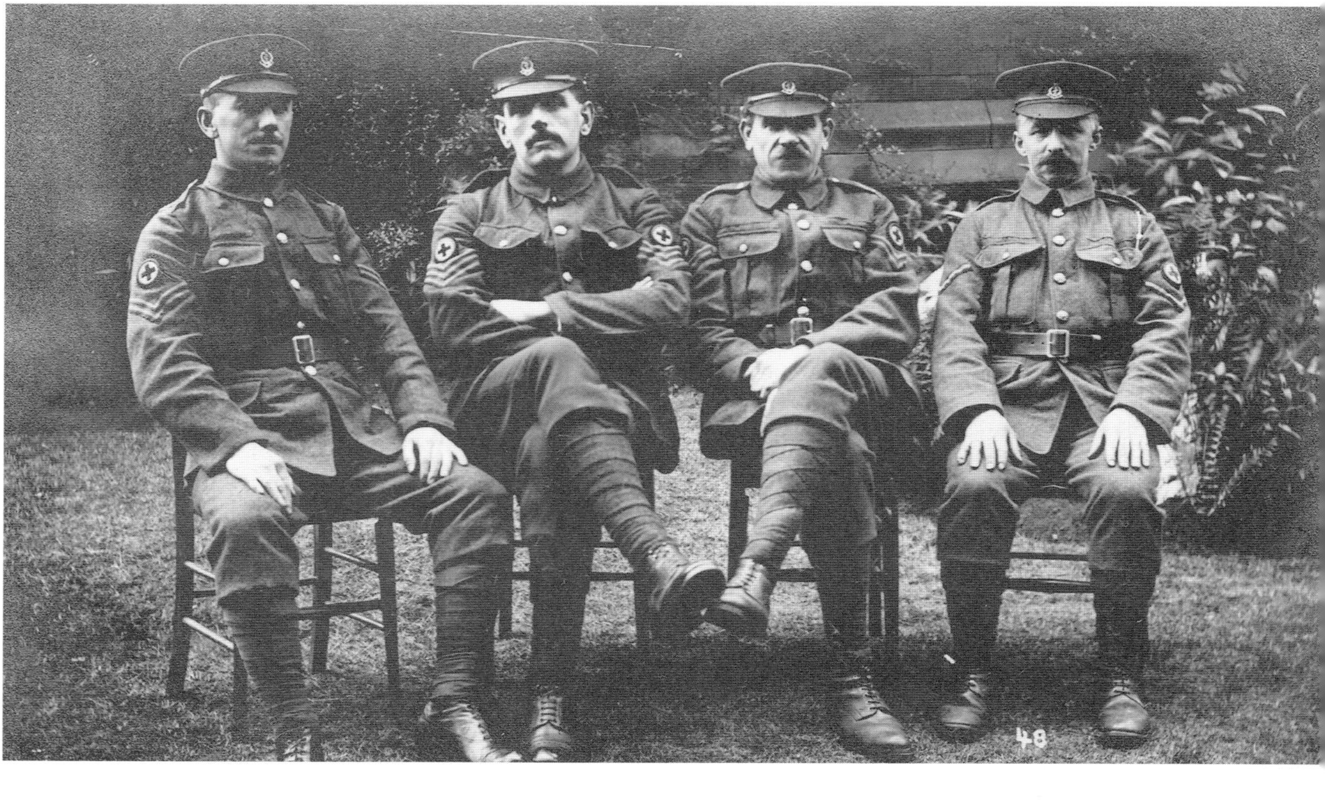

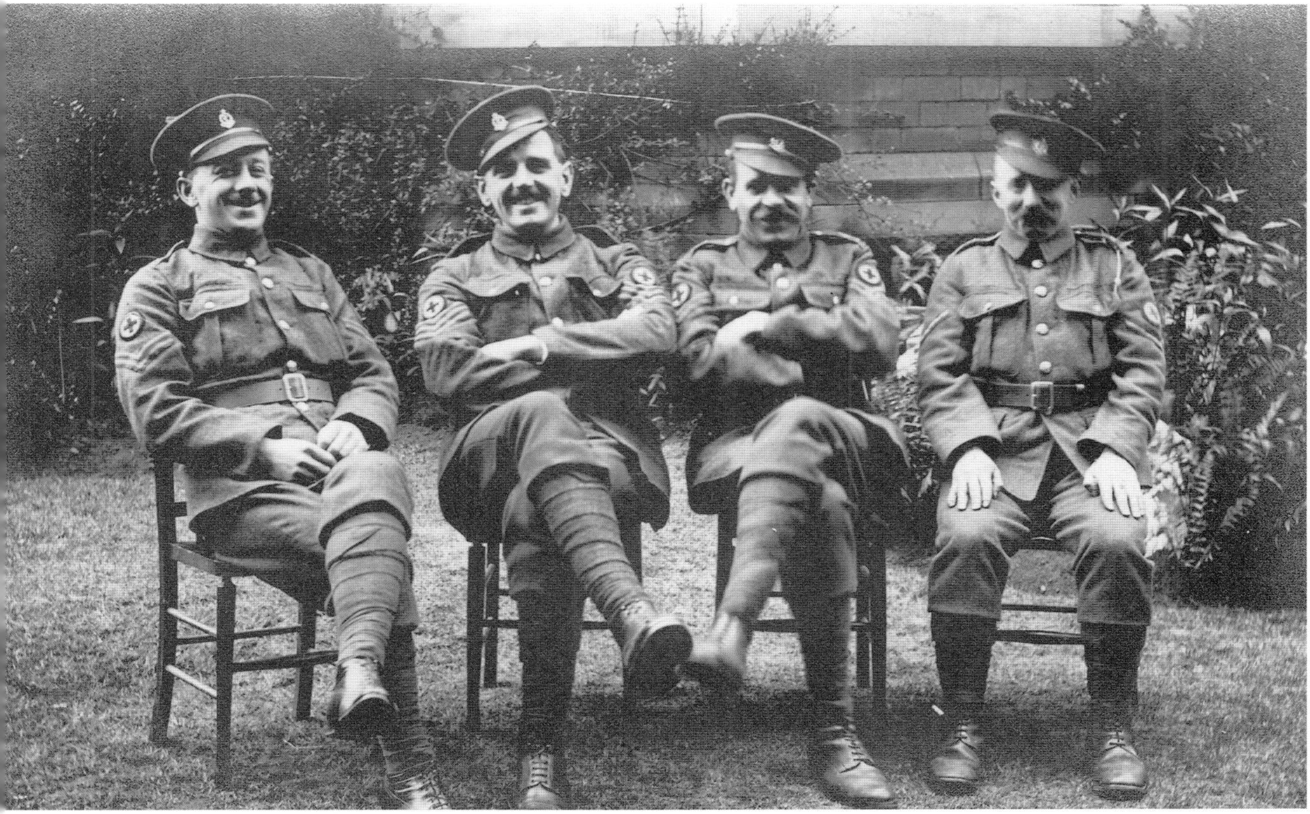

The same group of RAMC non-commissioned officers, photographed in an informal style on the same date.

Photographs were often taken at RAMC training camps. This group wear the insignia of a RAMC (TF) unit.

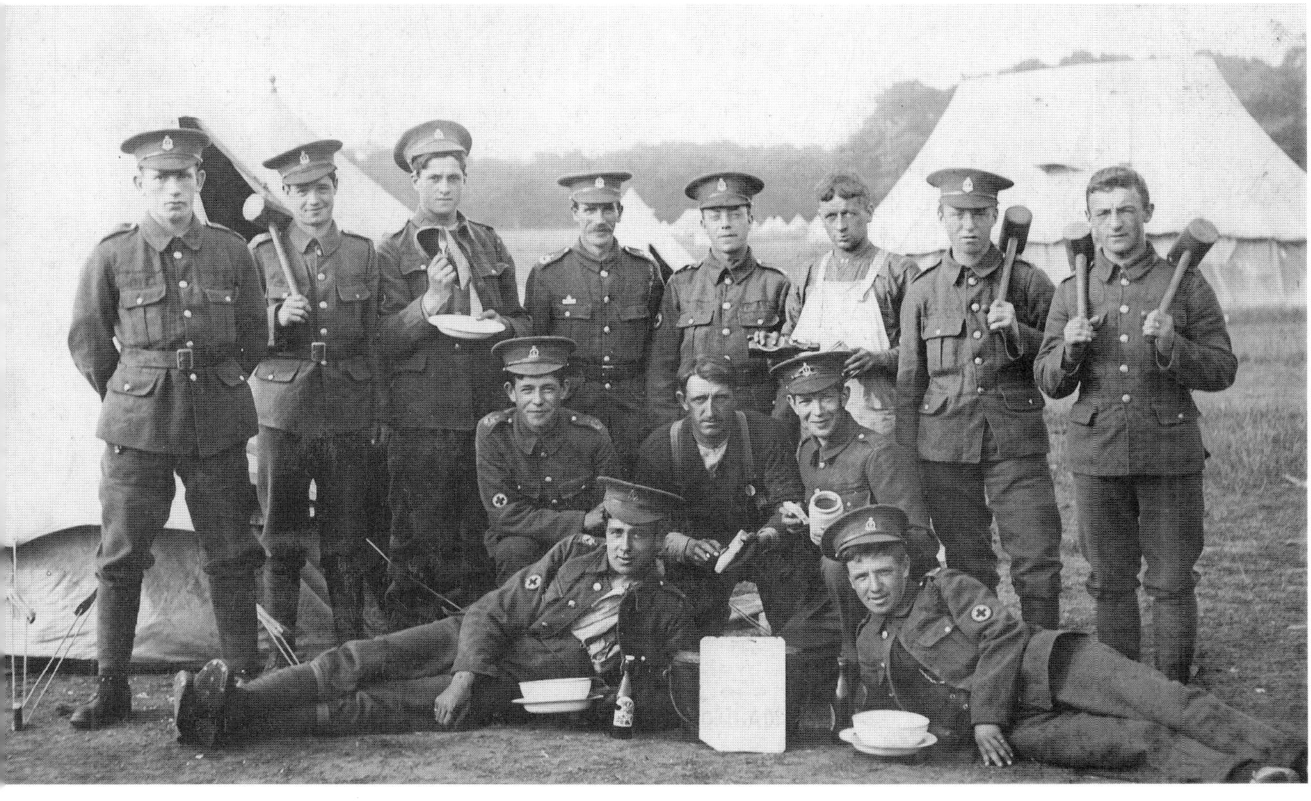

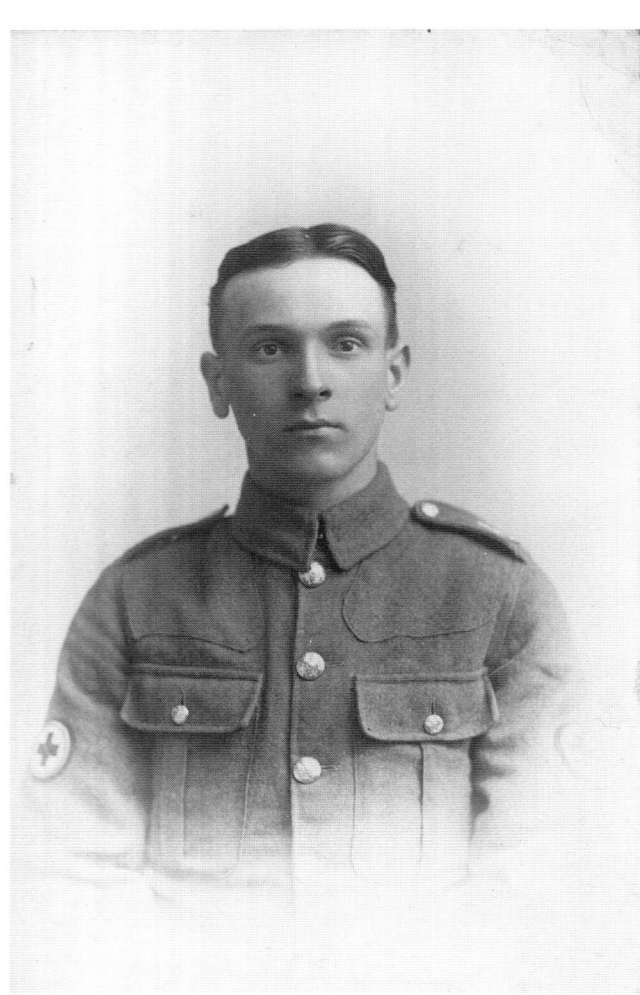 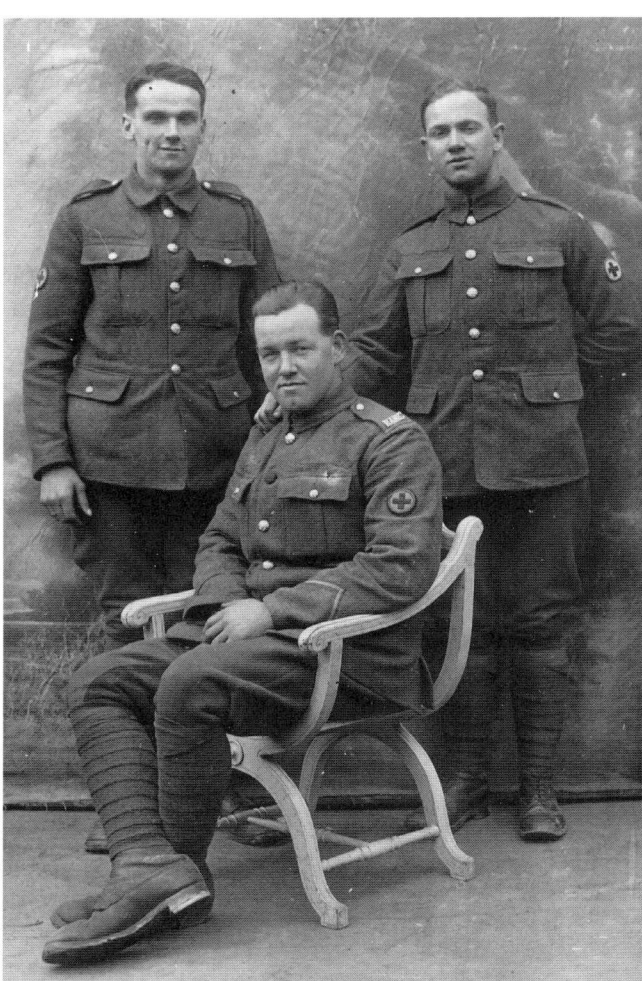

(**Above, left**) Some photographs have information written on them which helps to provide more about the subjects. Inscribed on the reverse of this photo is 'Charlie, Forest Row, 1914–15'.

(**Above, right**) A group of RAMC personnel in France; the seated private wears a black mourning button. Detail on service uniform such as this can help with photo interpretation.

(**Opposite, above**) The structures of buildings in the background of photographs can prove to be interesting. In this photo RAMC recruits are gathered in front of a prefabricated hut. During the First World War the increasing need for barracks resulted in a variety of building solutions.

(**Opposite, below**) Many types of vehicles were used to transport the injured and sick. In this photo, taken at a training camp, a group of RAMC personnel are in front of a horse drawn ambulance. In the foreground is a stretcher.

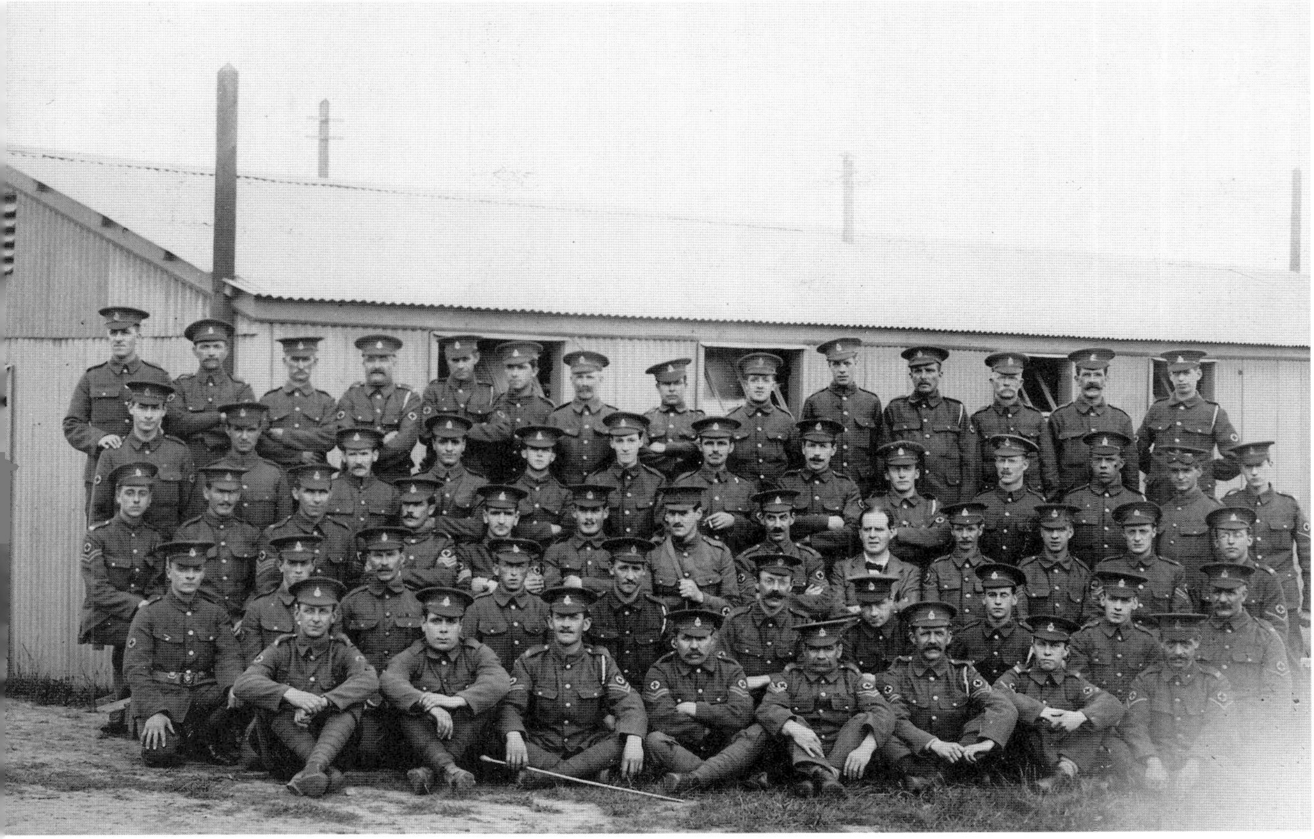

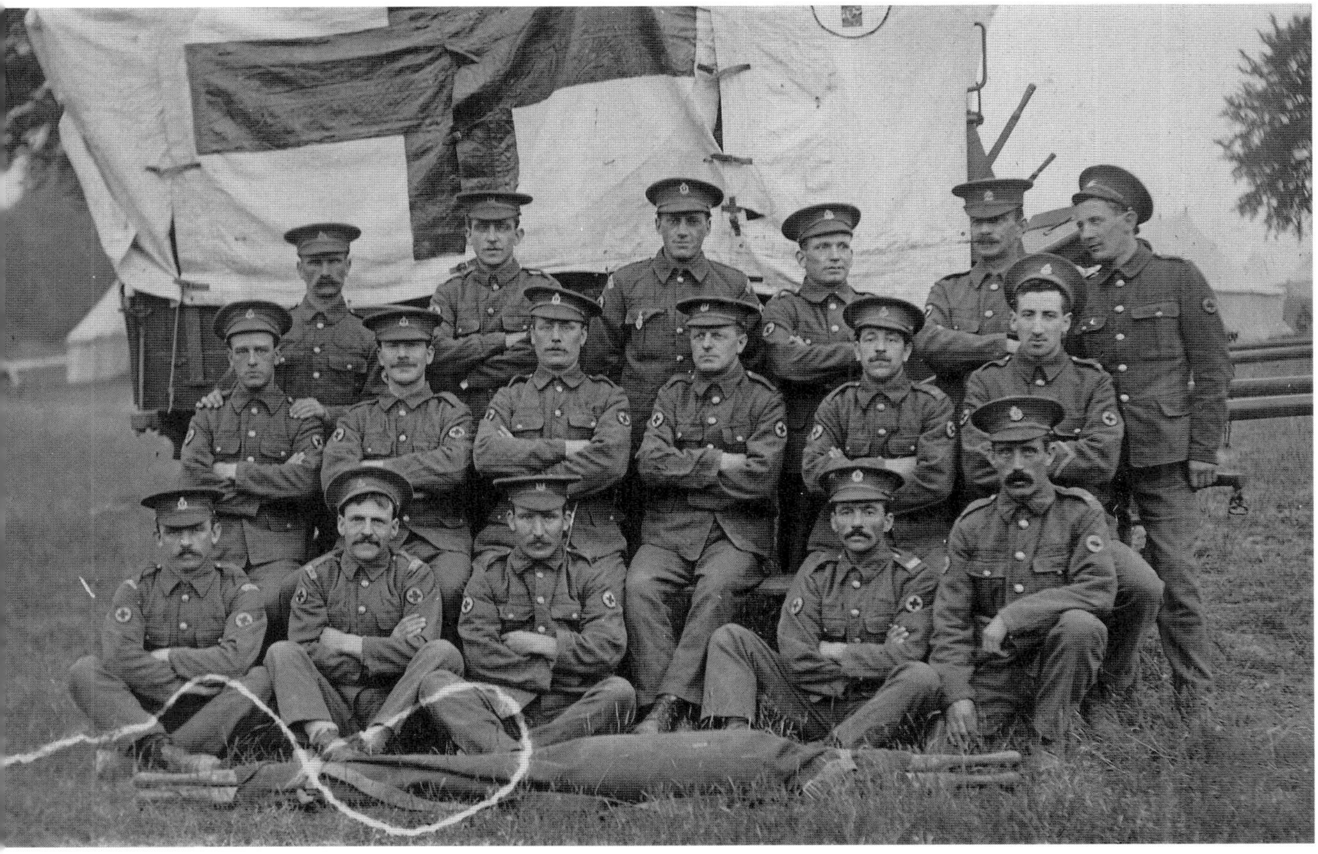

Medal ribbons worn on military uniform can help illustrate the previous service of photographed personnel. In this photo the RAMC soldier seated front right wears the ribbon of the Army Long Service and Good Conduct Medal.

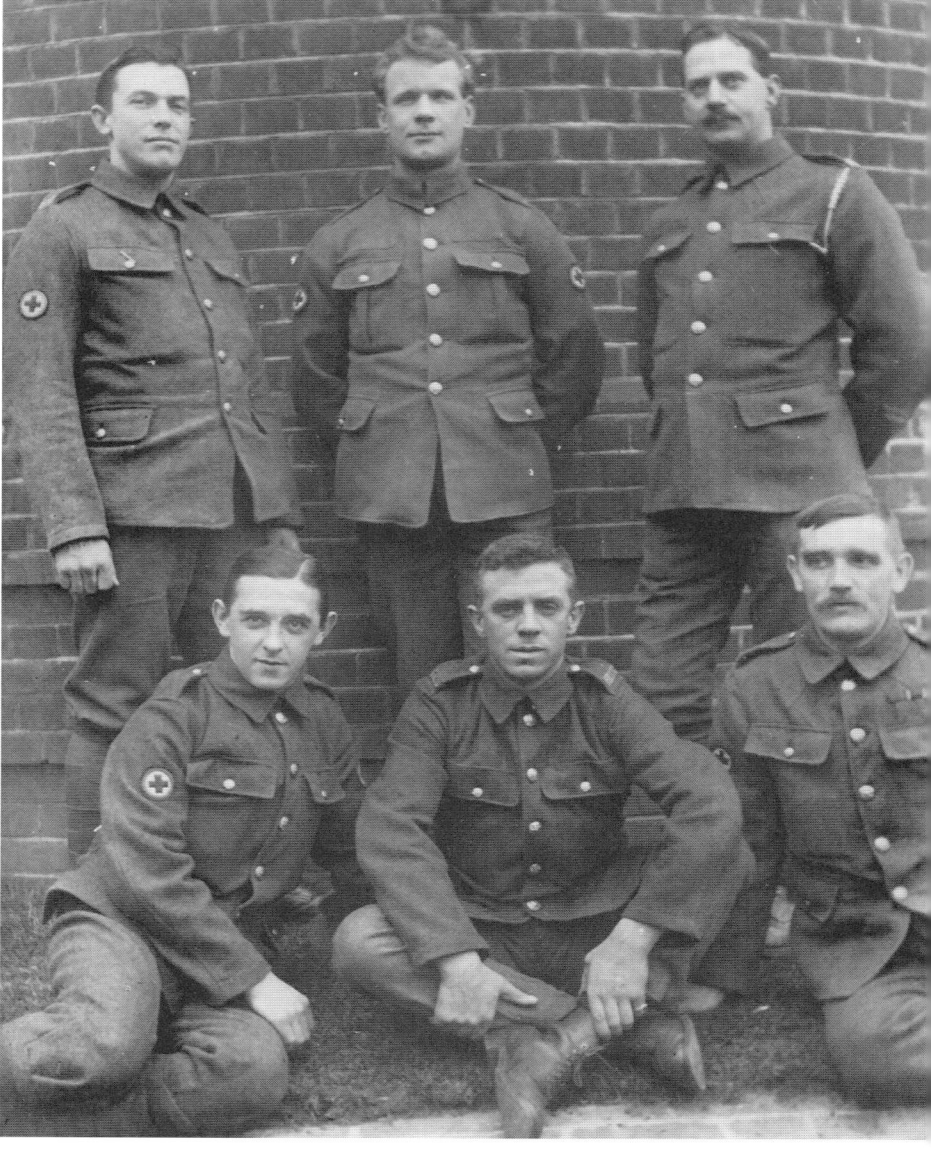

(**Opposite, above left**) Photographs taken overseas can be identified by the backing card of the photographs and also by regimental badges. In this photo a RAMC lance corporal, photographed overseas, wears unit battle patches over his round Red Cross badge.

(**Opposite, below**) Groups of RAMC personnel often chose to be photographed outside their billets and sometimes the locations can be identified. In this photo the RAMC soldiers seated left and second right wear wound stripes on the left cuffs of their uniforms.

(**Opposite, above right**) Studio photos were sometimes taken with family members and friends such as in this photo of a RAMC sergeant.

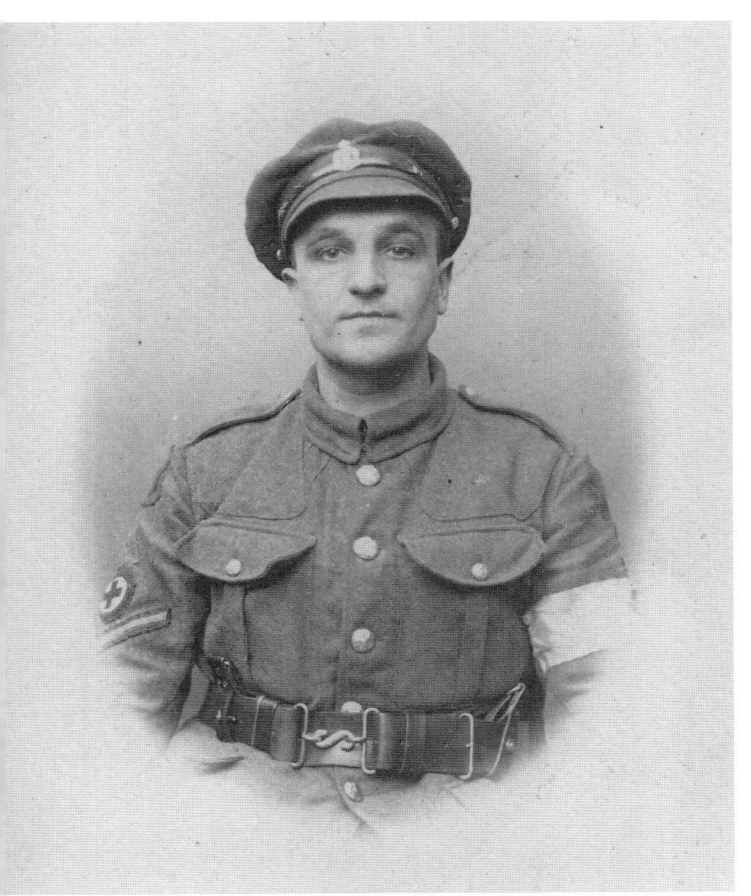
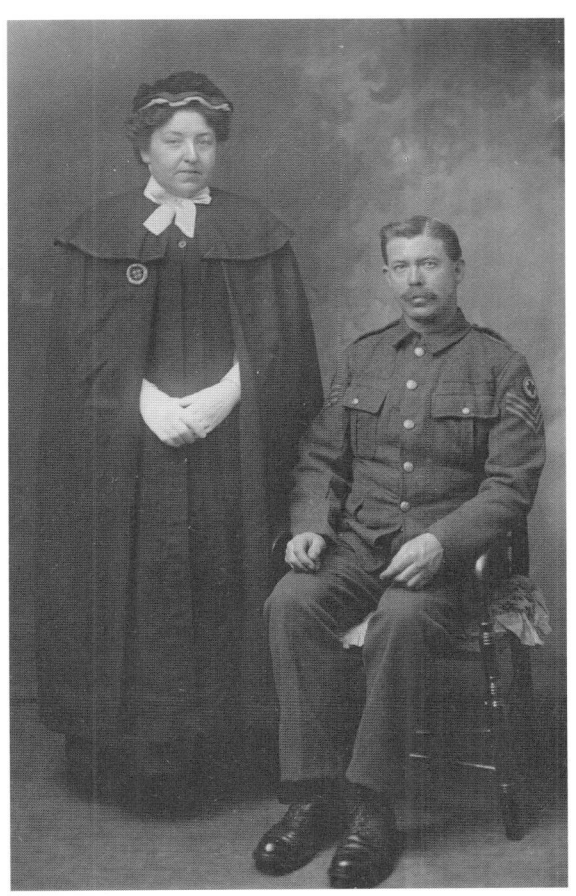

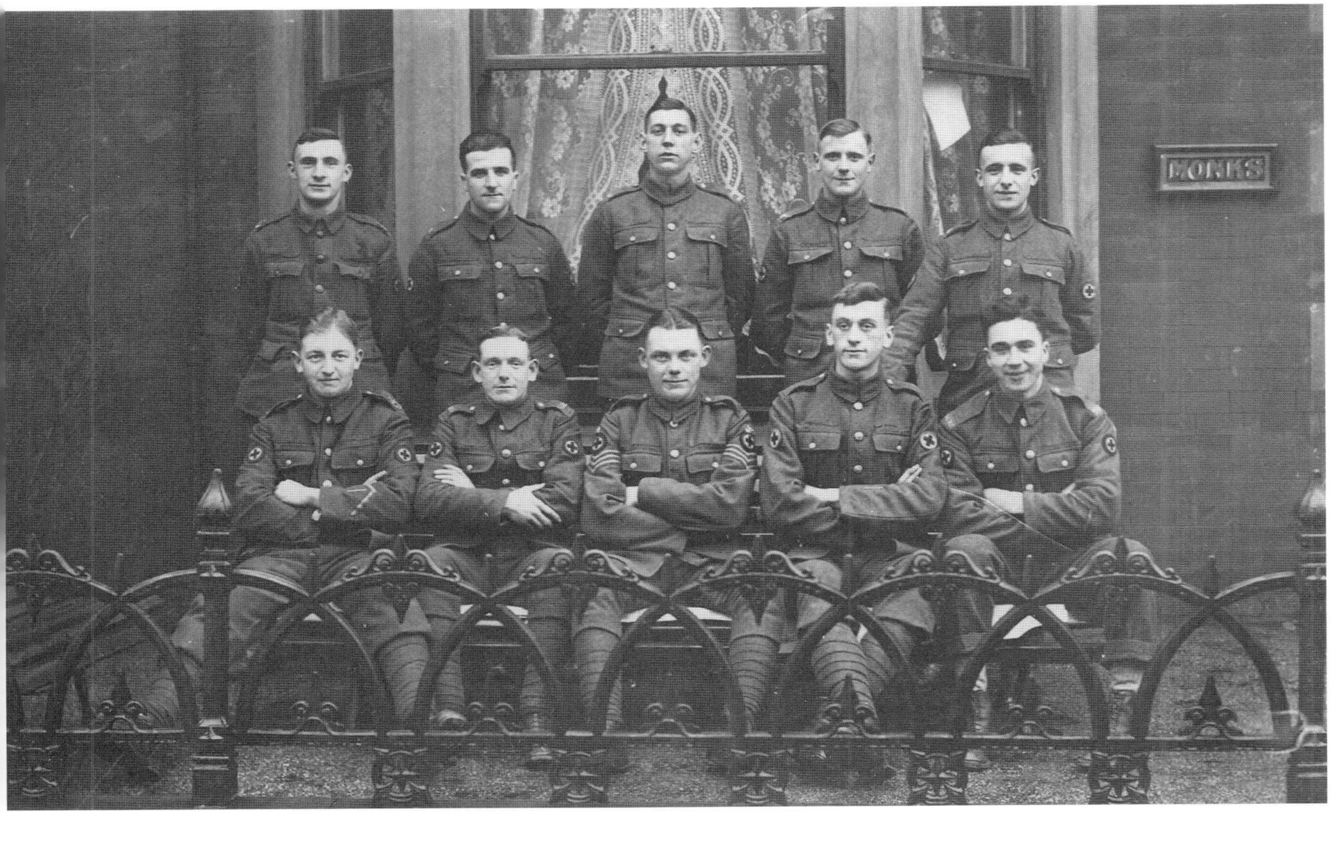

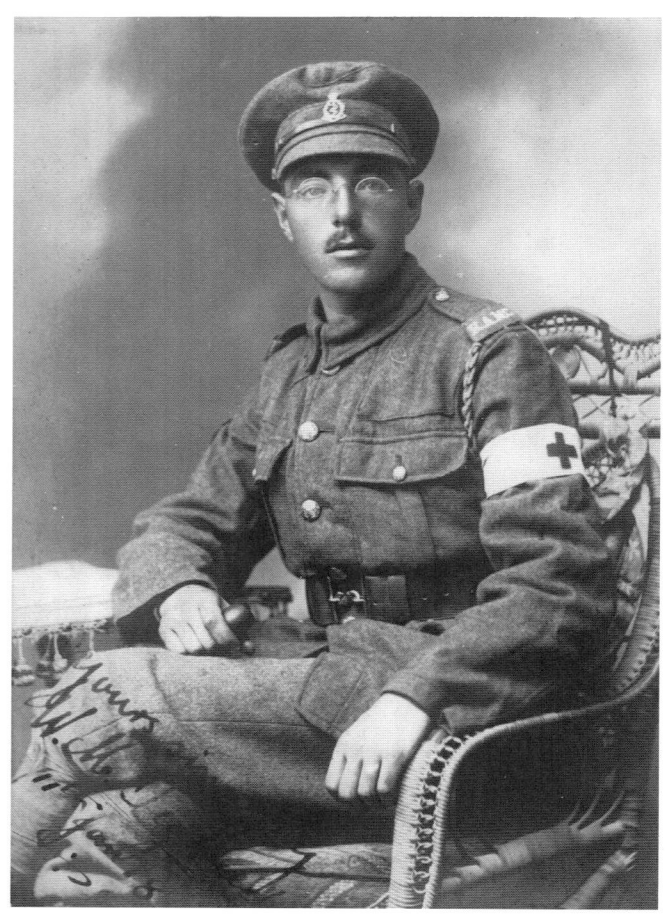

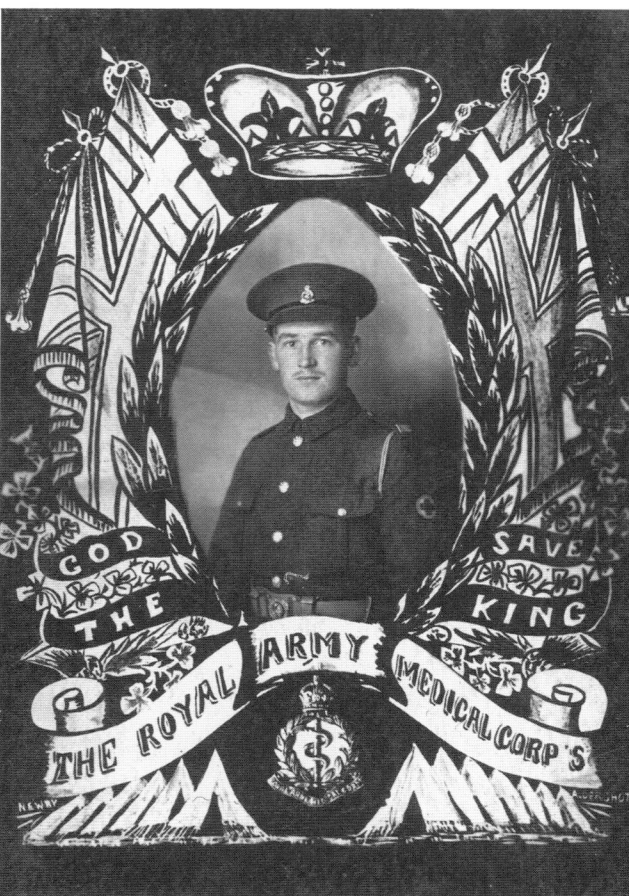

(**Above, left**) Sometimes those photographed signed and dated their photo. This is signed and dated 11 January 1918 by a RAMC private serving on the Western Front.

(**Above, right**) During the First World War photographers produced a range of regimental and patriotic style photo surrounds. This RAMC graphic design features the names of two military bases at each side of the tents, Aldershot and Newby.

(**Right**) Whilst serving overseas RAMC personnel sometimes took the opportunity to be photographed with their comrades. This group was photographed on the Western Front.

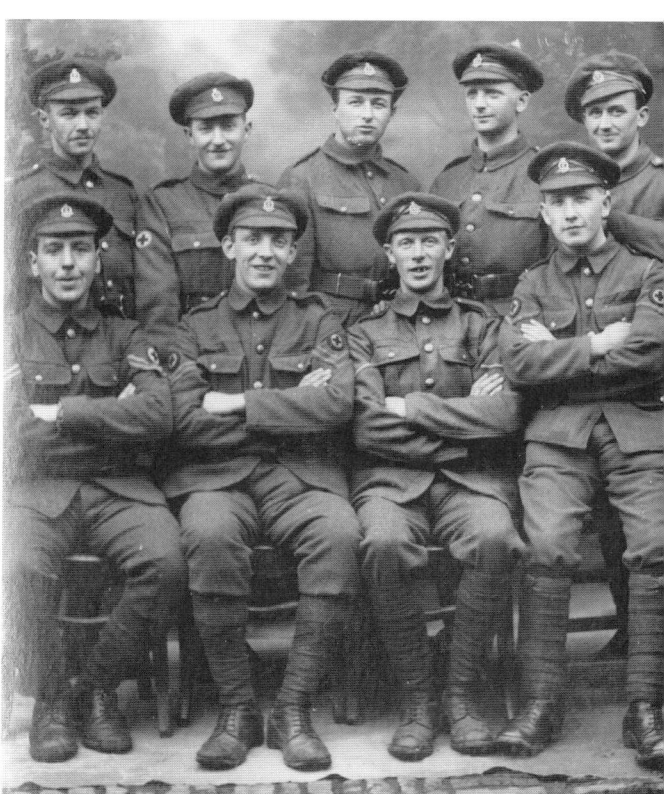

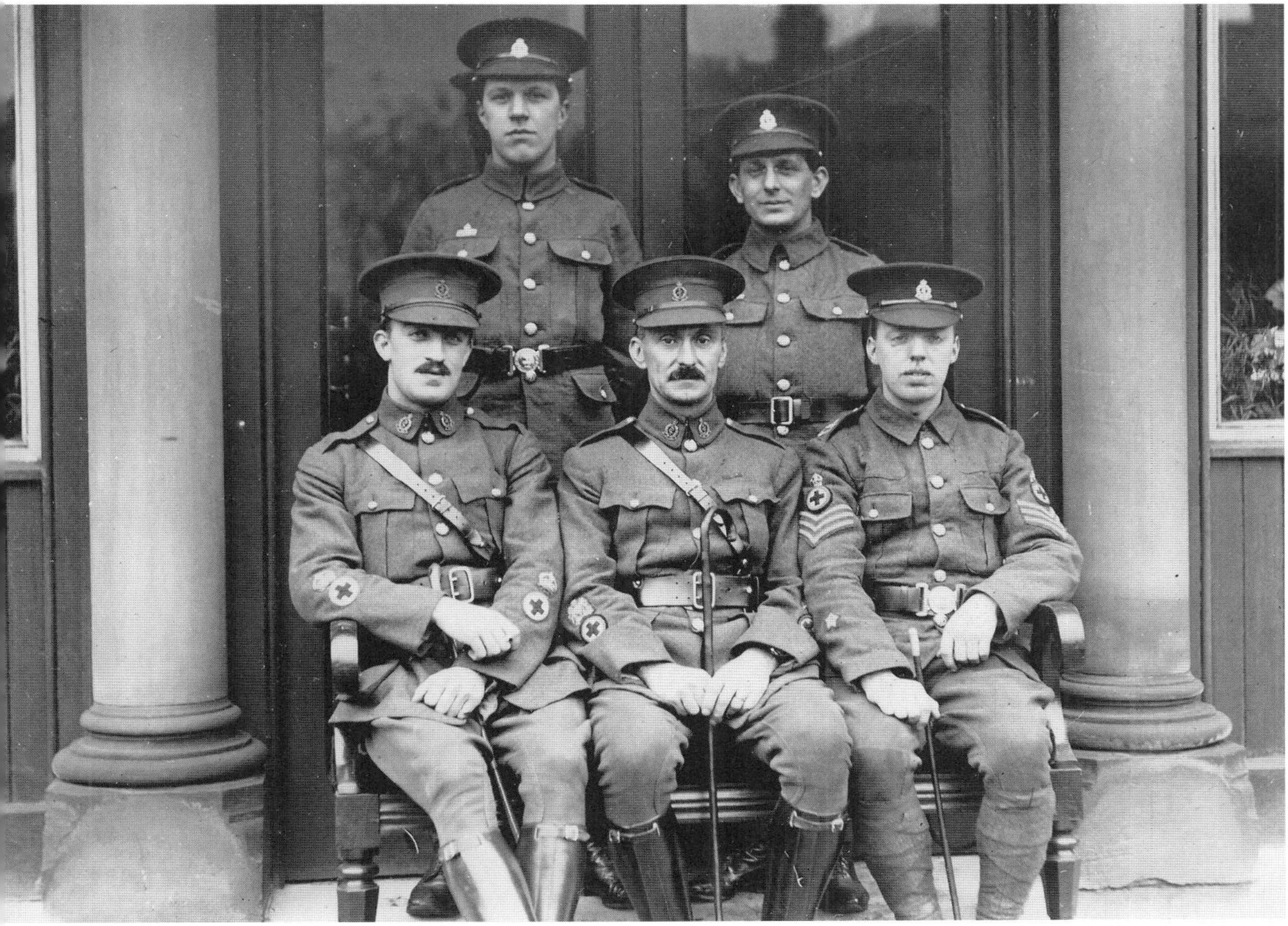

Rank badges can be helpful for identification. In this photo a RAMC warrant officer class 1 (WO1) is seated in the centre, with a warrant officer class 2 (WO2) seated on the left and a staff sergeant on the right.

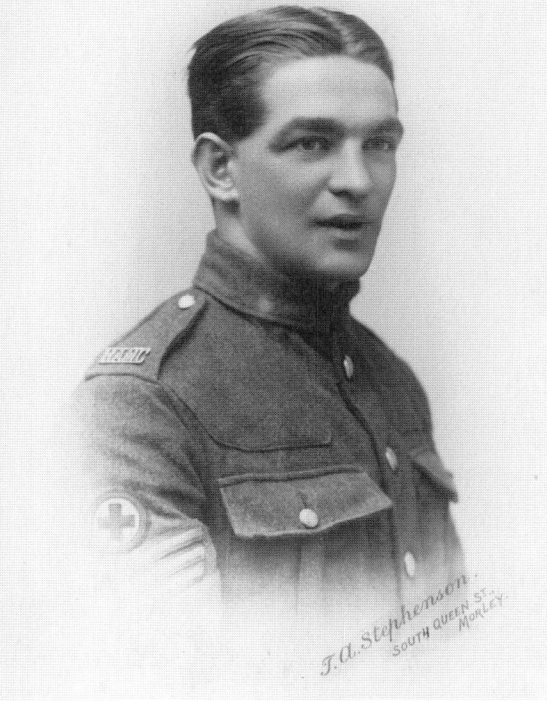

Unit shoulder badges can help to interpret those pictured. In this photo the sergeant's RAMC shoulder title can be clearly seen.

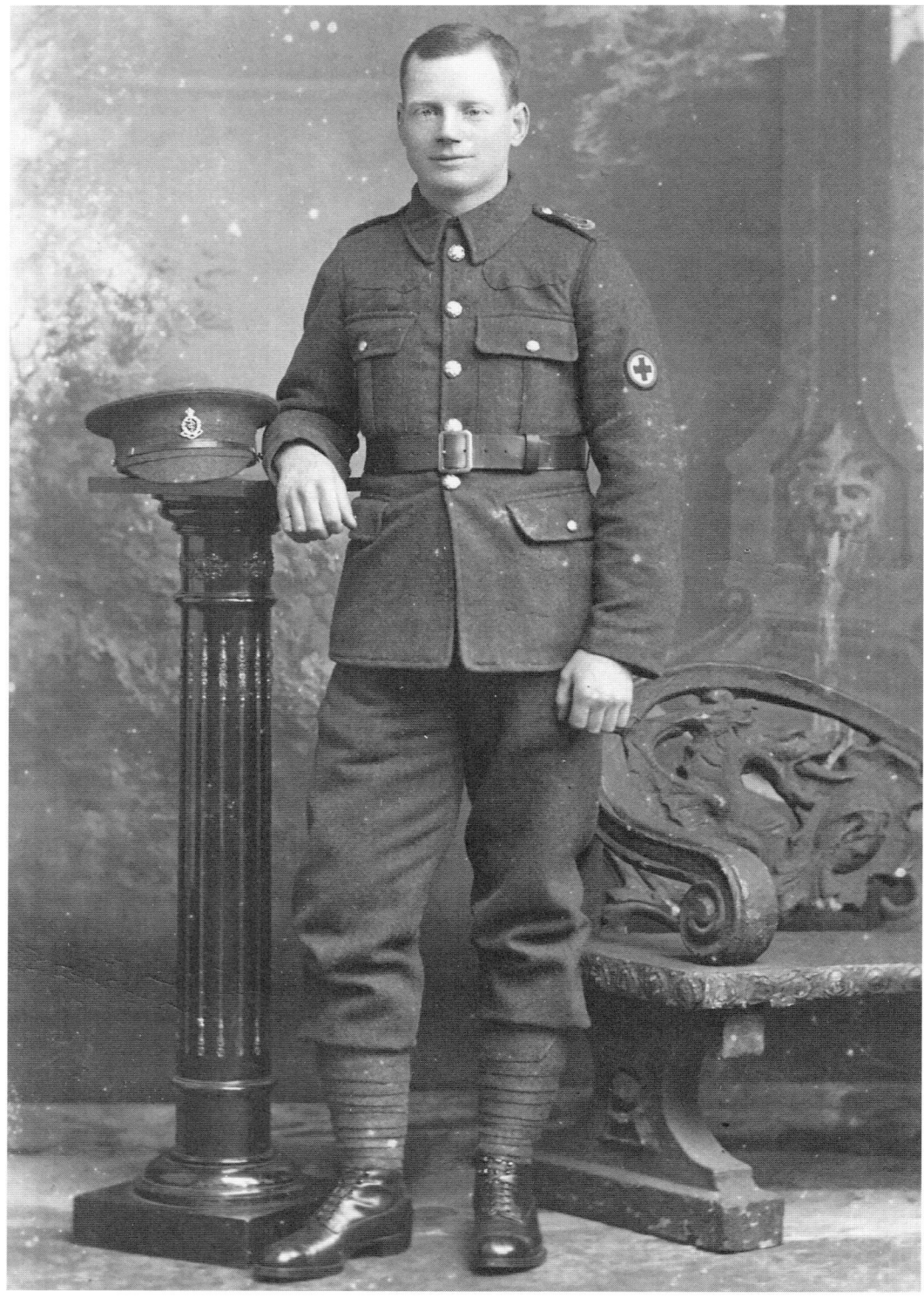

In this photograph, taken at Montrose, an RAMC Territorial Force soldier is identifiable due to the unit shoulder badges worn.

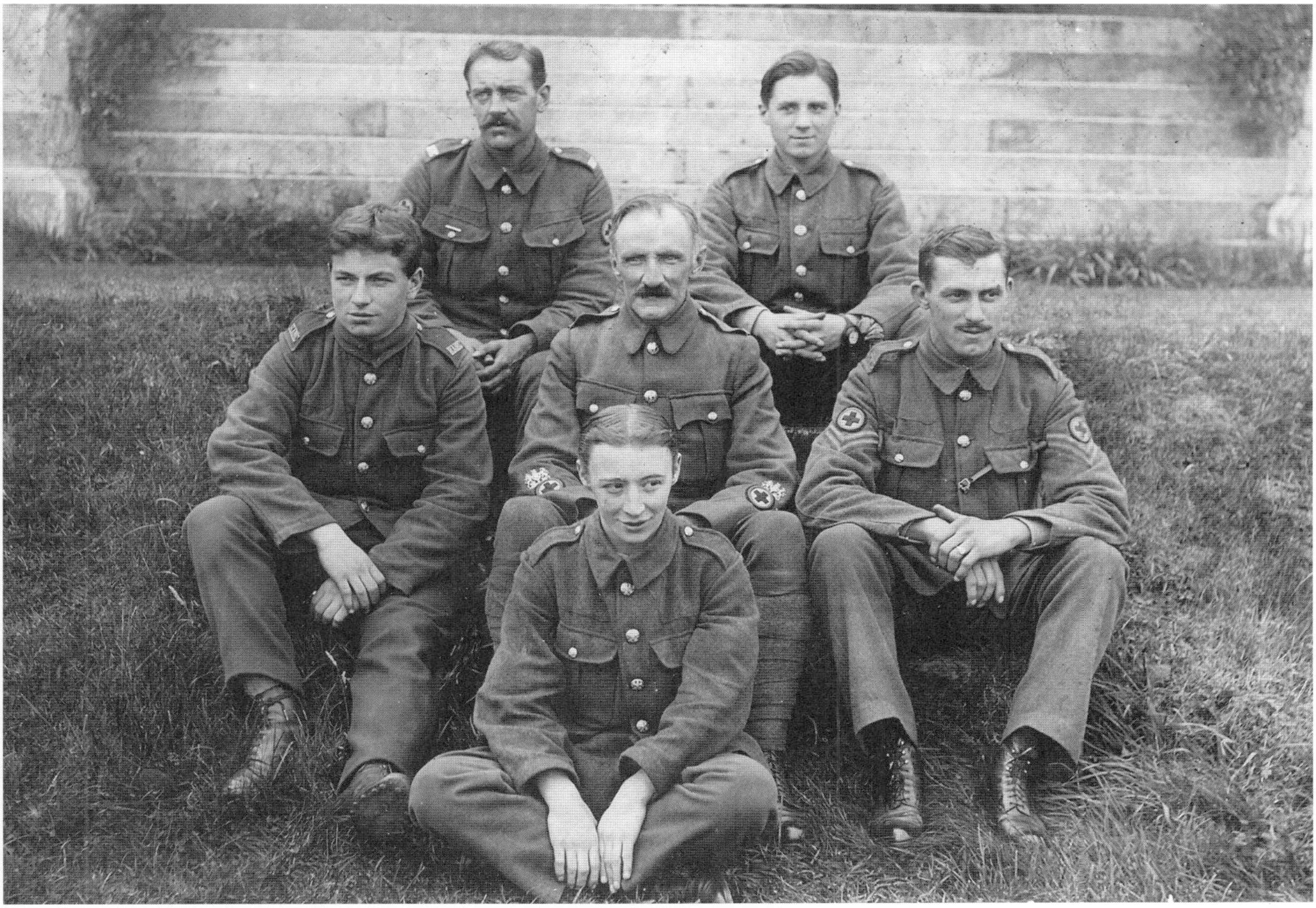

When photographed during the First World War, RAMC non-commissioned soldiers are usually pictured wearing round Red Cross badges on their uniform sleeves. However, as this photo shows, this was not always the case.

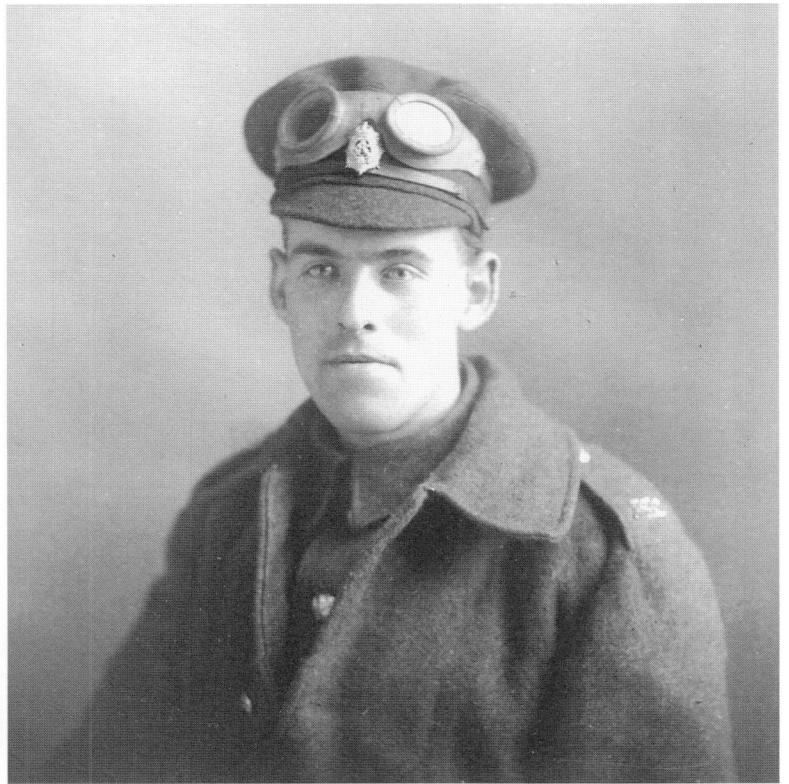

Personnel of the Army Service Corps (ASC) were attached to RAMC units in transportation roles, including horse drawn ambulance and motor ambulance drivers. This ASC driver is wearing driving goggles.

Chapter Two

The United Kingdom

In the United Kingdom RAMC personnel served in many medical units and military hospitals. Prior to service overseas RAMC recruits trained in a range of locations and new training centres were developed. As the conflict continued and the number of casualties grew, an increase in the number of medical facilities was required. Specialist treatments had to be developed to respond to casualties caused by new weapons, such as poison gas.

When hospital ships arrived in port, ambulance trains, staffed by RAMC personnel and nursing staff, transported casualties throughout the country for treatment. The hospitals were often located in buildings such as schools and colleges and each could treat a large number of patients. Once discharged from these hospitals, patients would often convalesce at smaller auxiliary hospitals staffed by local Voluntary Aid Detachments.

Photographs of RAMC personnel illustrate the preparations units made for service overseas and the range of locations where they trained. The images also illustrate a range of hospital locations, with patients from UK armed forces and also allied armies. Some of the photographs were taken as a memento for individuals and units prior to embarking for service overseas.

Apparent in several of the photographs is the vital role played by military nursing services and voluntary medical personnel in supporting RAMC medical units and hospitals, to ensure the effective treatment of casualties.

(**Opposite, above**) Personnel of the 2nd London General Hospital, RAMC (TF), at a training camp in Netley, August 1914.

(**Opposite, below**) Photograph of the Royal Victoria Hospital at Netley posted to Mrs Lippold by Sergeant Major Albert A. Lippold, 2nd London General Hospital, RAMC (TF). The photo was posted on the day war broke out, 4 August 1914. He noted that he was returning to London the following day and hoped to be home in the evening. Sergeant Major Lippold was commissioned during the First World War and later served as a captain and quartermaster with the 2nd London General Hospital. Prior to the First World War he was employed as an electrical engineer, in addition to serving in his spare time with the 2nd London General Hospital. Age 33 in 1911, he lived with his wife, son and brother at 172 Lambeth Road, London.

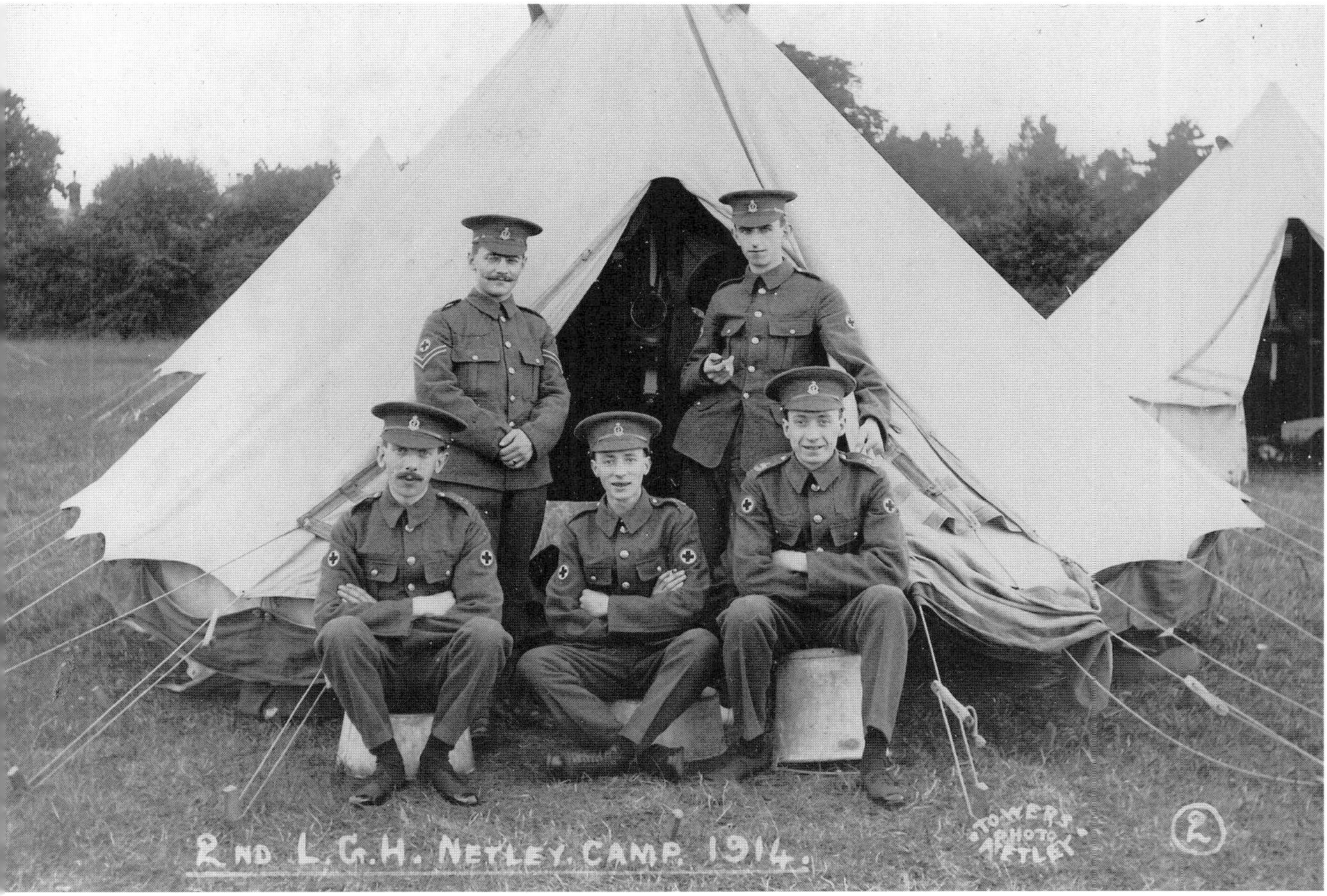

2ND L.G.H. NETLEY. CAMP. 1914.
TOWERS PHOTO NETLEY.
2

NORTH WING, R.V. HOSPITAL, NETLEY.
TOWERS, PHOTO, NETLEY.

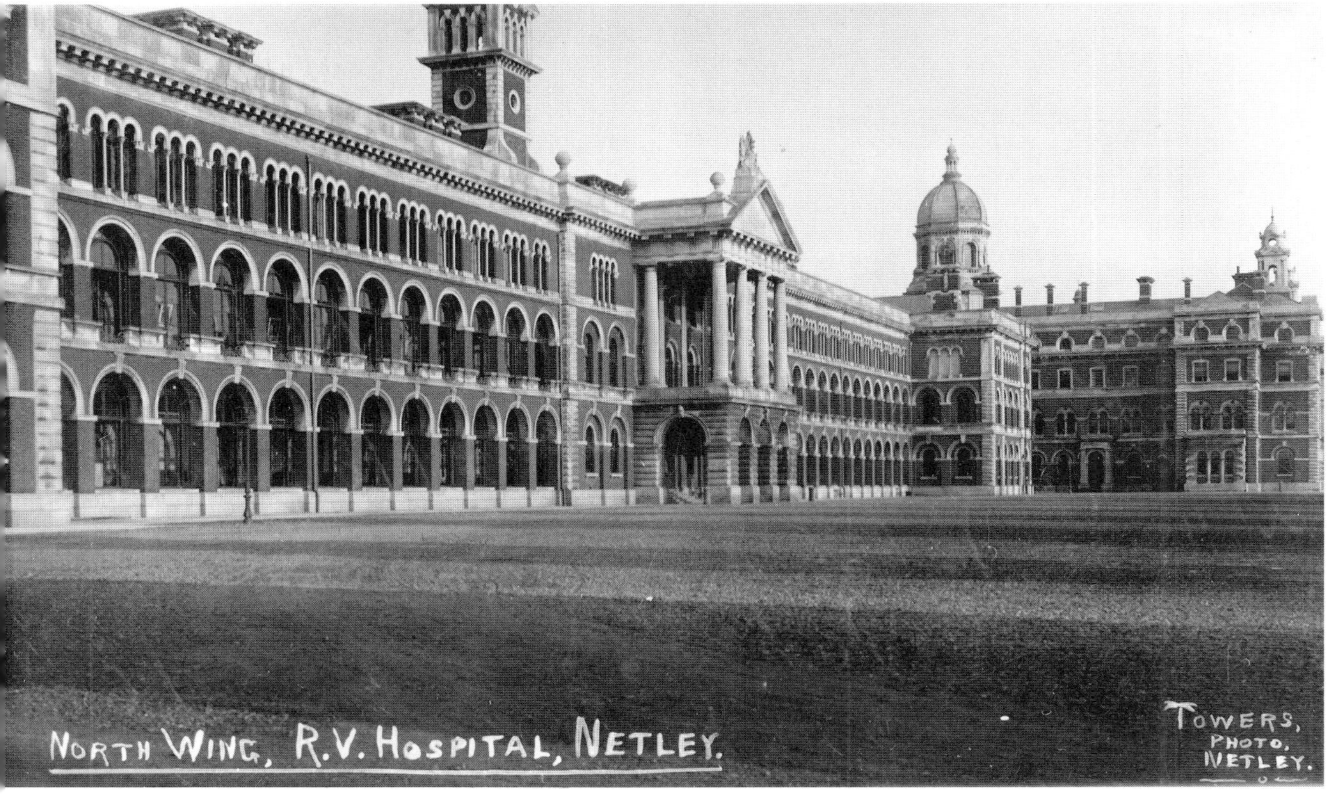

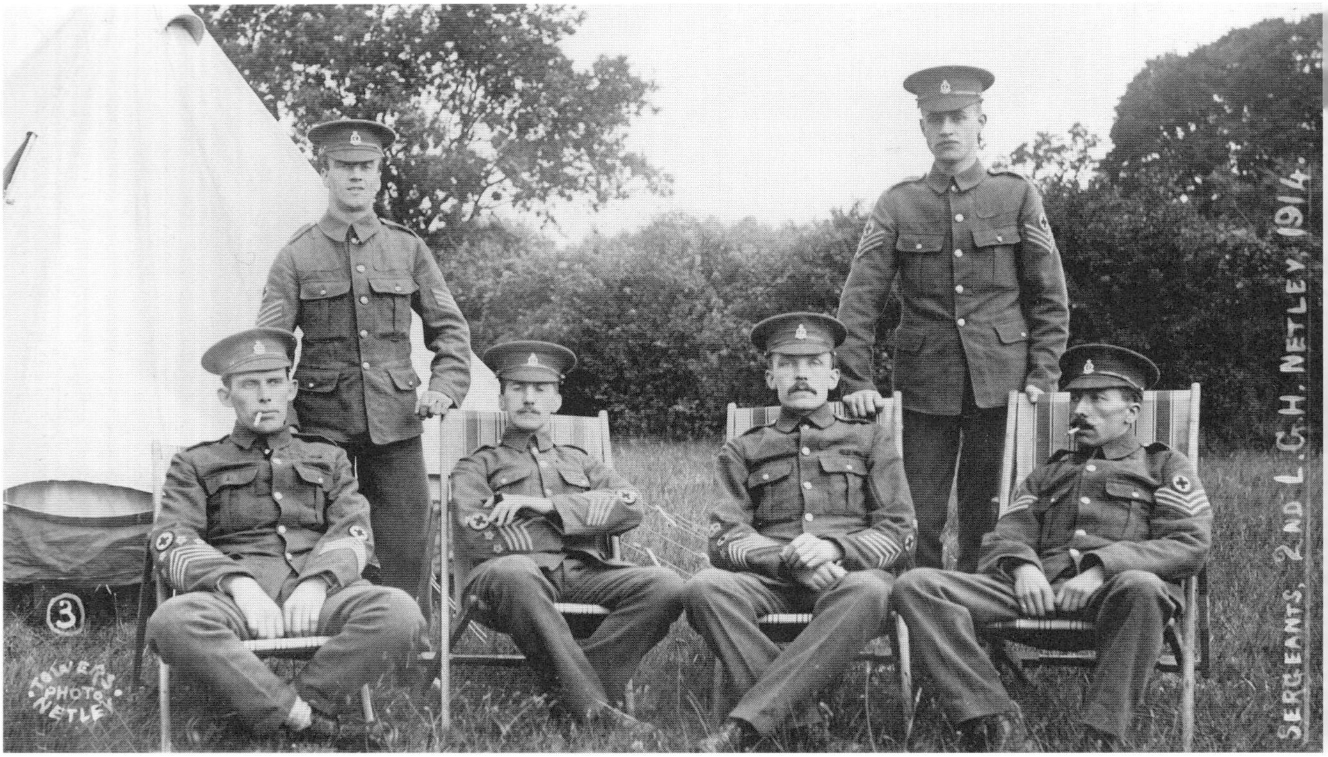

Warrant officers and sergeants of the 2nd London General Hospital, RAMC (TF) photographed at a training camp, Netley, in August 1914. Unfortunately the names of the soldiers are not noted on the photo, but it is likely Sergeant Major Albert Lippold is in this group photograph.

During the First World War the 2nd London General Hospital, RAMC (TF) was located at St Mark's College, Chelsea.

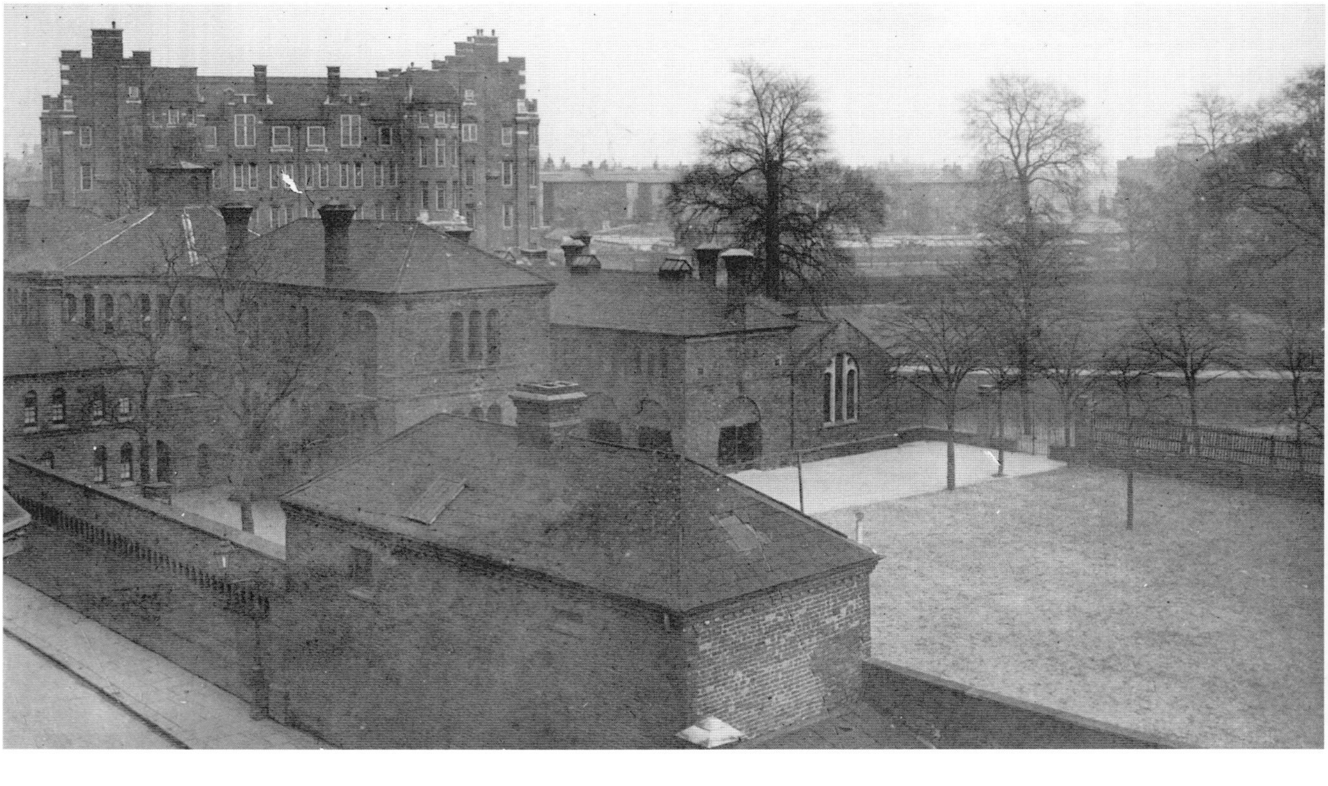

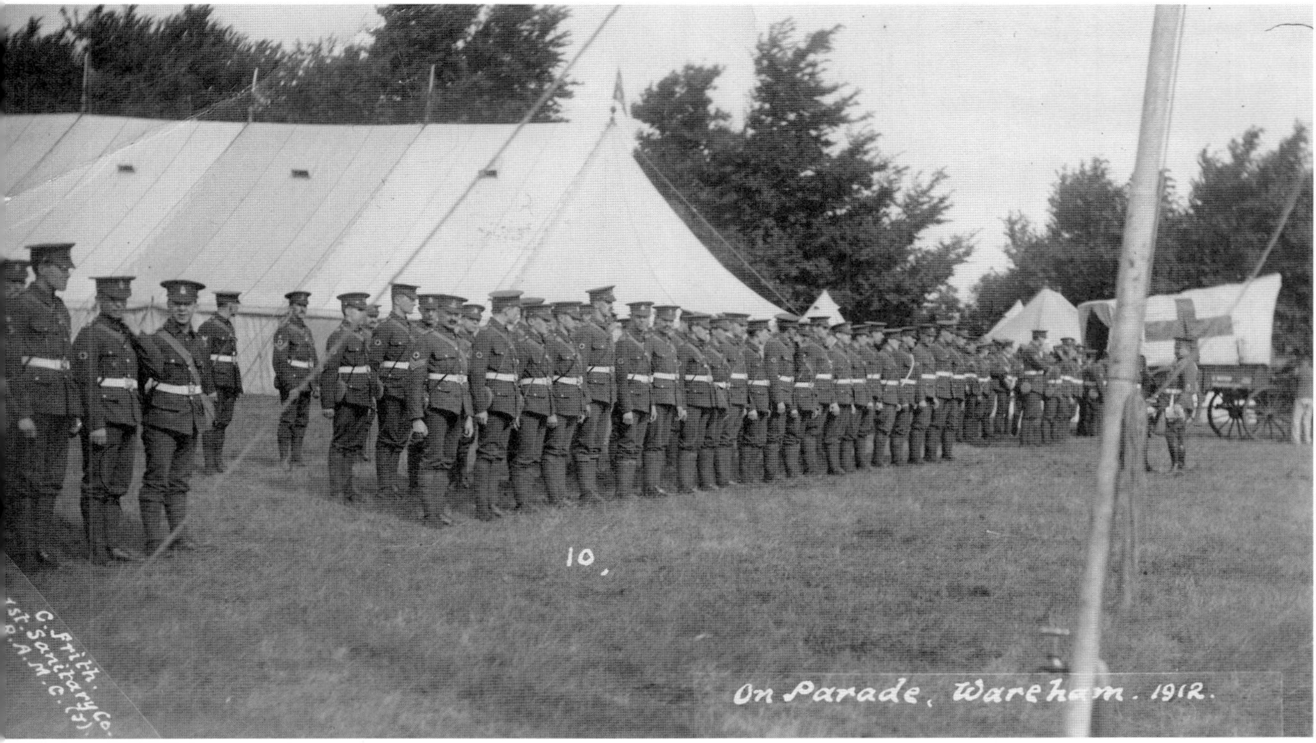

The 1st Sanitary Company, RAMC (TF). The unit is photographed at a training camp at Wareham in 1912. Personnel of this specialist unit helped to form the basis of Sanitary Sections during the First World War. A RAMC Sanitary Section was attached to each division from early 1915. Each section was responsible for maintaining clean water supplies, de-lousing stations, cooking facilities and billets. From March 1917 Sanitary Sections were detached from divisions and came under corps or army control.

A RAMC volunteer unit training at Bordon Camp, Hampshire, 1910.

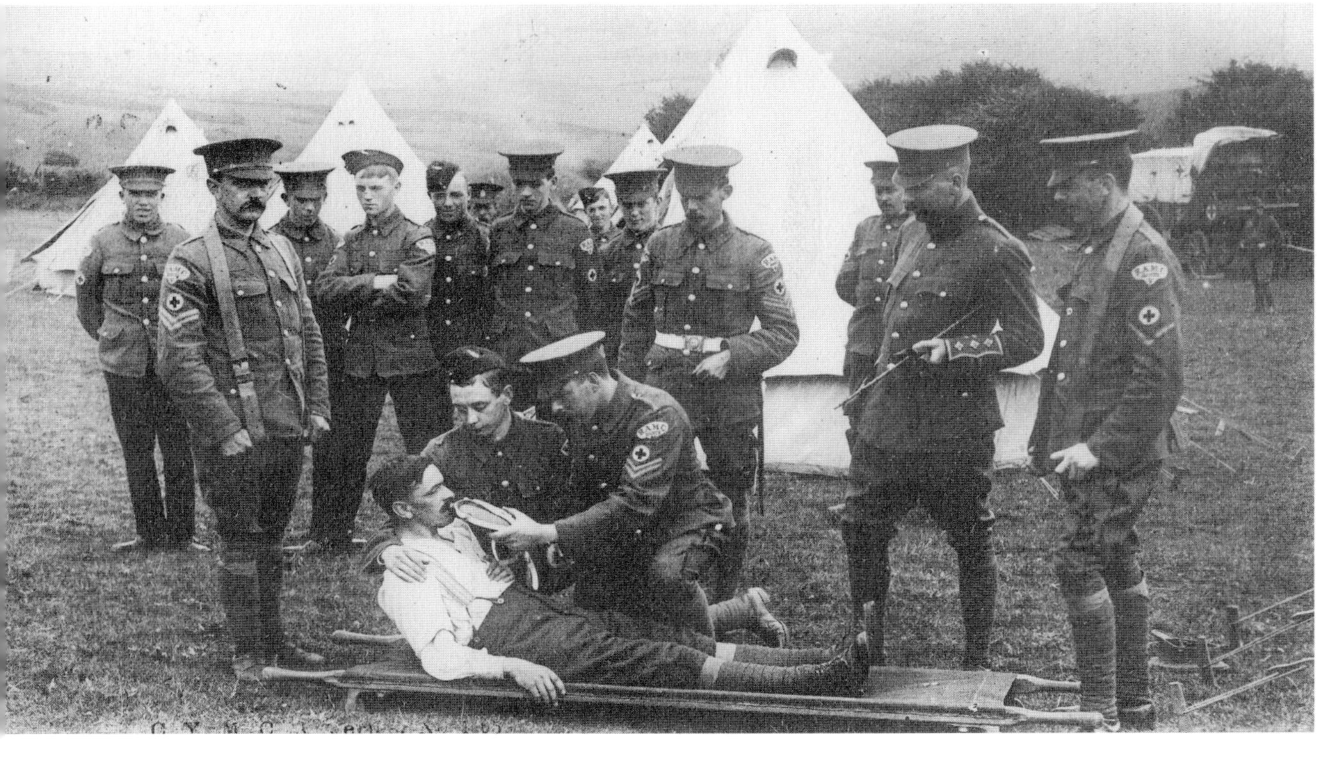

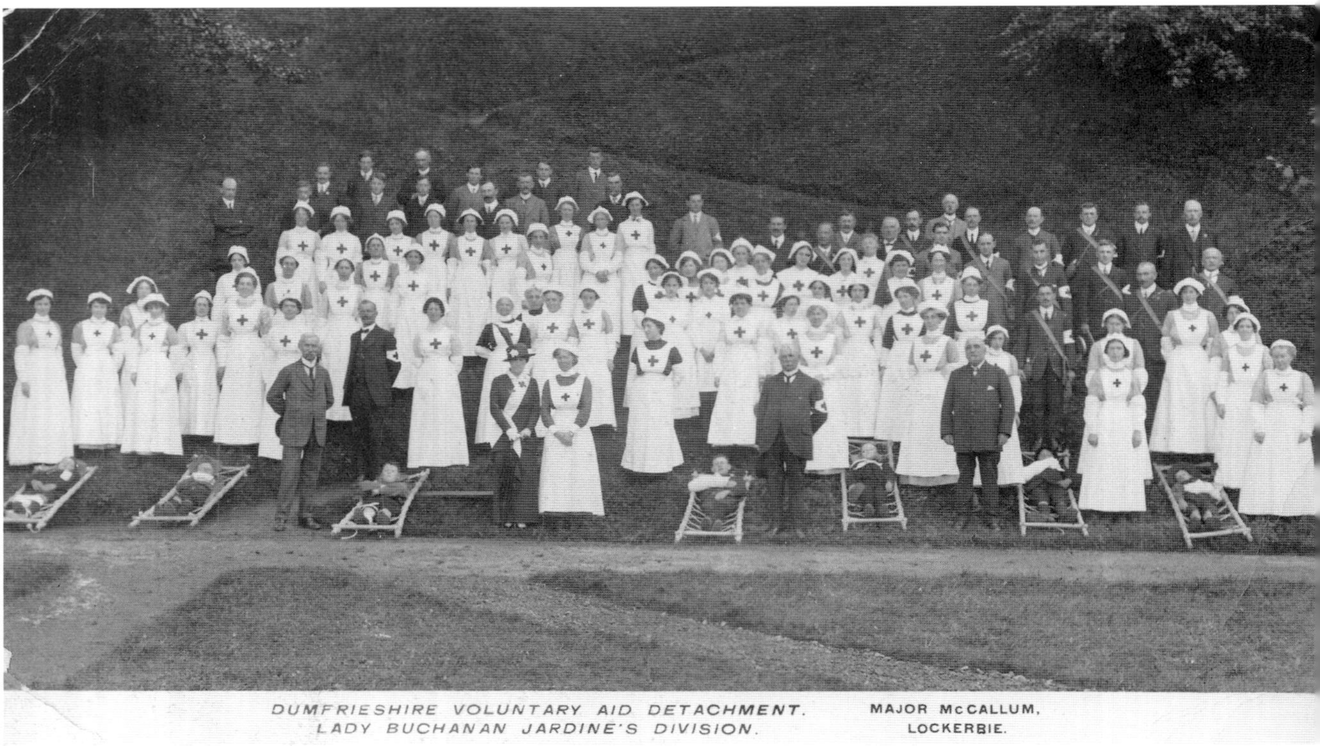

DUMFRIESHIRE VOLUNTARY AID DETACHMENT.　　MAJOR McCALLUM,
LADY BUCHANAN JARDINE'S DIVISION.　　LOCKERBIE.

A training event of a local Voluntary Aid Detachment, Lockerbie, Dumfriesshire. During the First World War VAD personnel supported the army medical services at home and overseas in a variety of roles including nursing and ambulance driving.

No. 1 Section, F Company, RAMC, Redan Hill, Aldershot, November 1914. All of the recruits, except the sergeant seated in the middle of the front row, wear 'Kitchener's Blue' uniform. This emergency blue uniform was issued to recruits before enough khaki uniforms became available.

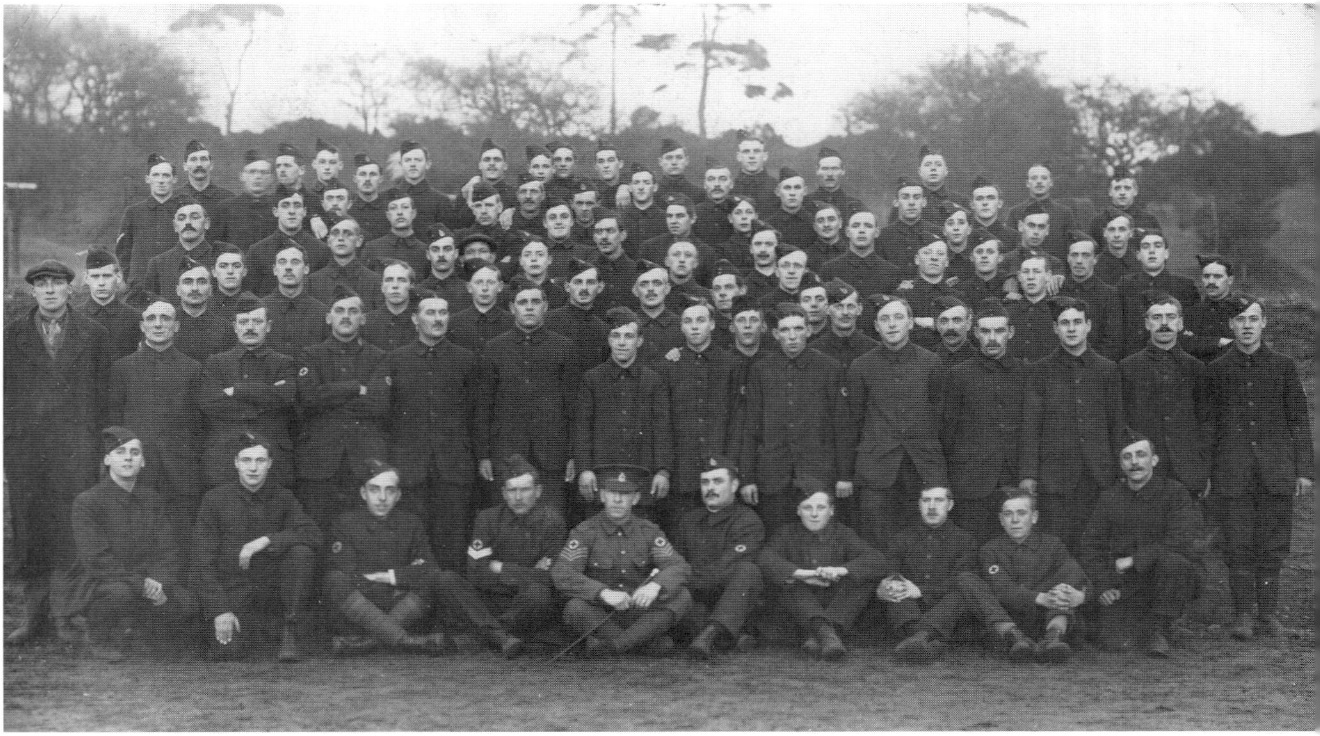

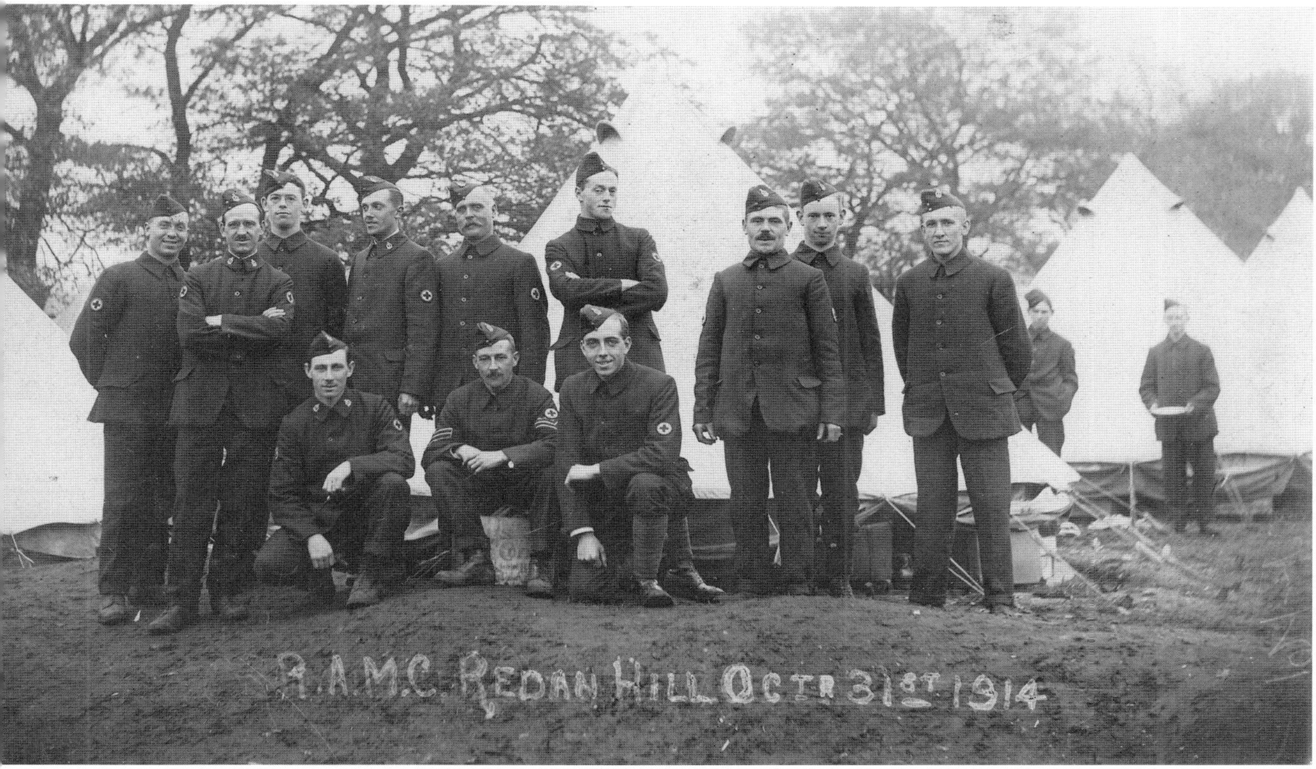

A RAMC group at Redan Hill, Aldershot on 31 October 1914. All wear 'Kitchener's Blue' uniform.

A group of St John's Ambulance Brigade personnel, photographed at a training camp in Kettering. During the war the St John's Ambulance Brigade supported the RAMC in a variety of roles and personnel also volunteered for service in the RAMC on the outbreak of war.

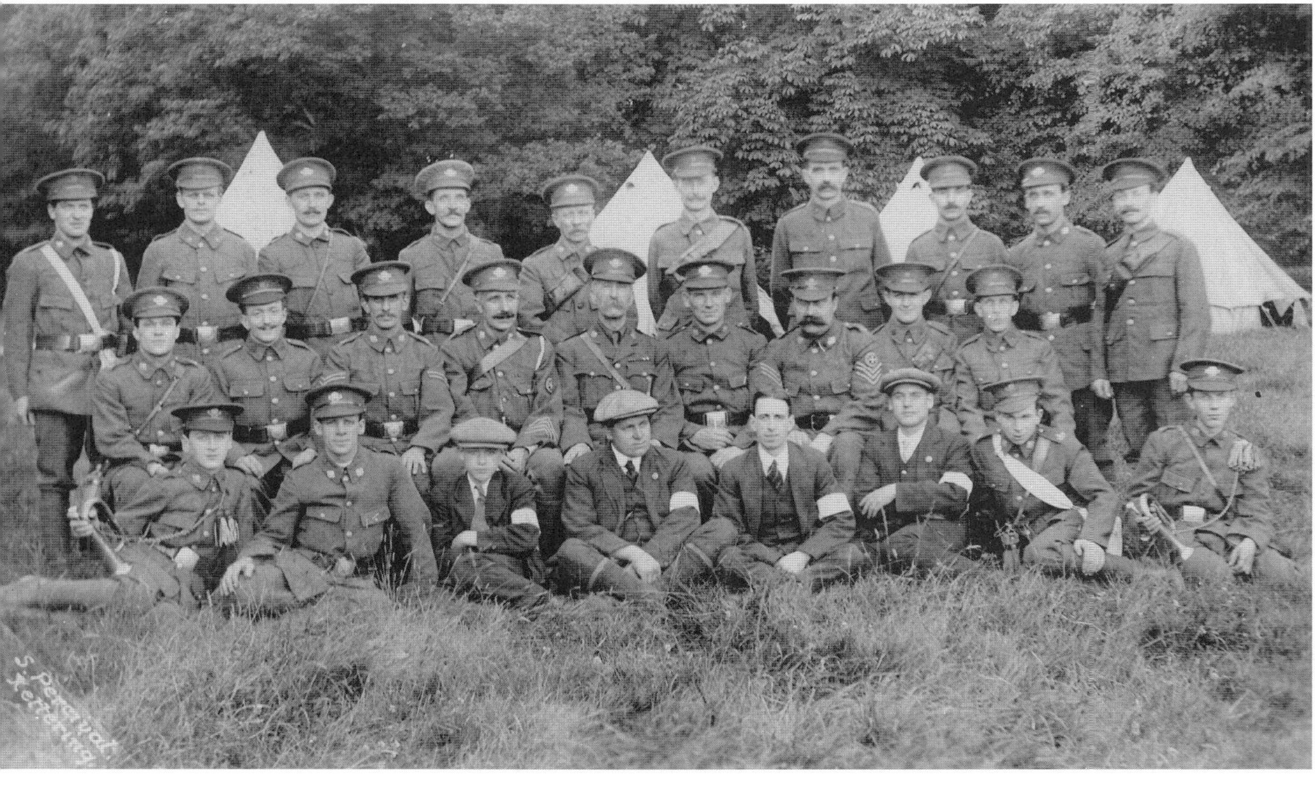

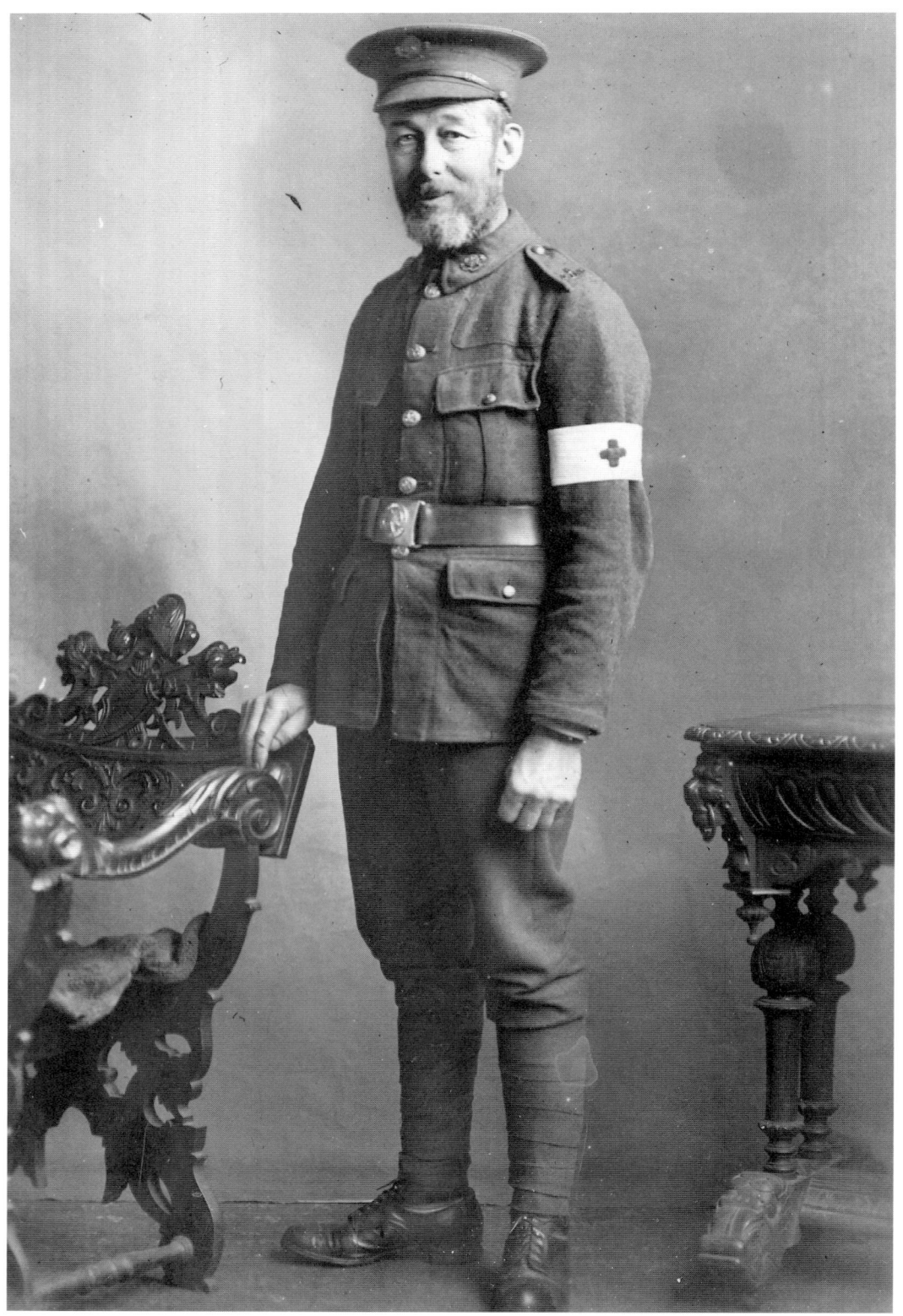
A St John's Ambulance Brigade volunteer.

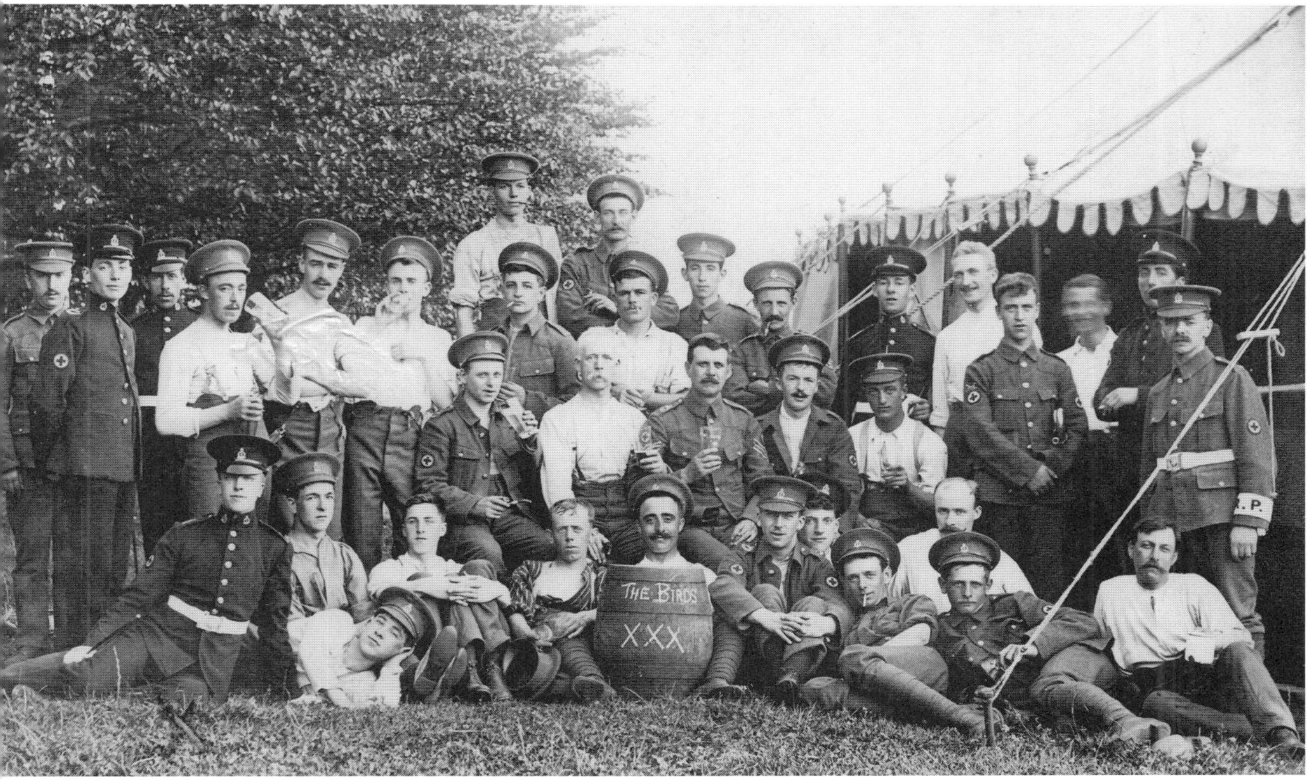

An RAMC (TF) unit training camp; a mix of dress and khaki uniform is being worn. The photo was posted from Hampstead on 30 August 1909.

An RAMC (TF) unit parade, Crickhowell, Wales.

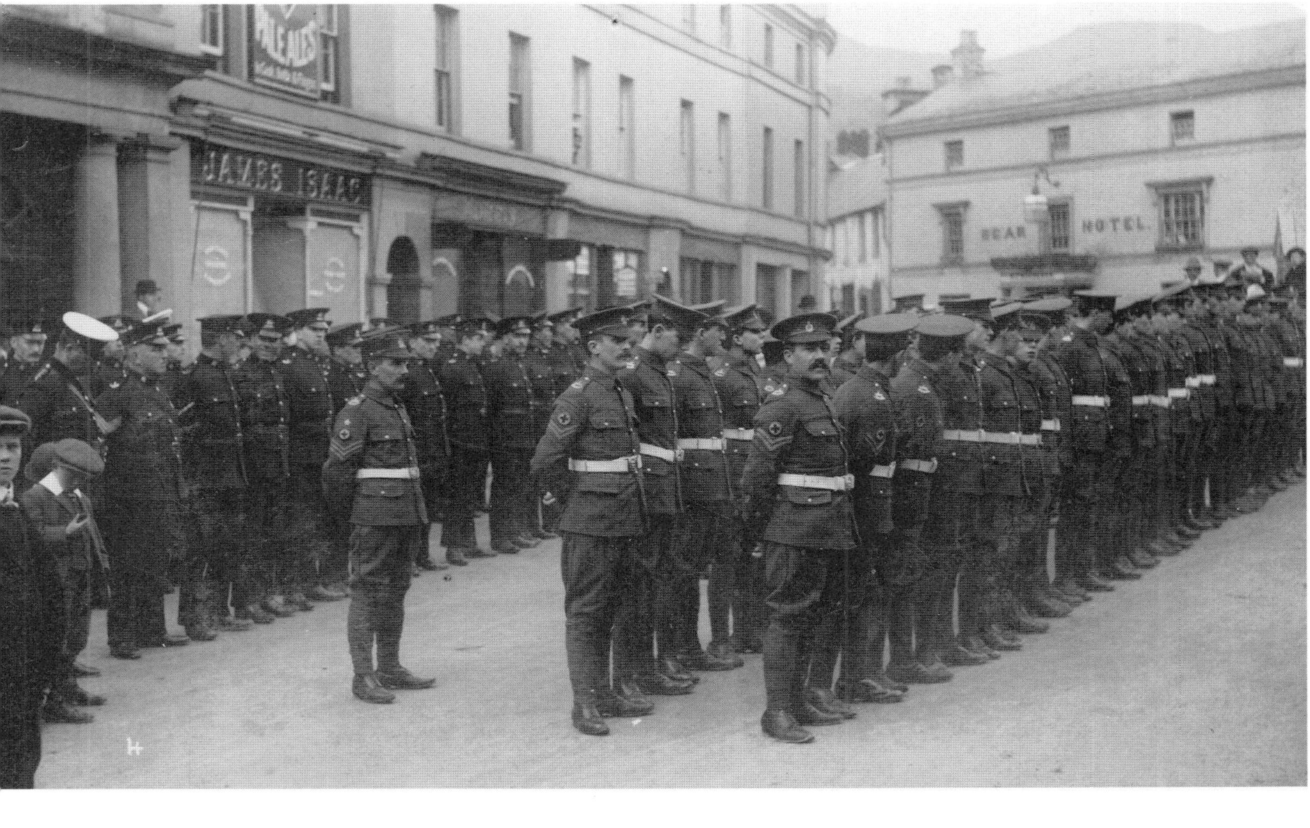

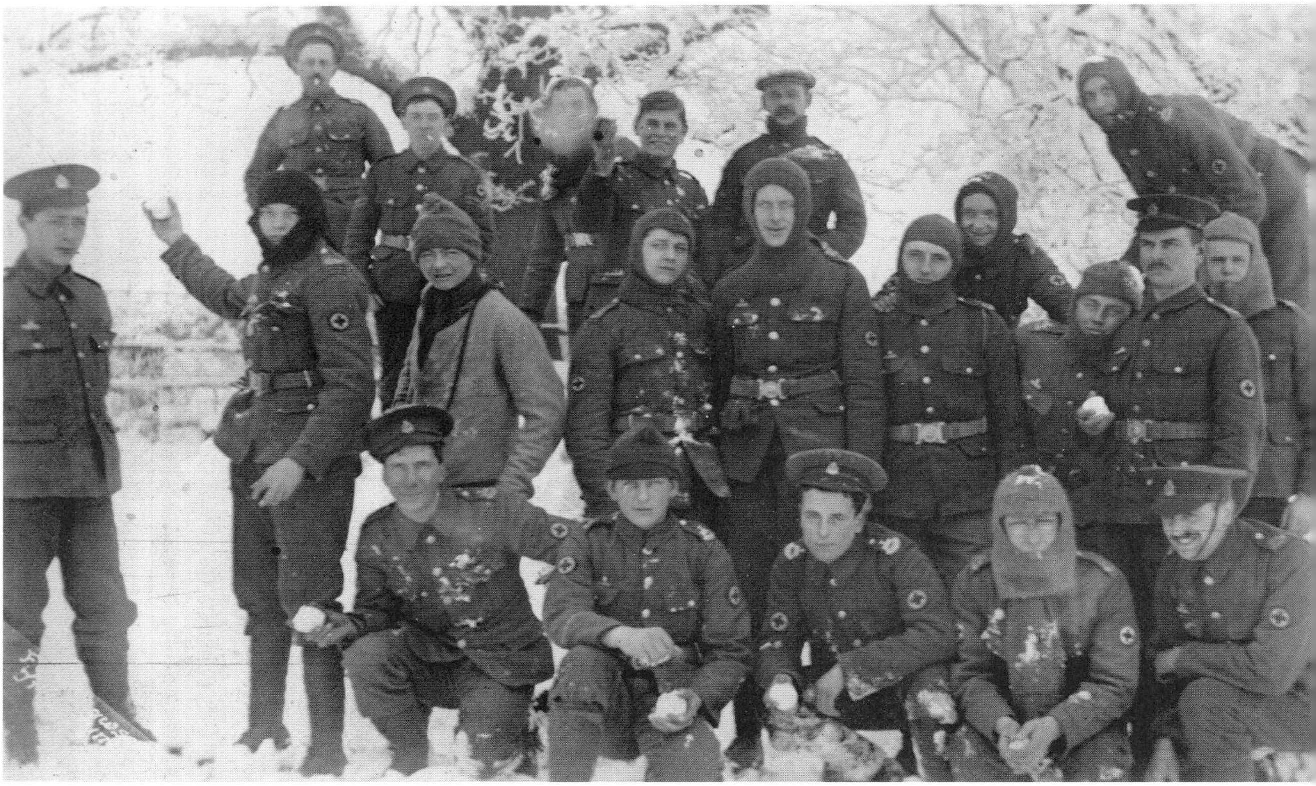

RAMC (TF) personnel training in winter.

RAMC soldiers, with the property owning family, photographed in front of their billet in Blackpool, April 1918. From early in 1917, a Royal Army Medical Corps training centre was located at Blackpool.

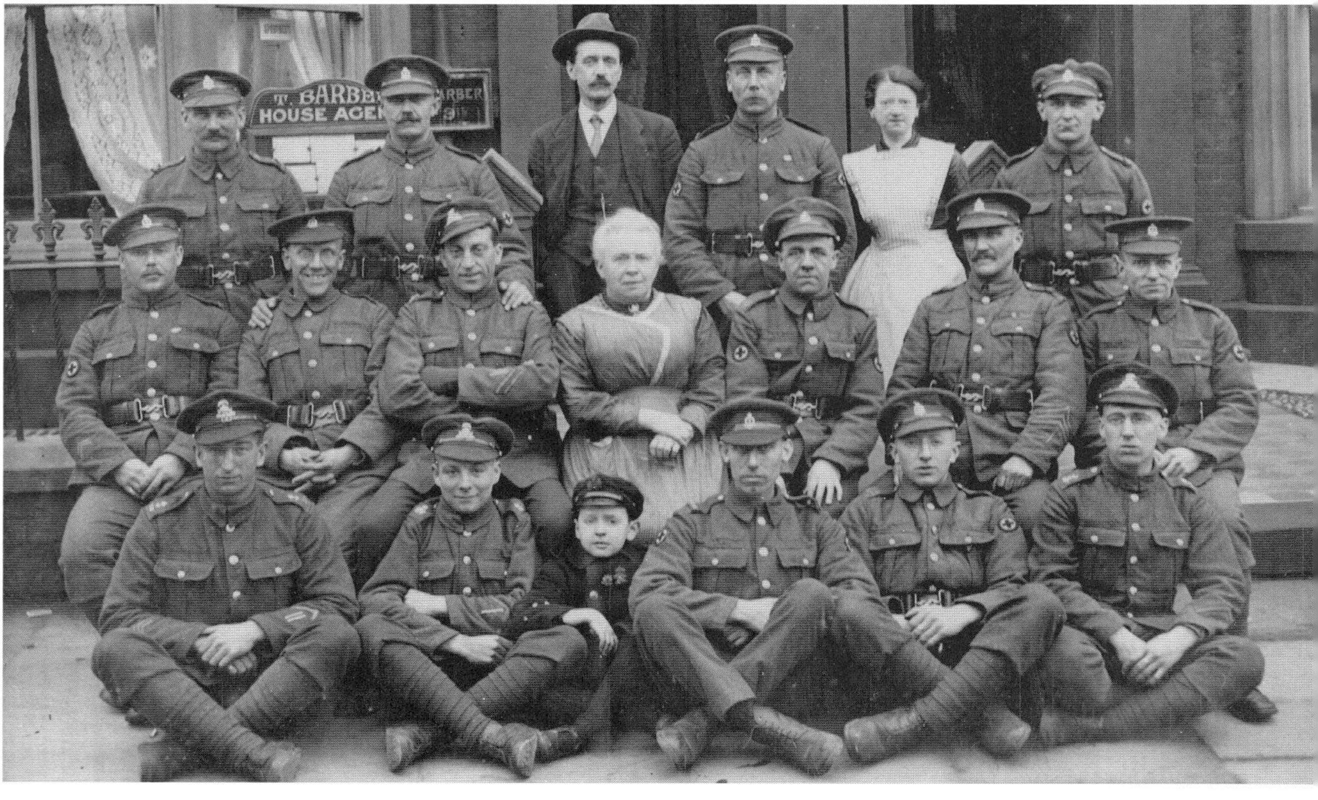

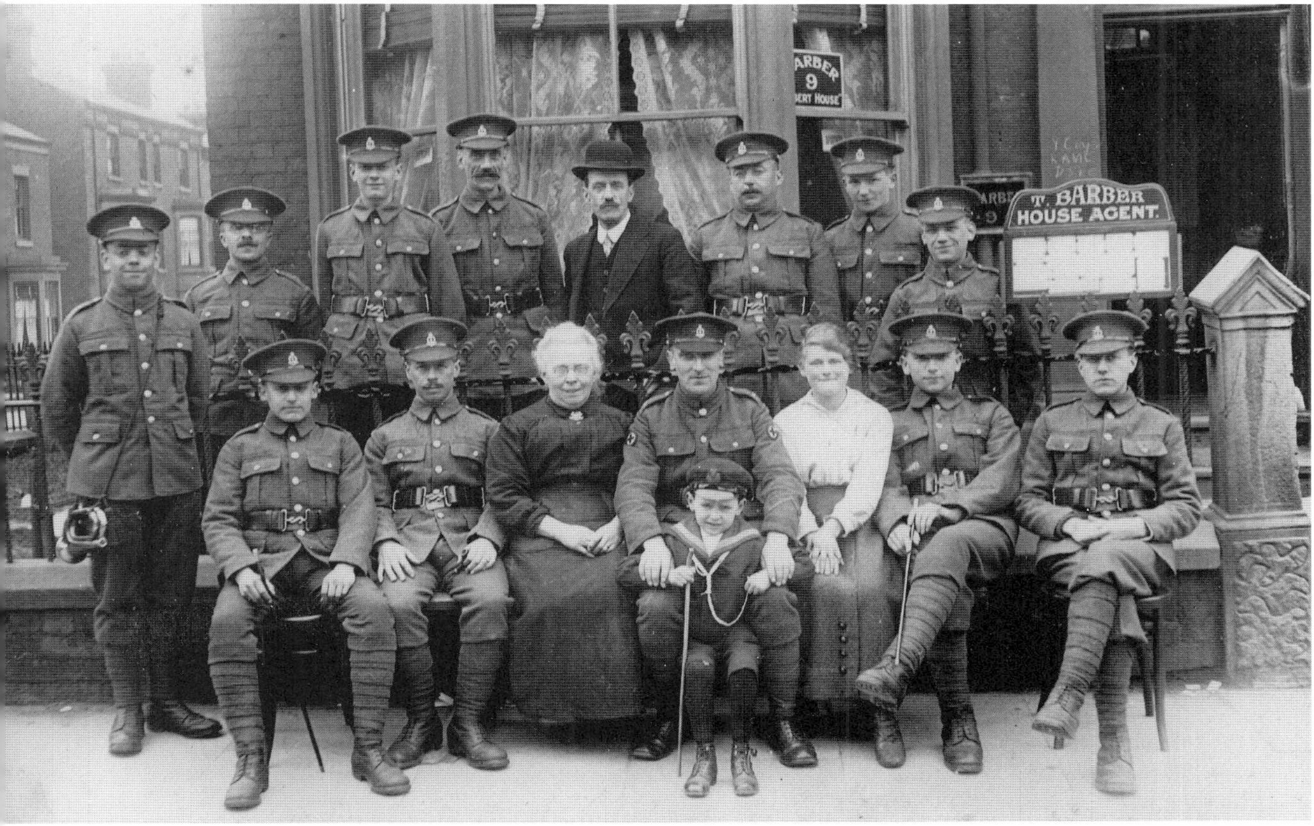

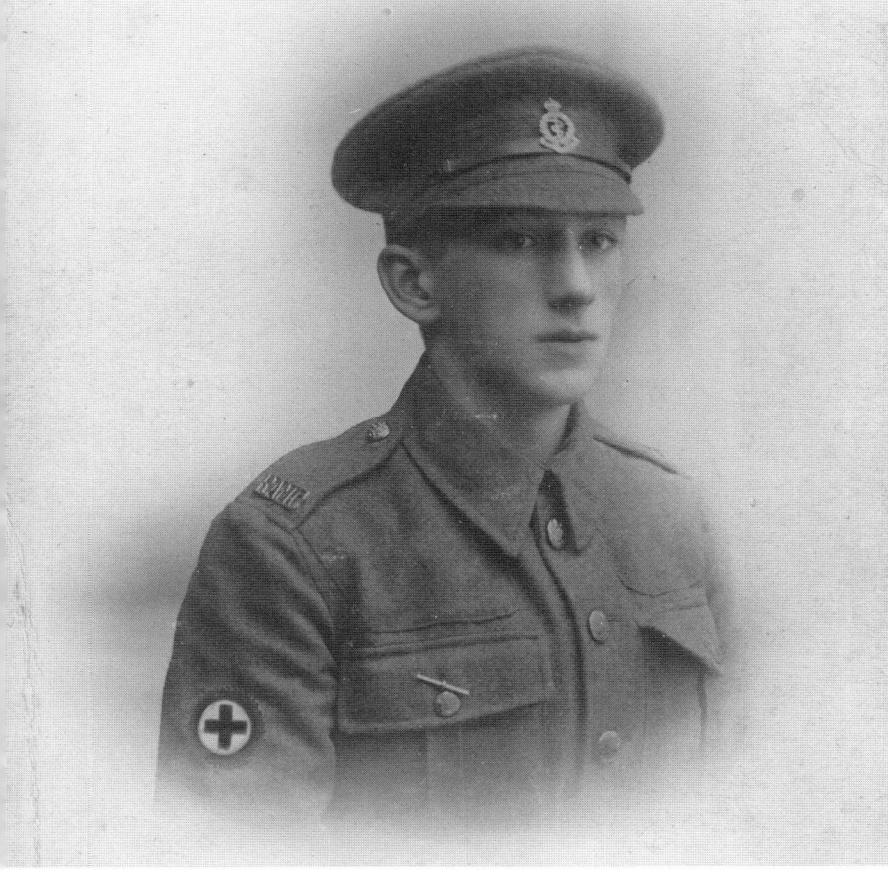

RAMC personnel, with the property owning family, outside their billet in Blackpool. Chalked on doorway is, 'Y Coy, RAMC, D Section'.

Photo of a private serving with the RAMC in Blackpool. Unusually, the photo includes colour tinting.

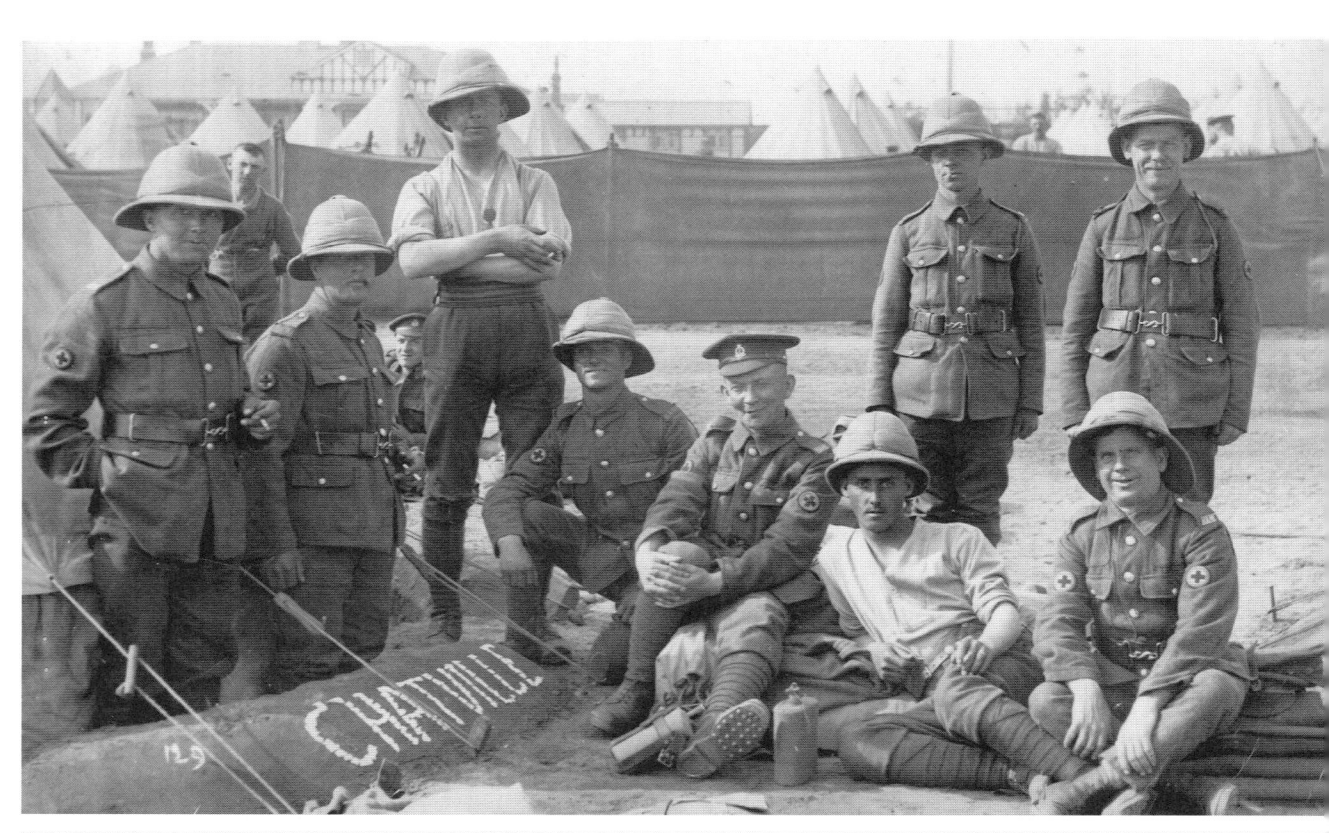

(**Right**) An RAMC private photographed at Warminster. The town is located close to Salisbury Plain military training area.

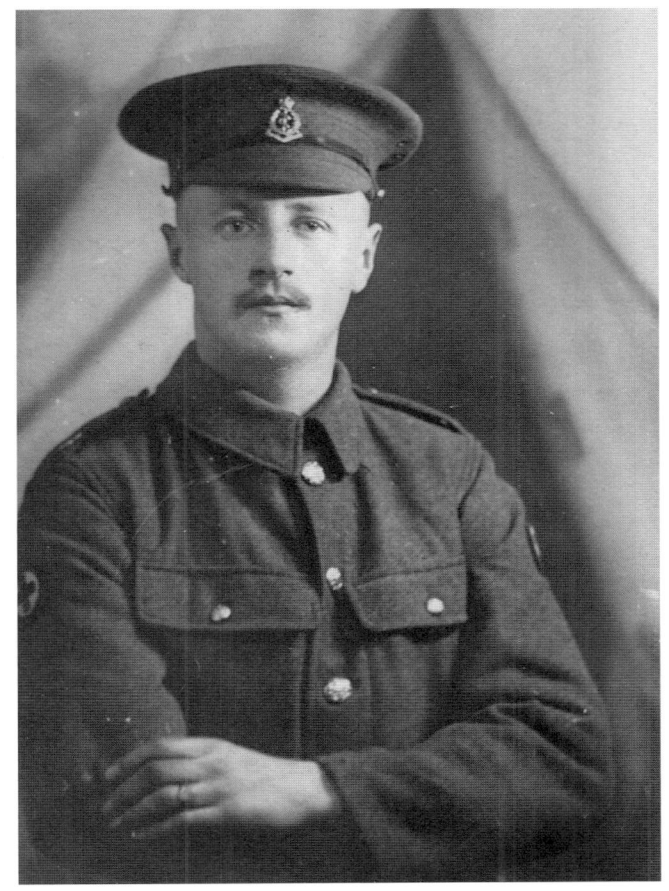

(**Opposite page**) Royal Army Medical Corps personnel at Squires Gate Camp, Blackpool. An RAMC training centre was located at Squires Gate. Most of the soldiers wear Wolseley Sun Helmets, which suggests they were waiting to proceed overseas, possibly to the Middle East or Salonika. It was thought the Wolseley Sun Helmet was effective in protecting the wearer from sunstroke. The reverse of the photograph notes their tent, 'Chatville', was named due to the large number of lice at Squires Gate Camp.

(**Below**) Haig Hutments, RAMC Training Centre. The card was posted on 28 August 1915.

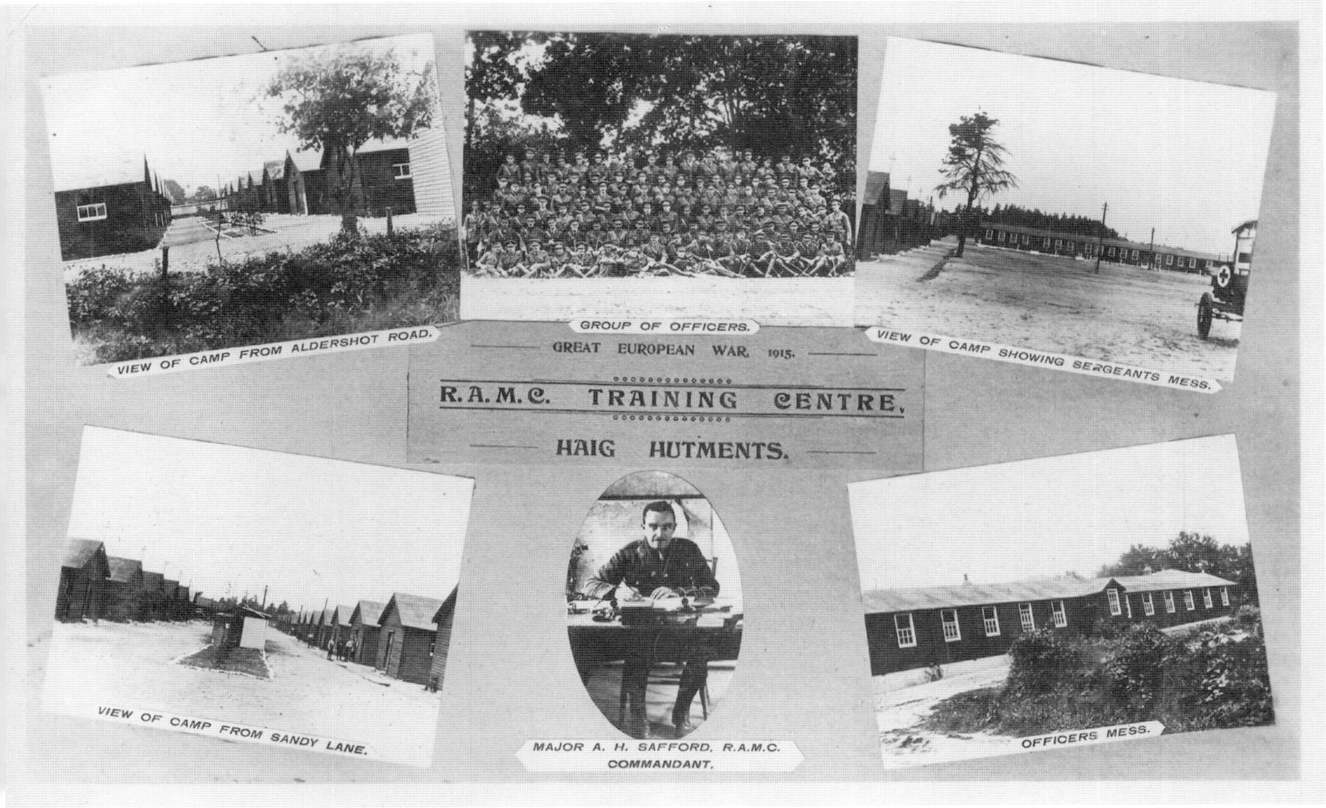

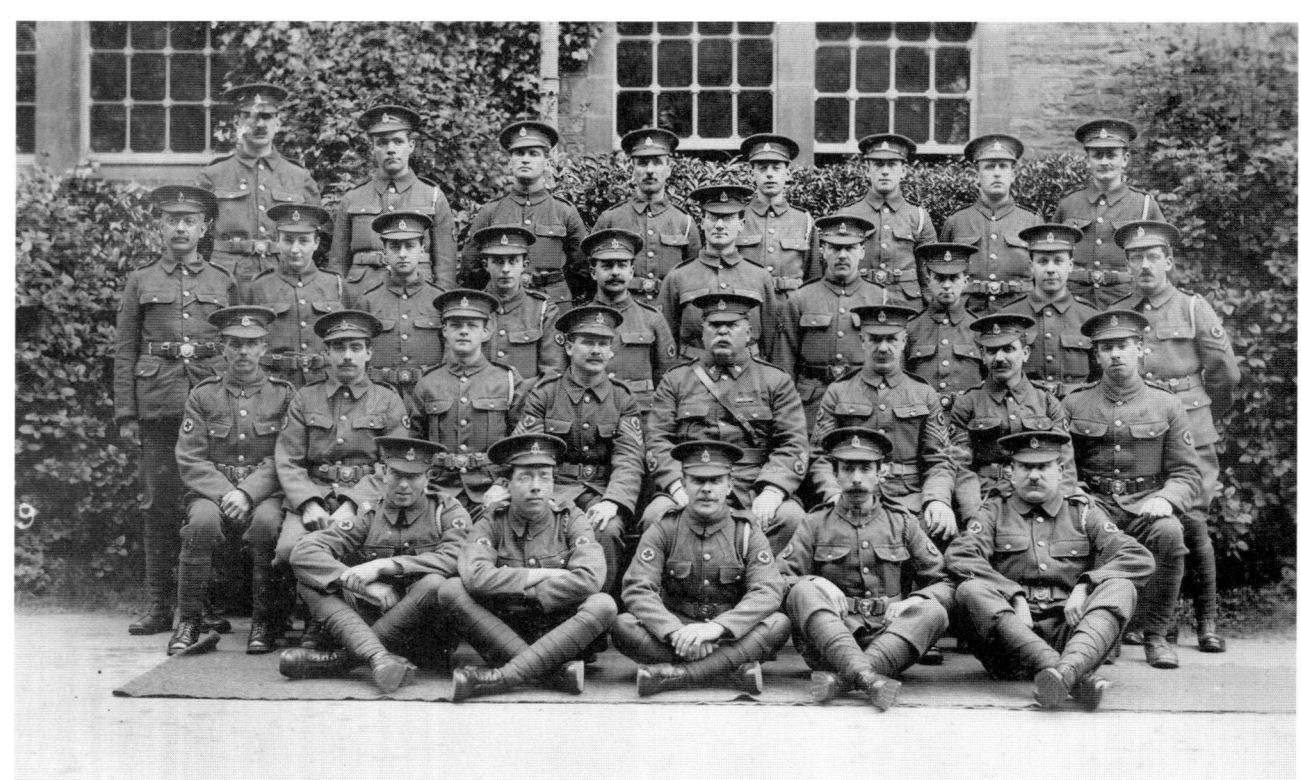

Photographic postcard taken at a RAMC training centre for recruits who would be serving in the UK. They are photographed with their training RAMC non-commissioned officers. Interestingly, all the soldiers are named on the reverse of the photograph.

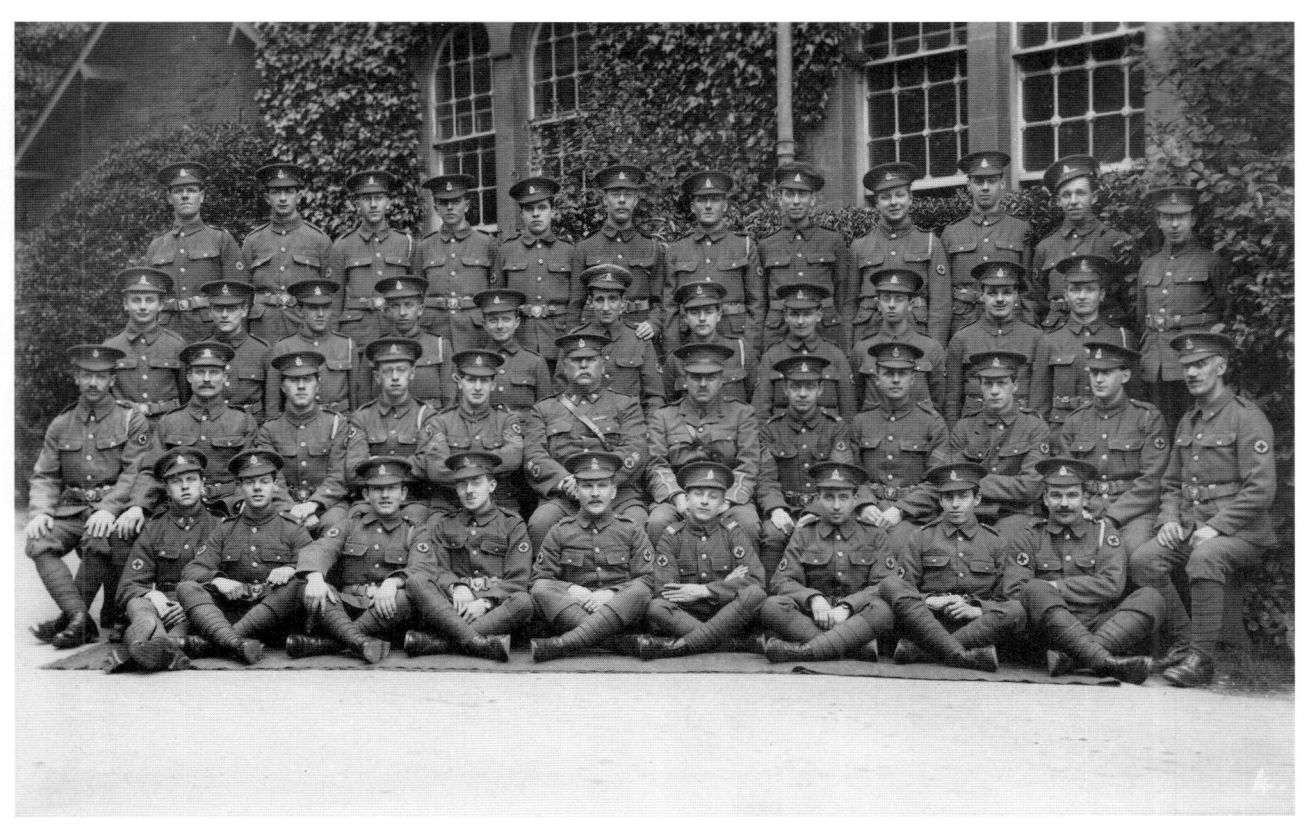

Photographic postcard taken at a RAMC training centre of personnel who would be serving overseas. They are photographed with their training RAMC major and non-commissioned officers. Again, unusually, all are named on the reverse of the photo.

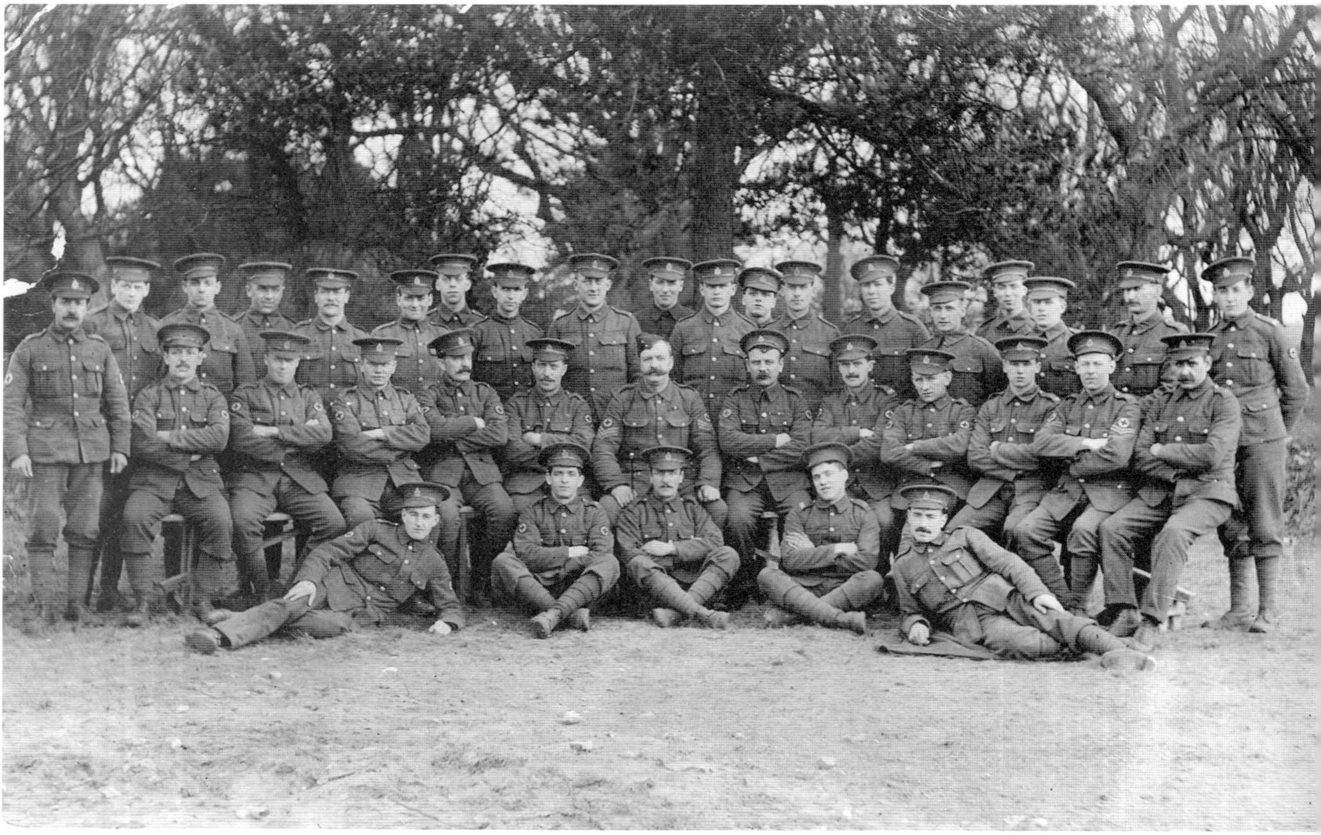

Personnel at the RAMC Training Centre, Crookham, Hampshire.

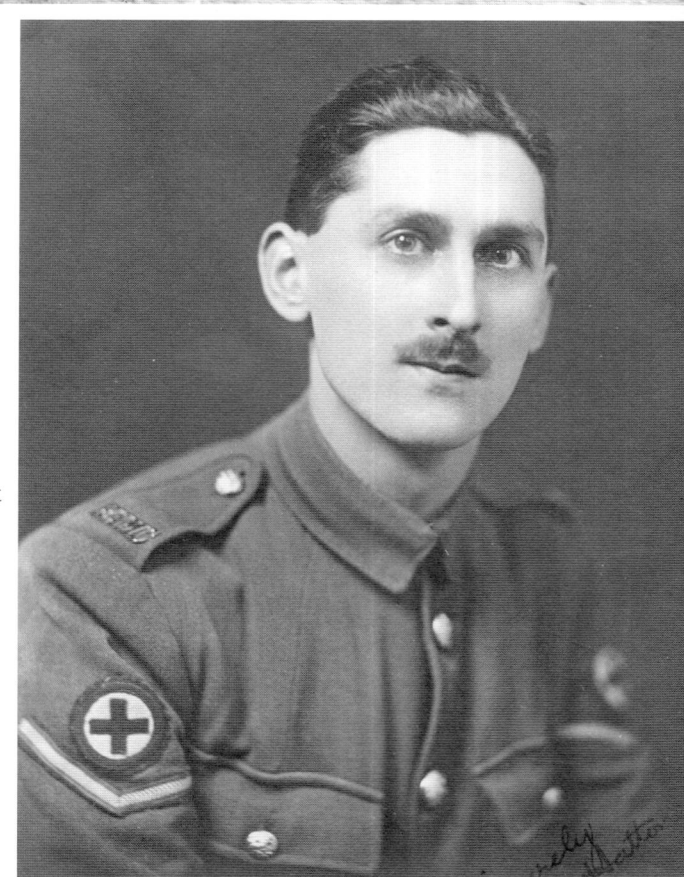

99002 Lance Corporal (later Sergeant) Horace Reginald Hatton, RAMC, who served with medical units in the UK. Horace Reginald Hatton was born at New Barnet, Hertfordshire in 1892. He enlisted on 30 August 1916 at Ripon. On enlistment he was a shipping clerk, residing at 115 Stroud Gardens Road, Finsbury Park. His next of kin was his father, Martin Southwell Hatton. He originally served with T Company RAMC and was then posted to 319 (East Anglian) Field Ambulance on 24 January 1917 and later to 20th Company, RAMC, at Durrington on 28 June 1919. He married Iris Christiana Smith on 5 May 1917. On demobilisation his address was given as 90 Wilberforce Road, Finsbury Park. He died at Amersham, Buckinghamshire, in 1971.

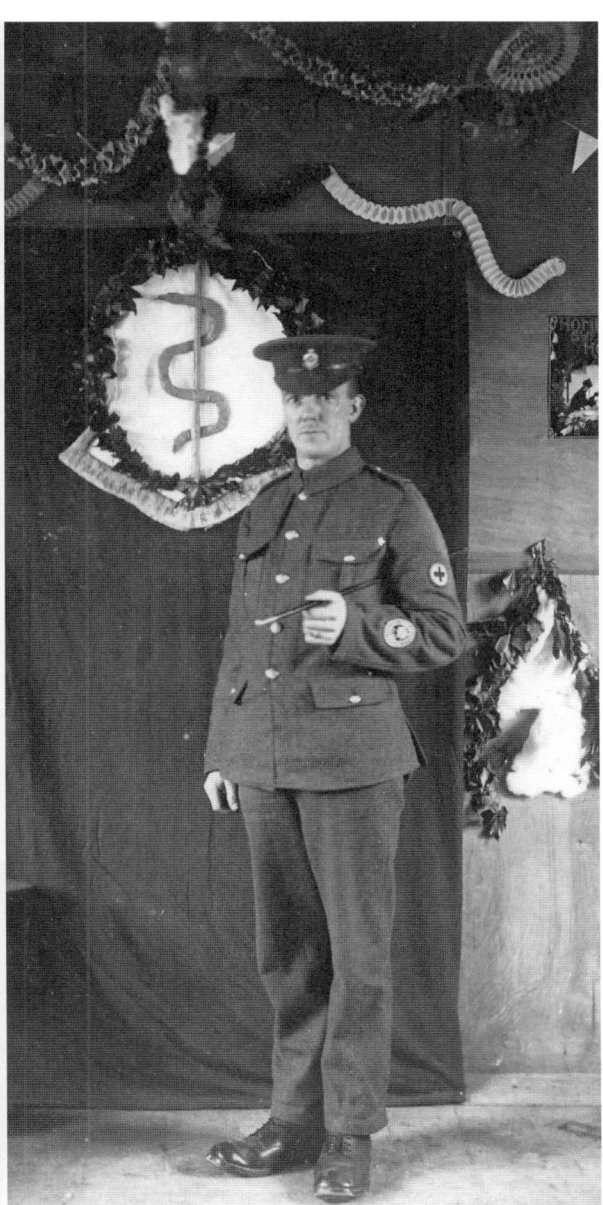 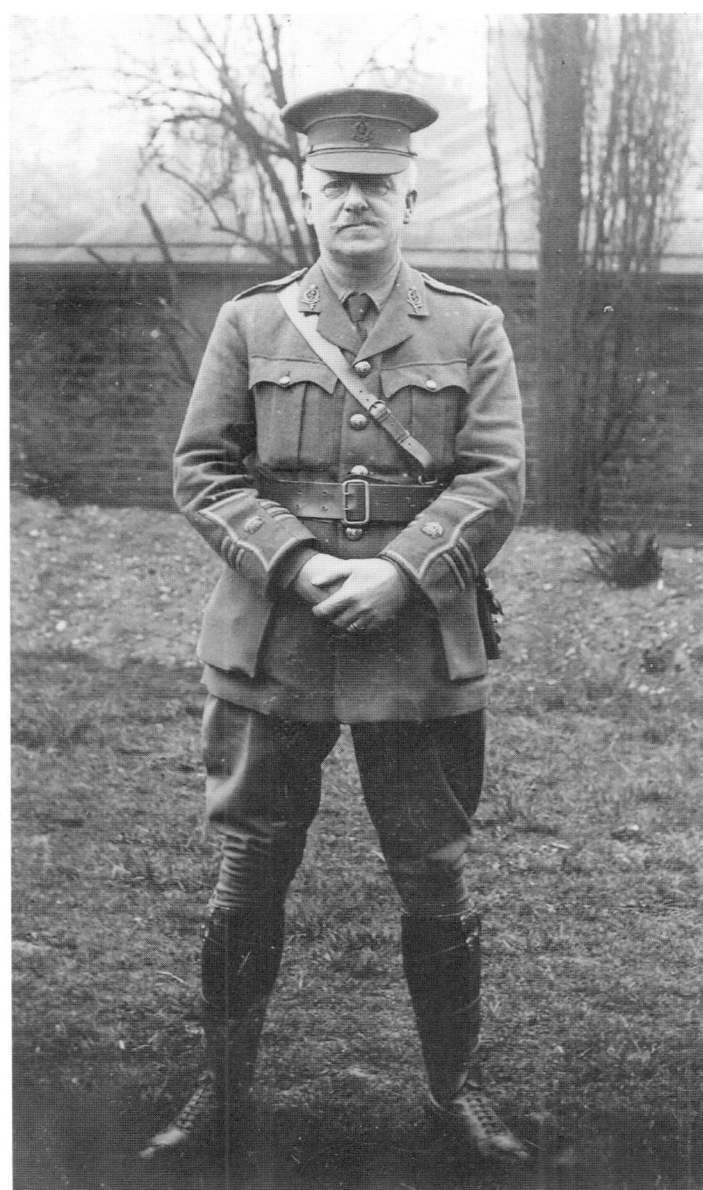

(**Left**) 101064 Private John Henry Abrahams RAMC, serving at Bulford Camp. Note the RAMC badge made from paper and textiles in the background.

(**Right**) Major Robert James William Oswald (later Lieutenant Colonel) serving with the 1st City of London General Hospital, RAMC (TF). In 1880, in Edinburgh, he qualified as a Licentiate of the Royal College of Practitioners and in 1881 as a Member of the Royal College of Surgeons. He served throughout the war in the UK and his home address was 185, Clapham Road, London. He was awarded an OBE for his services during the First World War.

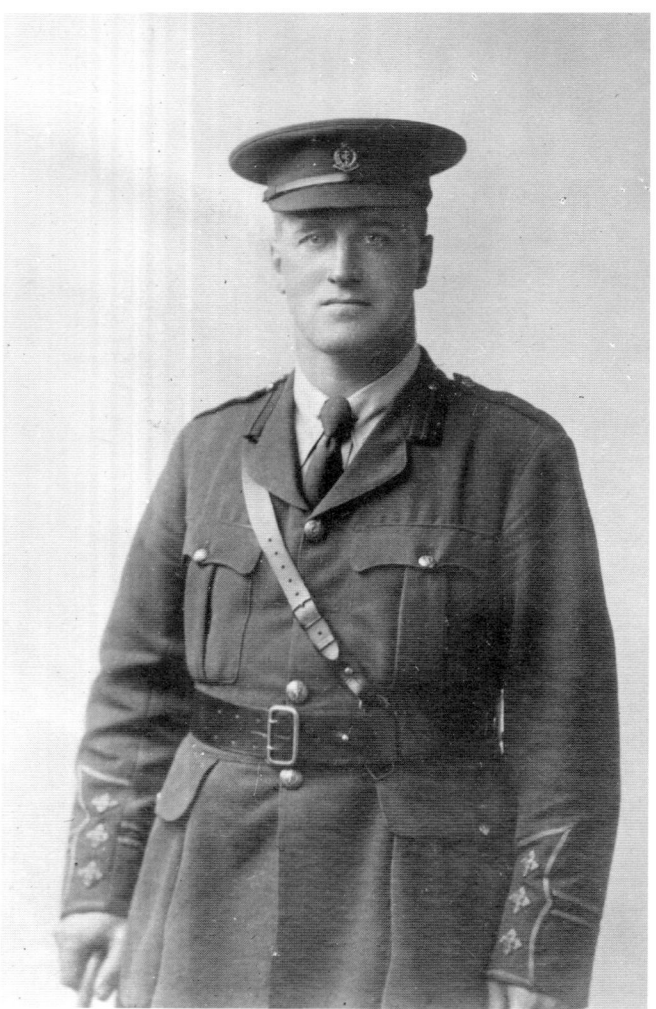 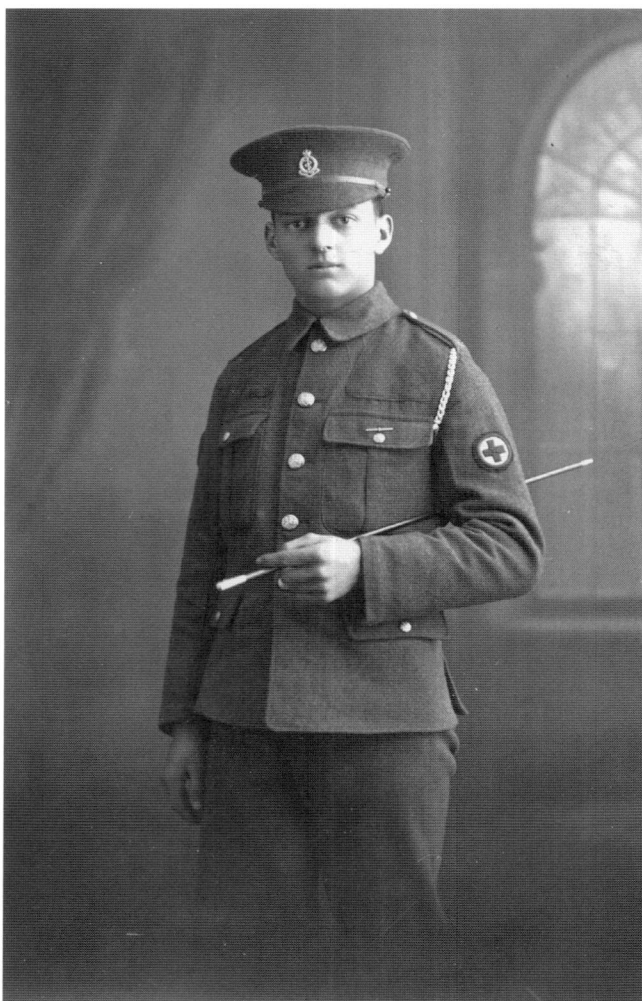

(**Left**) Captain Robert Arthur Lyster, RAMC. He wears staff officer collar patches. Robert Arthur Lyster was an expert in Hygiene and was employed as a Specialist Sanitary Officer for the Winchester area, Southern Command, 1914–1918. He died in 1955. He had a very distinguished career in Public Health, holding a number of positions including: Lecturer in Public Health and in Forensic Medicine at St Bartholomew's Hospital (London University), 1911–41; Member of Faculty of Medicine and Board of Studies in Hygiene in the University of London; Vice President Medical Defence Union, 1911–42; Member Medical Board, Lord Mayor Treloar's Hospital, Alton; Chairman National Society for Prevention of Venereal Disease; Member Public Health Advisory Committee of the Labour Party; County Medical Officer, Hampshire; also Chief School Medical Officer and Chief Tuberculosis Officer, 1908–29; Editor of *Public Health*, 1918–25; President of the Association of County Medical Officers of Health, 1926–27; Specialist Sanitary Officer for Barracks and Camps and Venereal Diseases Officer; Member Advisory Com. for the Welfare of Blind Persons (Ministry of Health); Member of Ministry of Health Committee on Sewage Disposal.

(**Right**) This photograph was posted by an RAMC private from New Barracks, Limerick, Ireland. The message describes a good Christmas dinner provided for his unit by his officer, Limerick races held on Boxing Day and being somewhat homesick after leaving Sheffield. The photo is signed 'Cecil'.

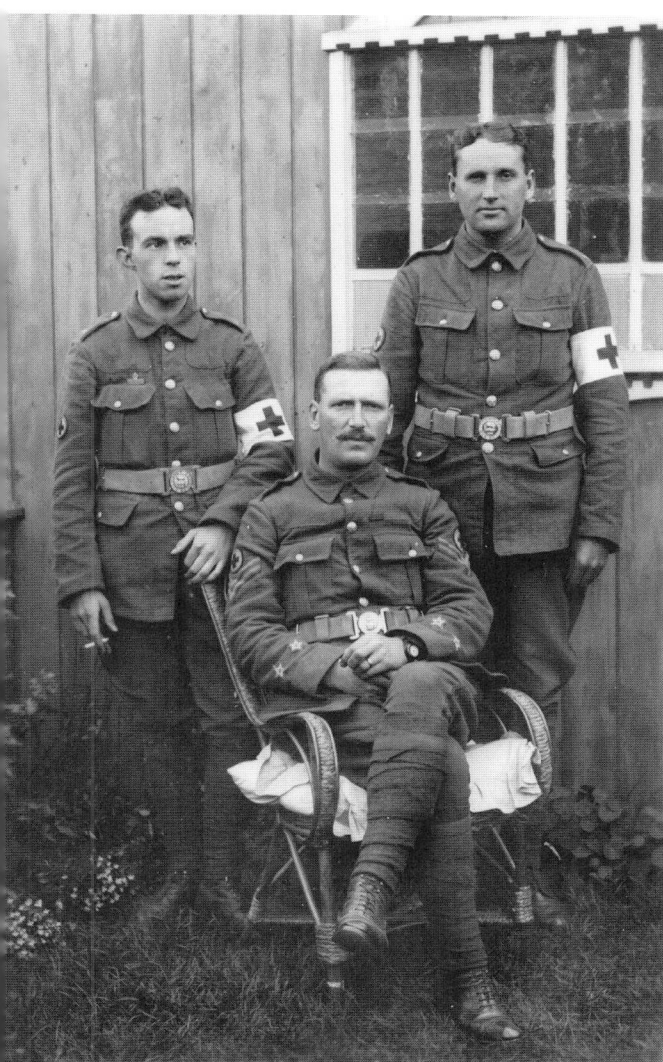 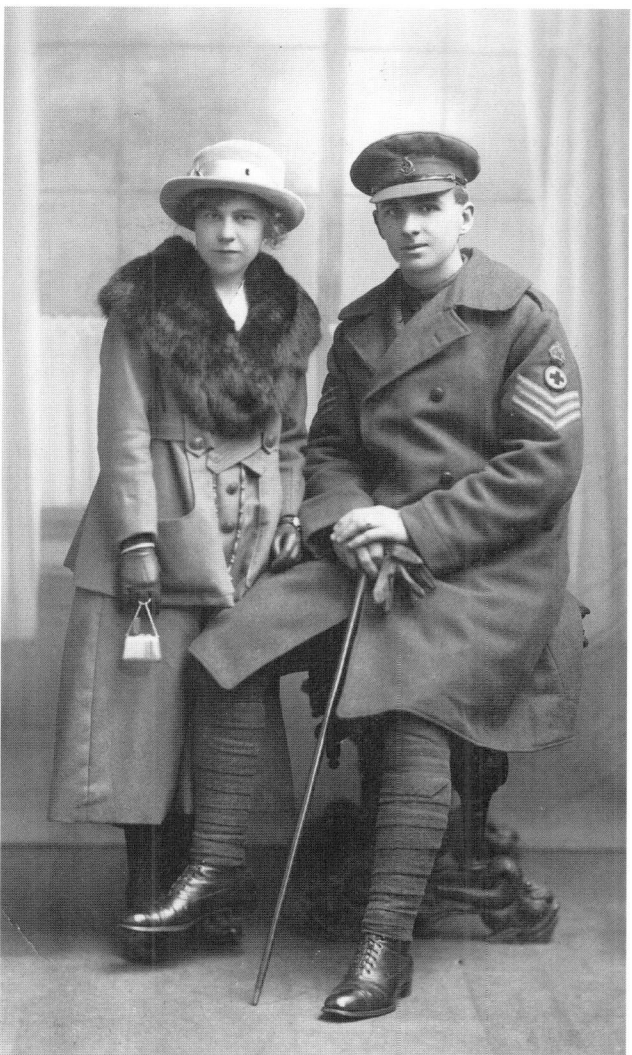

(**Left**) A corporal and two privates serving with an RAMC (TF) unit. The private (back left) wears an Imperial Service Badge above his right pocket which indicates service in a unit which had volunteered for overseas service. The corporal wears two qualification stars on each cuff and the ribbon of the Queen's South Africa Medal, above his left pocket, denoting service in the South African War of 1899–1902.

(**Right**) An RAMC staff sergeant photographed with a member of his family. Family photographs were often taken prior to overseas service. The reverse of the photograph, taken in Margate, is inscribed 'To Lil, With Love & Best Wishes, from Ernie and Gertie'.

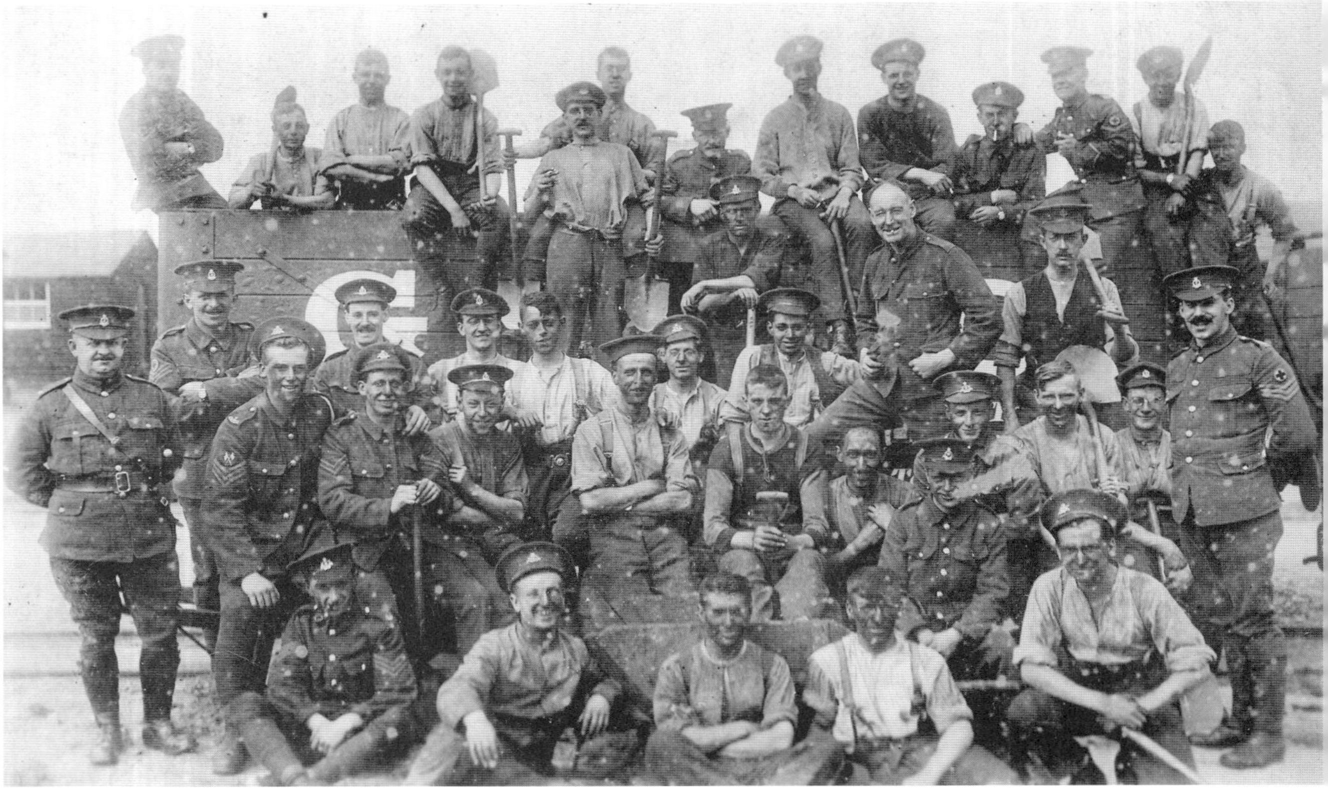

RAMC and Cyclist Corps personnel photographed at Mansfield. They appear to be on fatigue duty, sitting on a railway wagon.

An RAMC corporal and his section at a military camp or medical facility. They appear to be working to improve drainage or to dig the foundations for another hut.

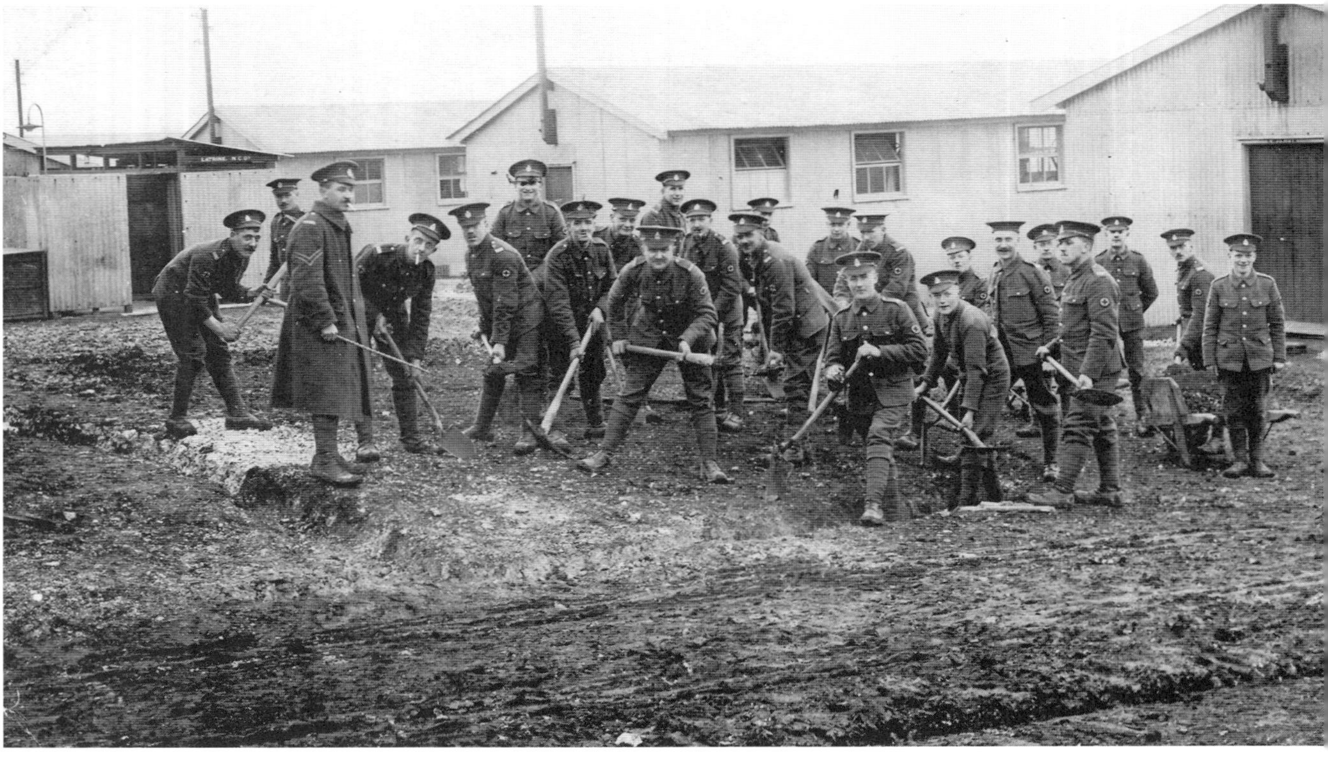

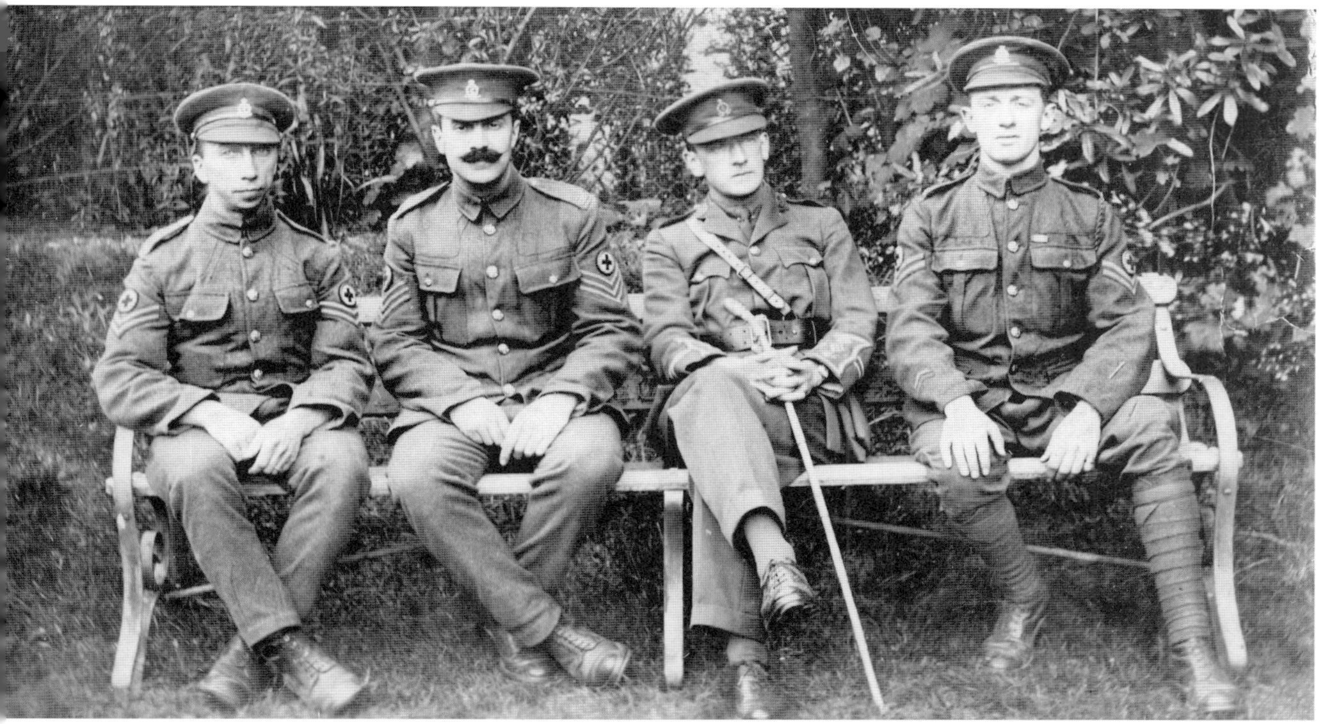

A captain, sergeant and two corporals serving with the RAMC. The corporal, seated right, wears a wound stripe and two overseas service chevrons.

RAMC (TF) personnel in Newcastle upon Tyne. Several of the servicemen wear Imperial Service Badges.

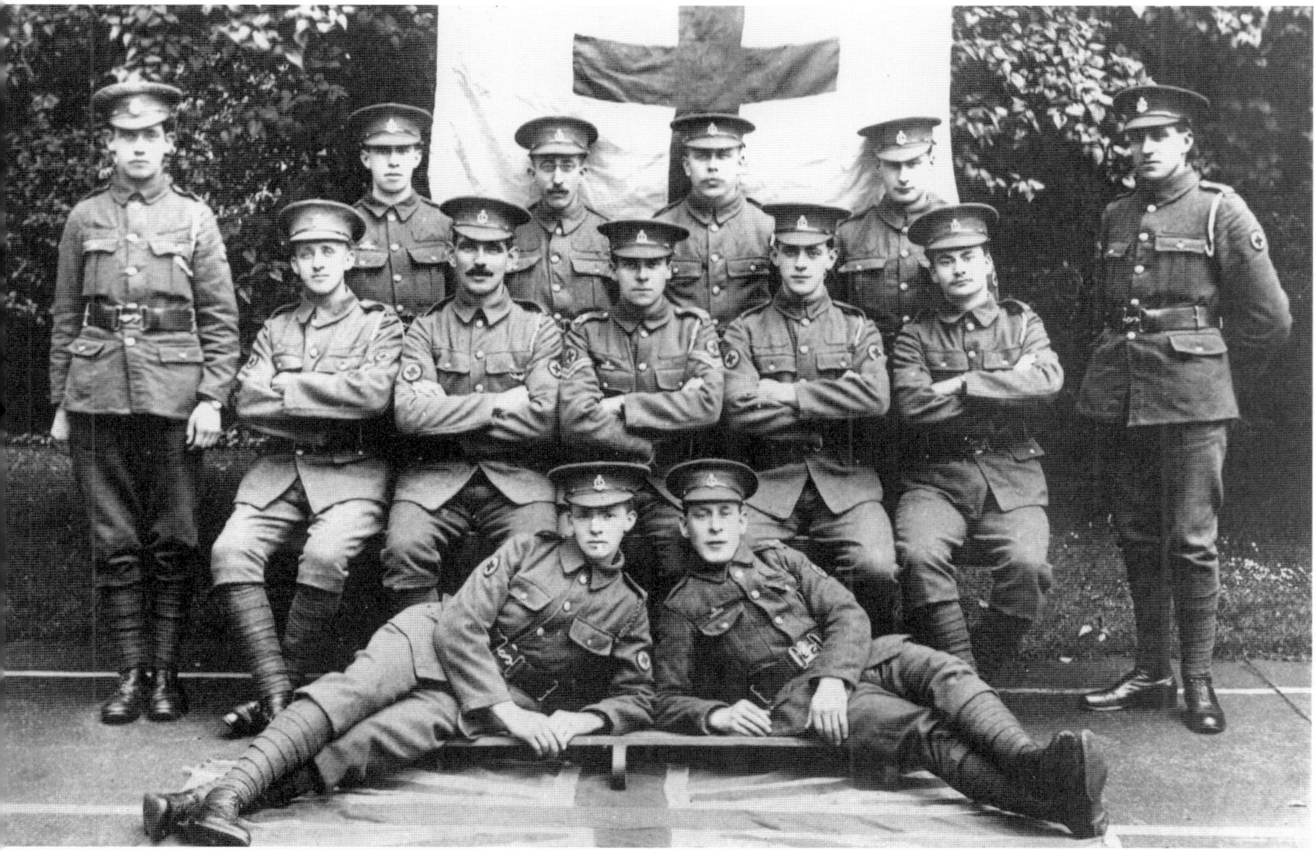

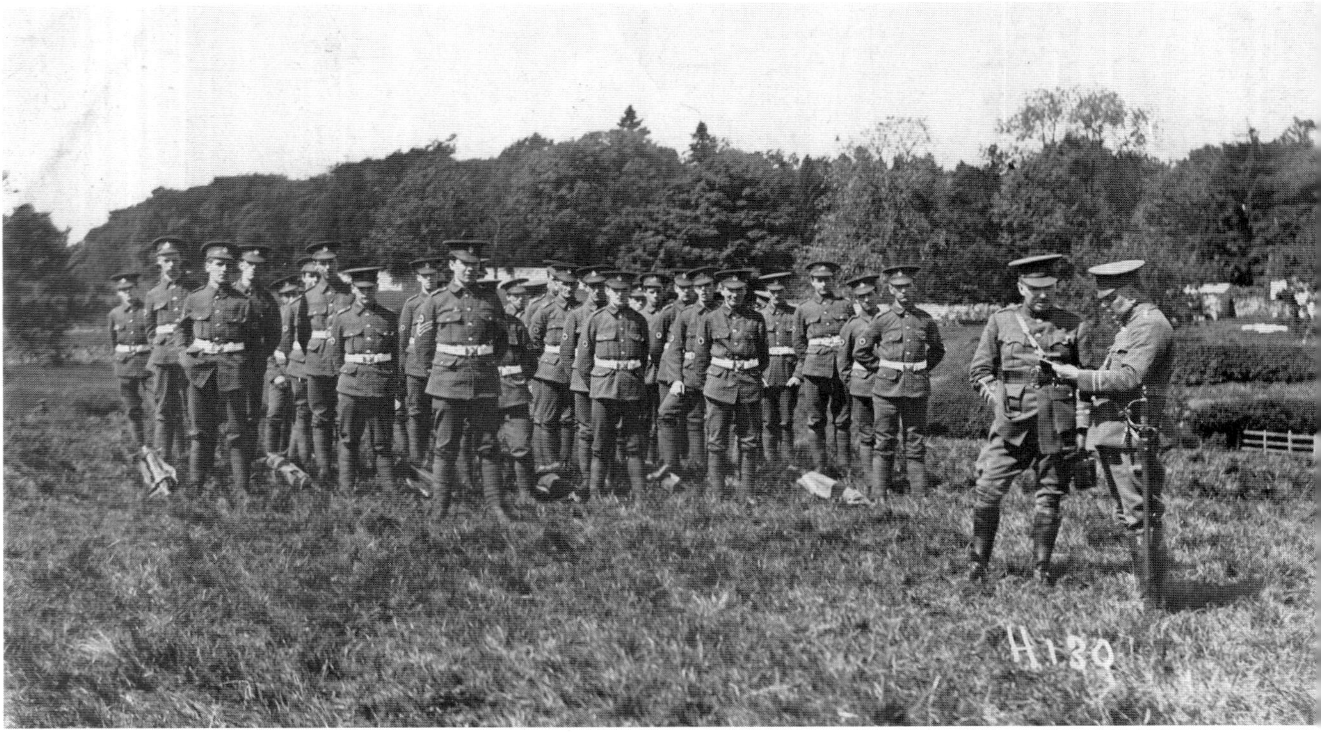

(**Above**) RAMC personnel training with stretchers. This photograph was posted from Newcastle upon Tyne to Maryport, Cumbria, on 10 October 1914.

(**Opposite page**) A private serving with a RAMC (TF) unit photographed in Gateshead.

(**Below**) RAMC personnel serving with a RAMC (TF) unit photographed at Cowes, Isle of Wight.

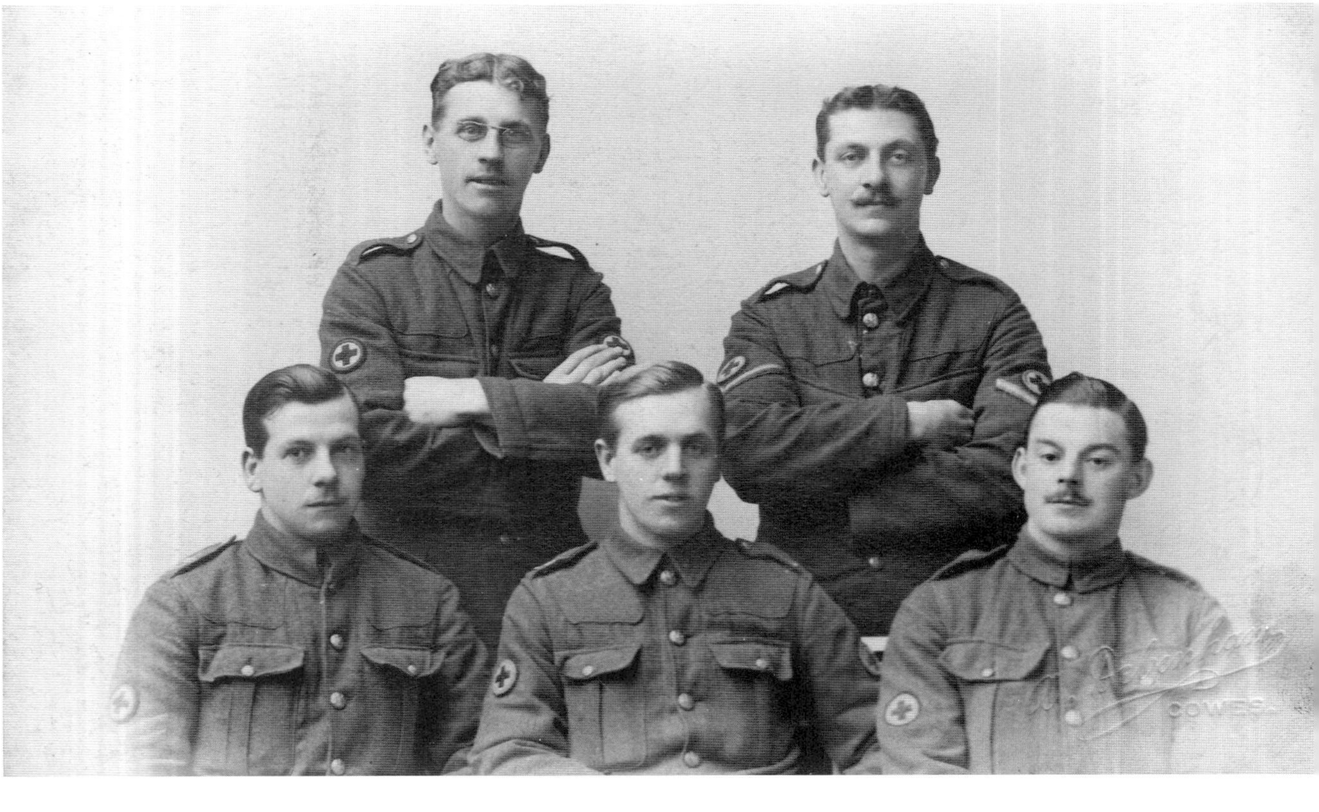

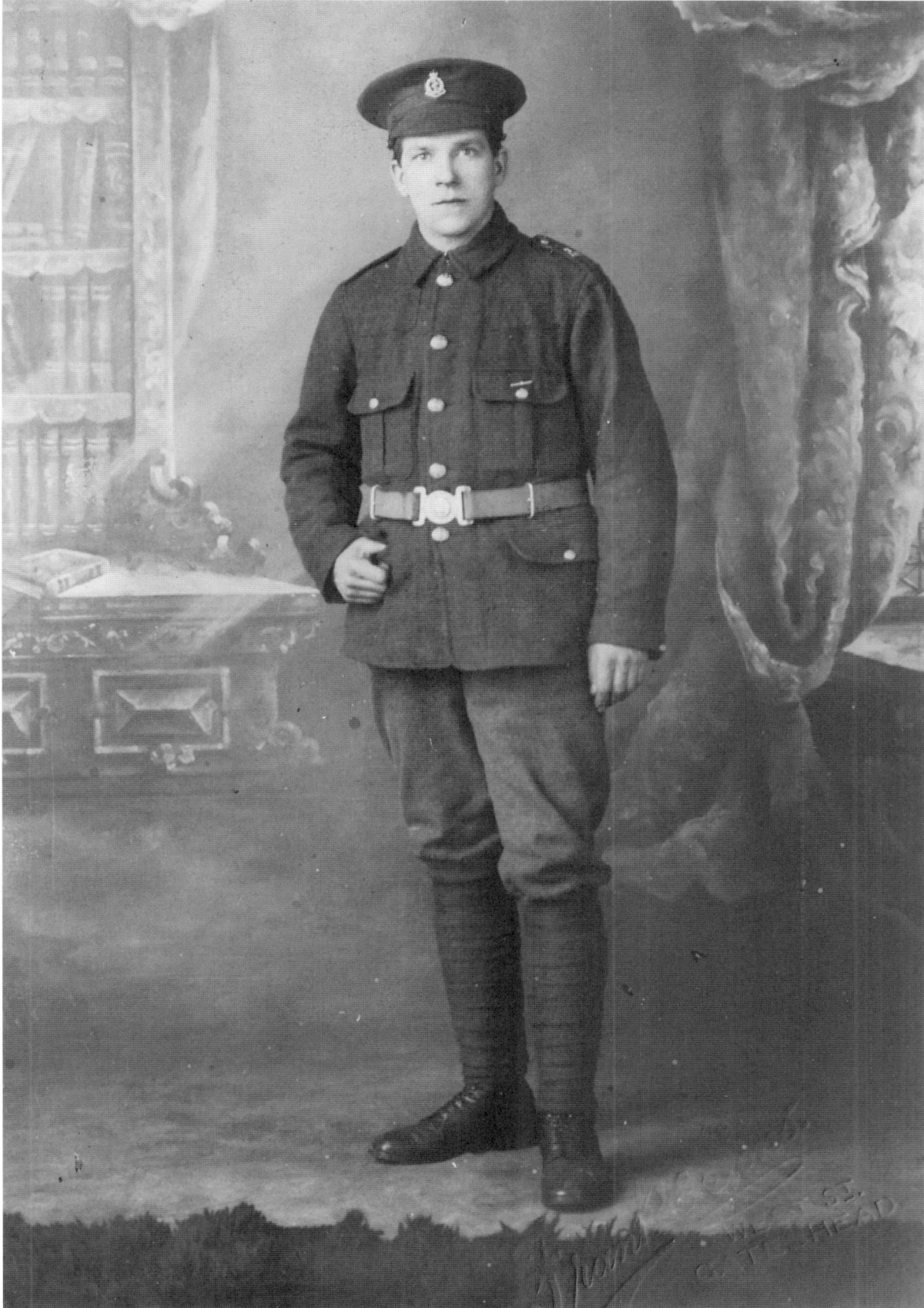

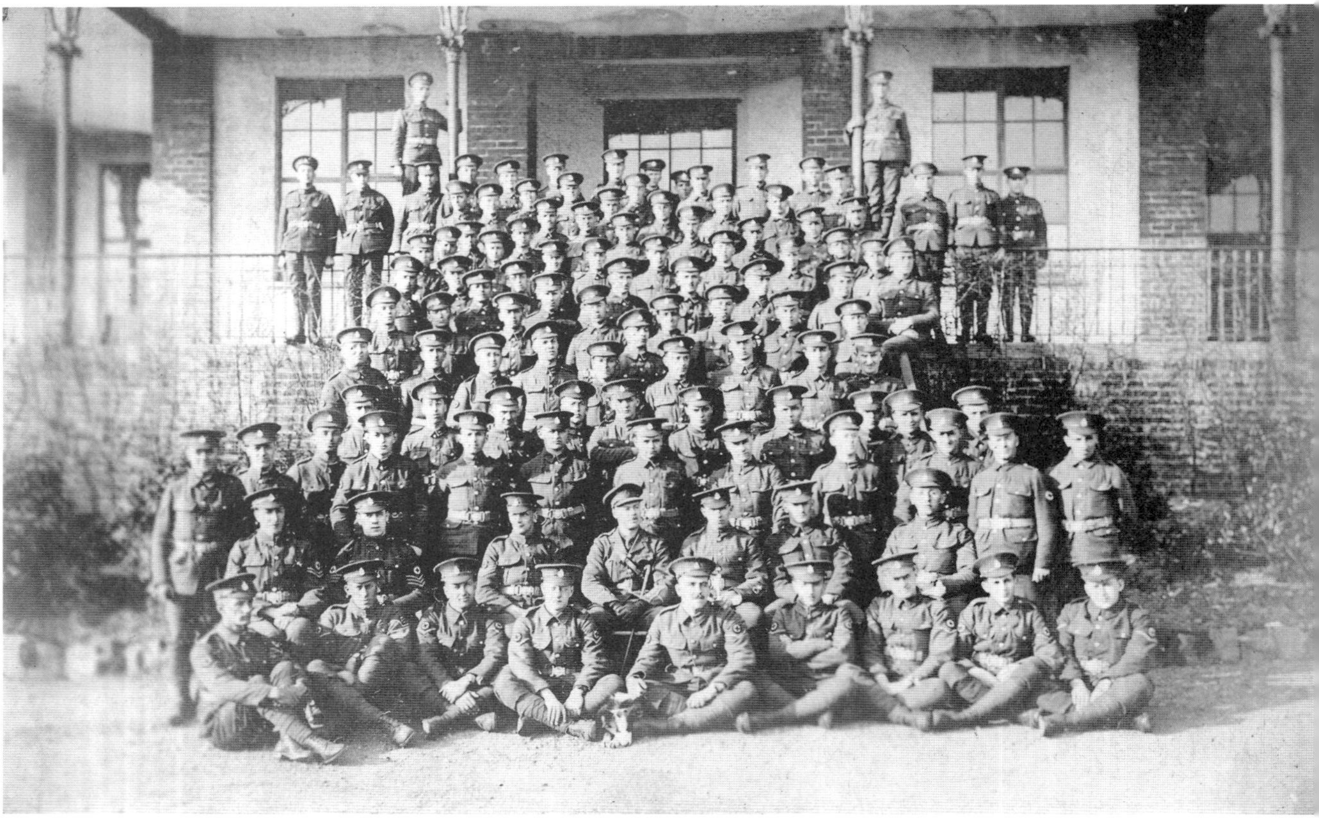

(**Above**) A RAMC unit photographed at Llandrindod Wells, Powys.

(**Opposite page**) Personnel of a RAMC (TF) unit, photographed in Doncaster on 17 March 1917.

(**Below**) RAMC personnel at Herne Bay, Kent.

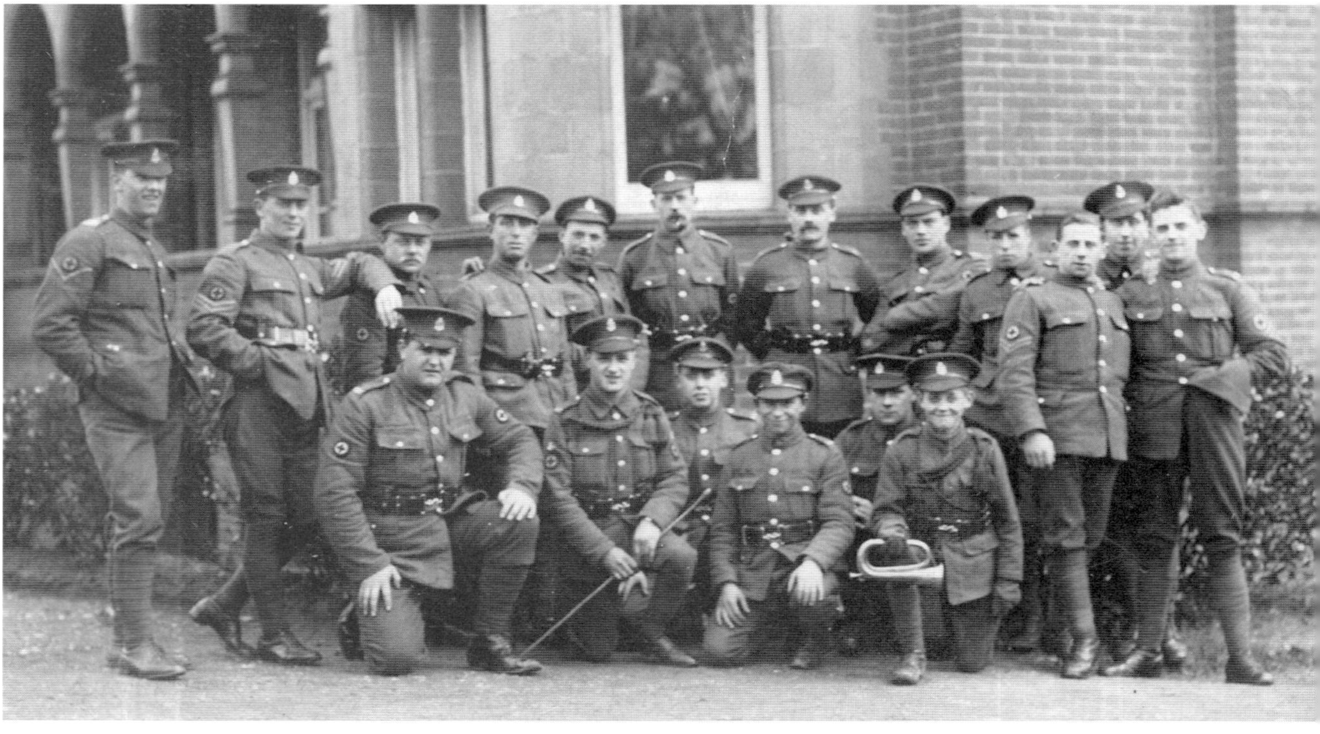

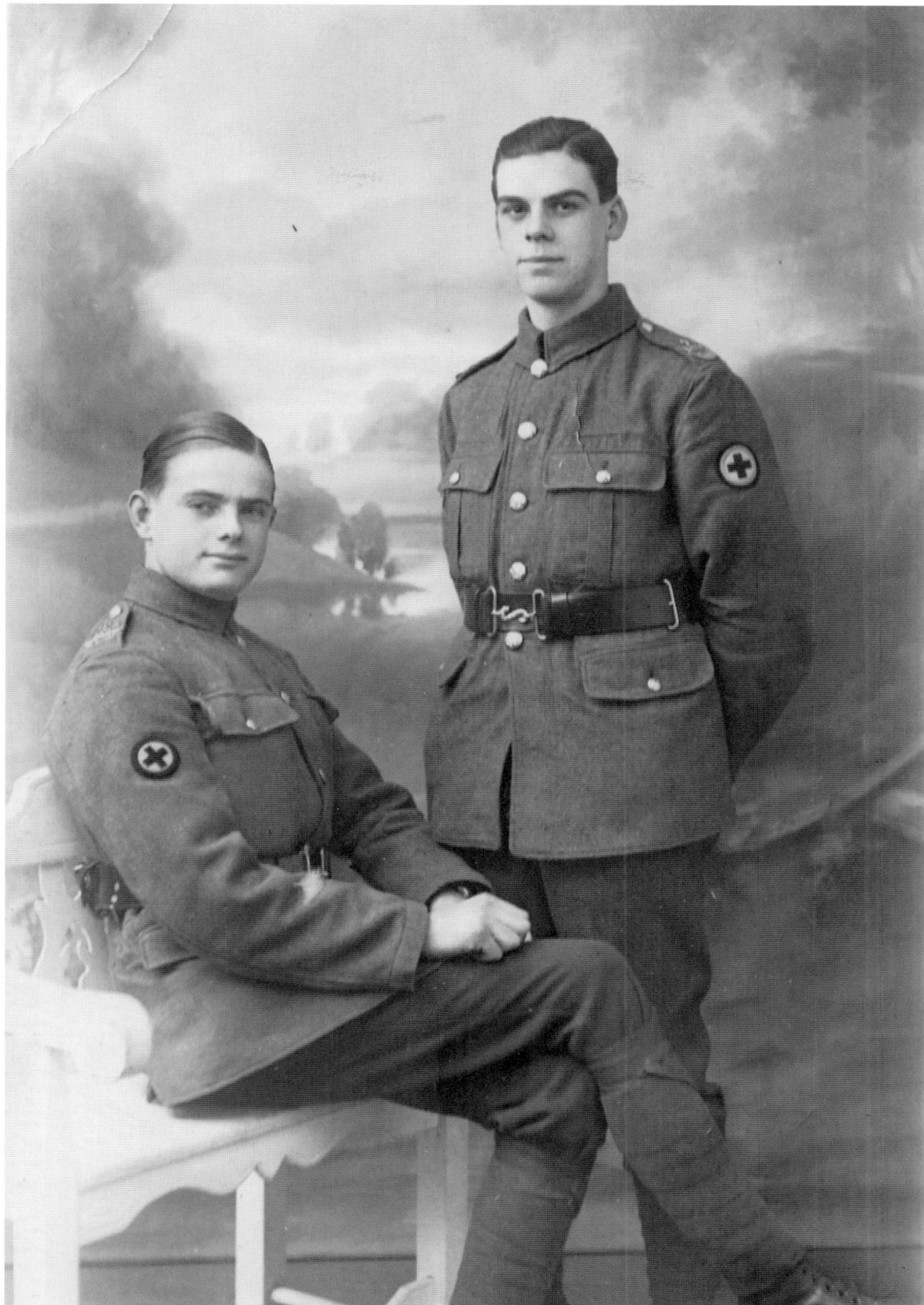

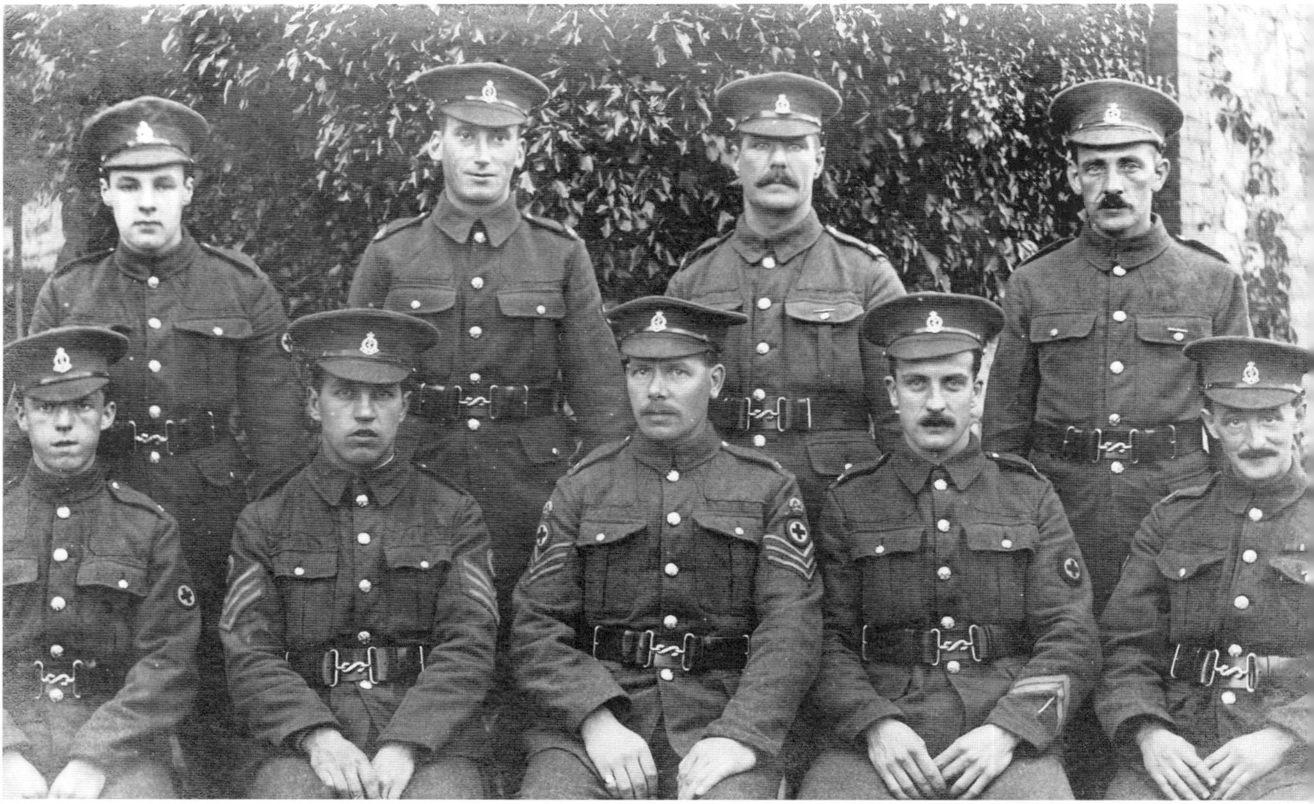

14th Company RAMC Detachment, Military Orthopaedic Hospital, Blackrock, County Dublin, August 1917.

RAMC unit sports; a warrant officer watches in the background.

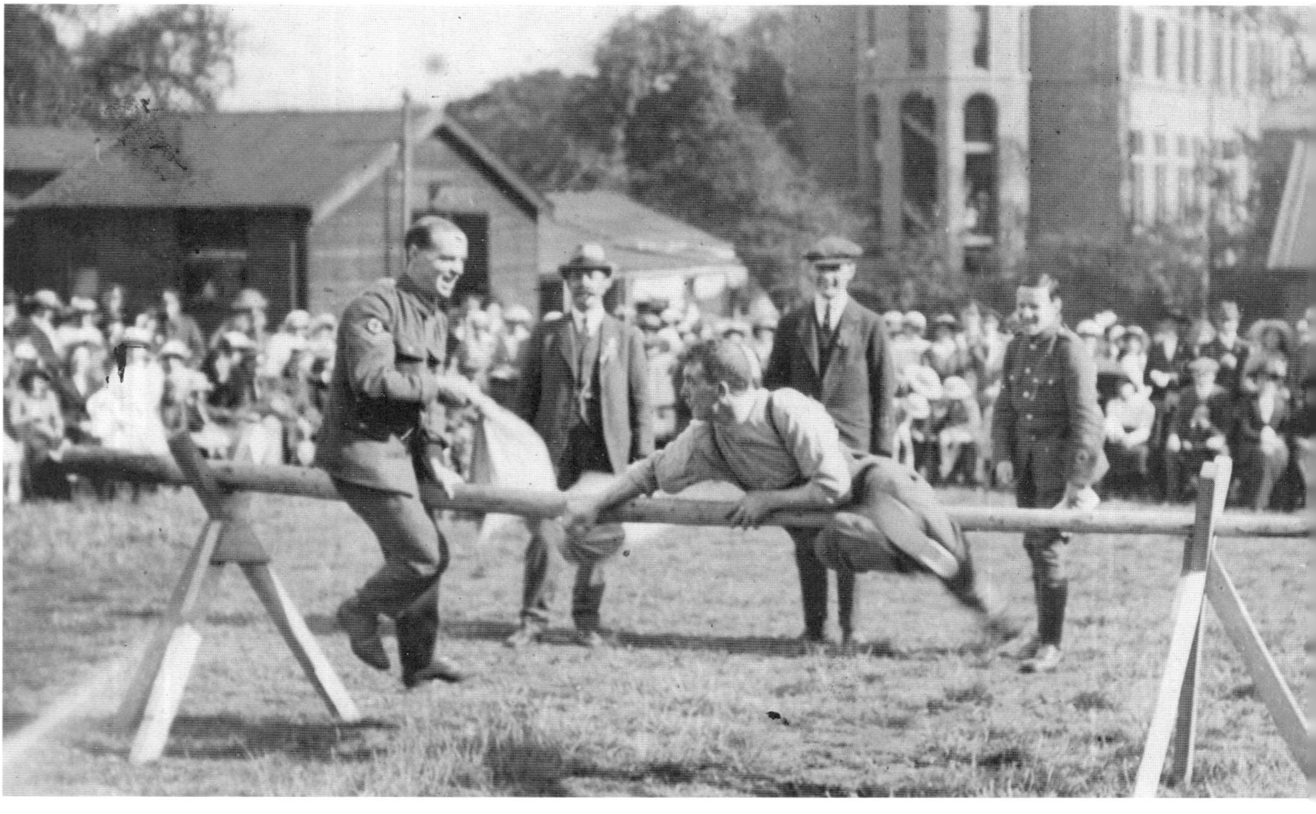

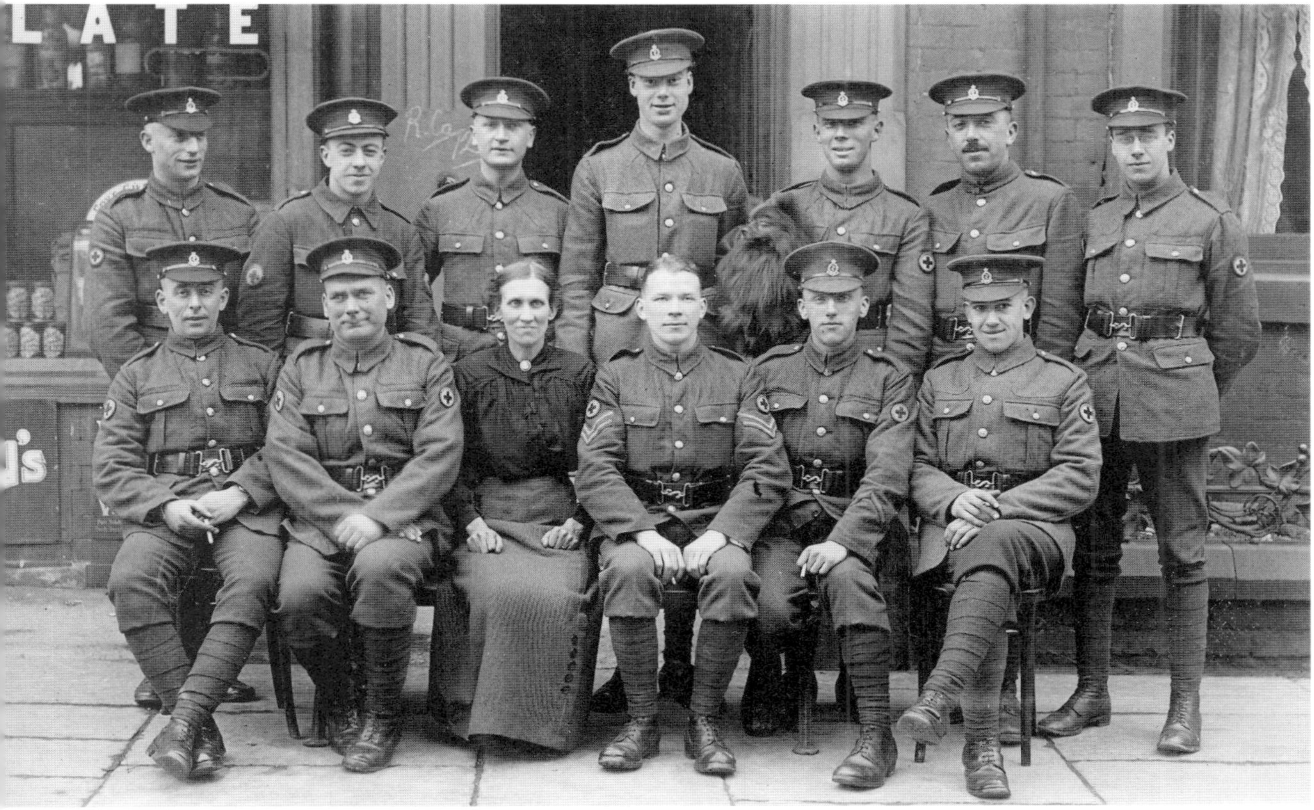

RAMC personnel photographed, with the property owner, outside their billet. Note the chocolate advertising display in the window.

RAMC personnel photographed at Aldershot. Two of the recruits wear St John's Ambulance Brigade Badges on the left cuff of their uniform.

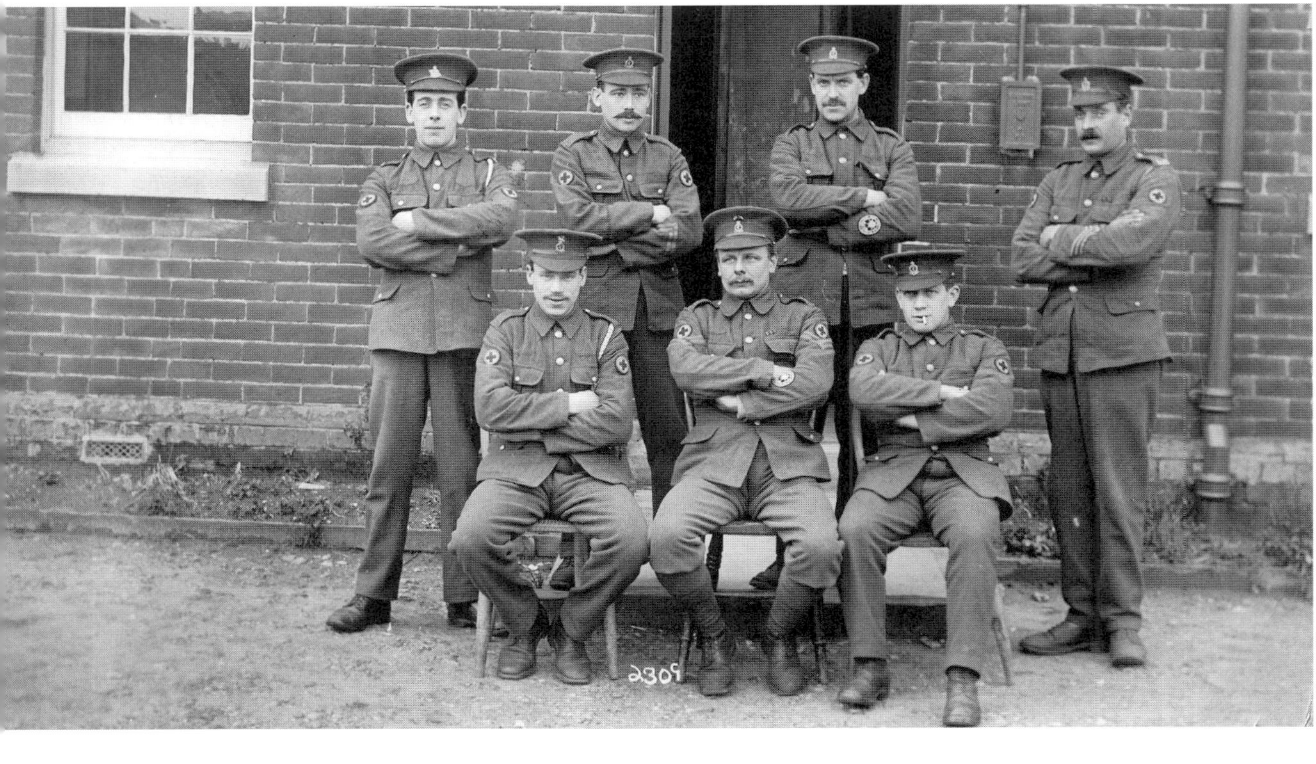

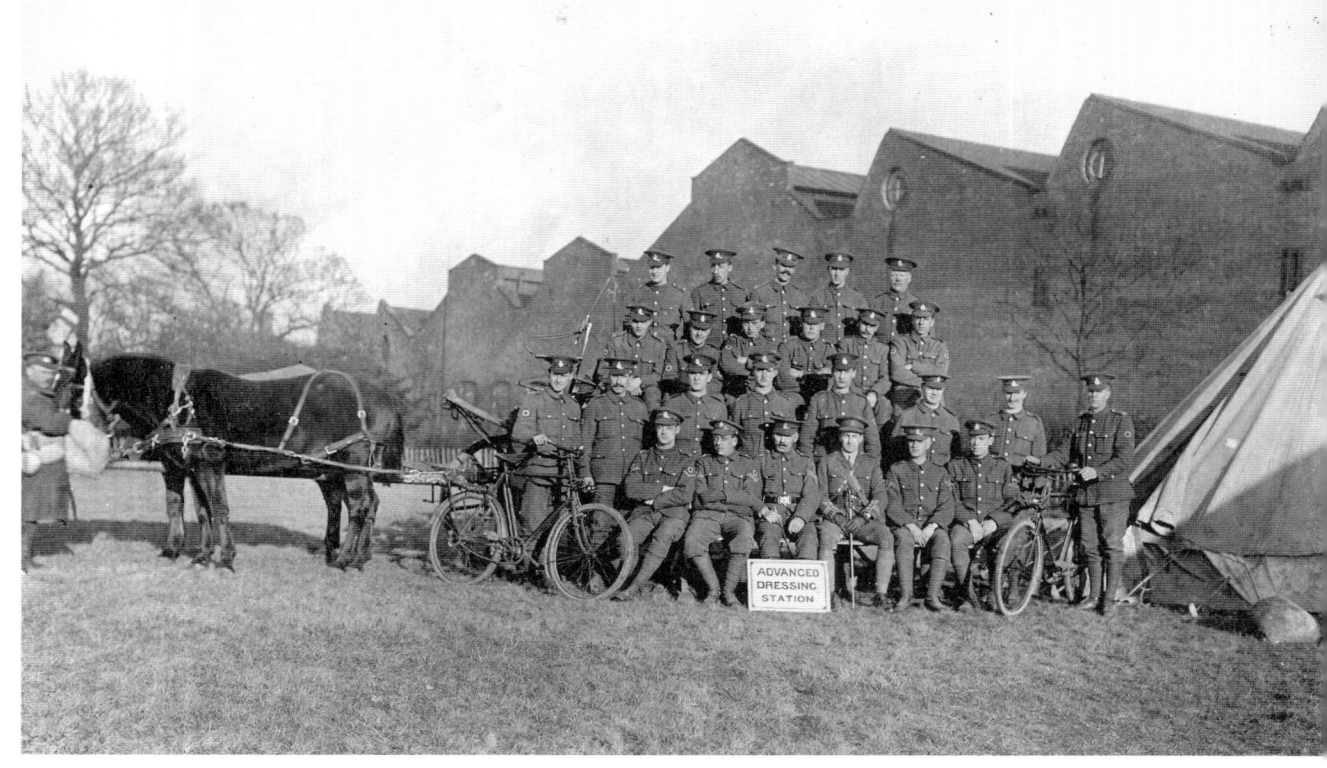

RAMC personnel of an advanced dressing station training at Bury St Edmunds. Interestingly all the personnel, including the two horses, Norah and Peggy, are named on the reverse of the photograph.

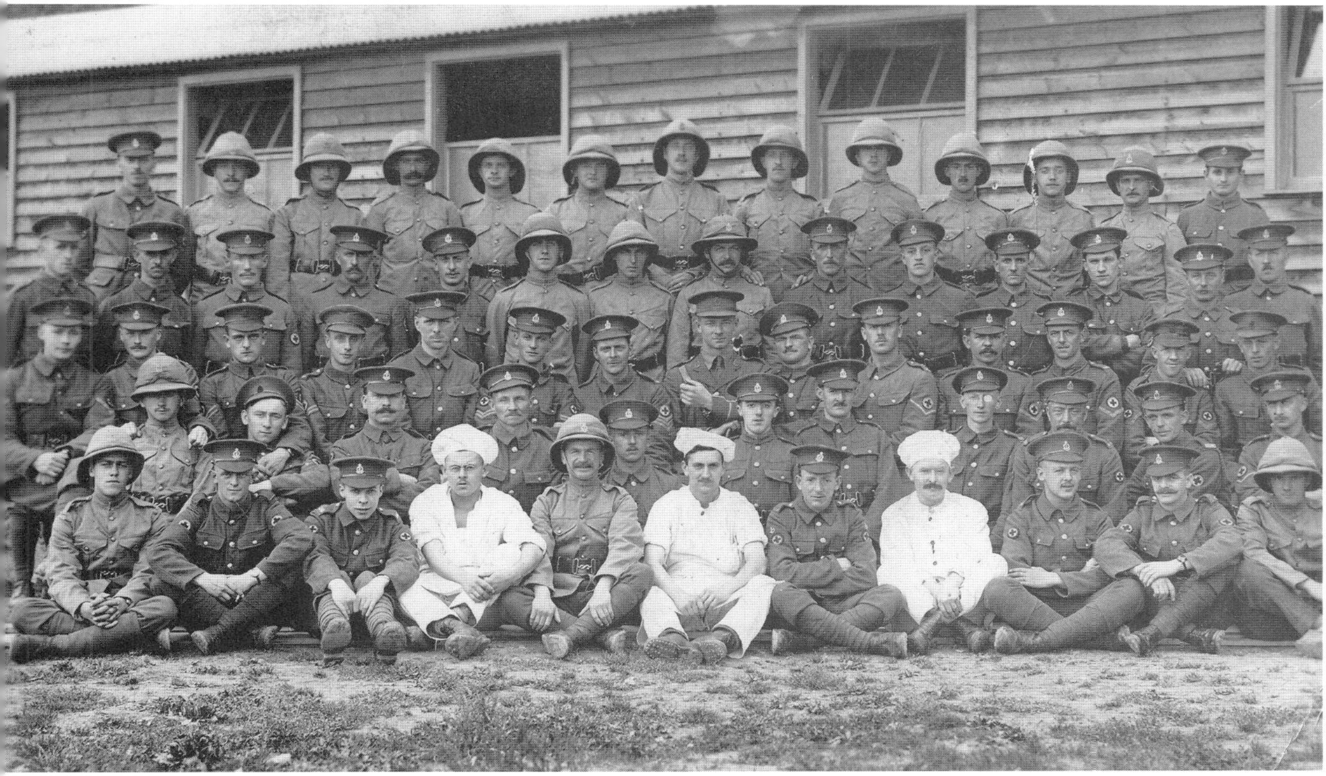

RAMC recruits training, some wearing warm weather uniforms and others, kitchen clothing.

A draft of the 4/3rd Home Counties Field Ambulance, RAMC (TF).

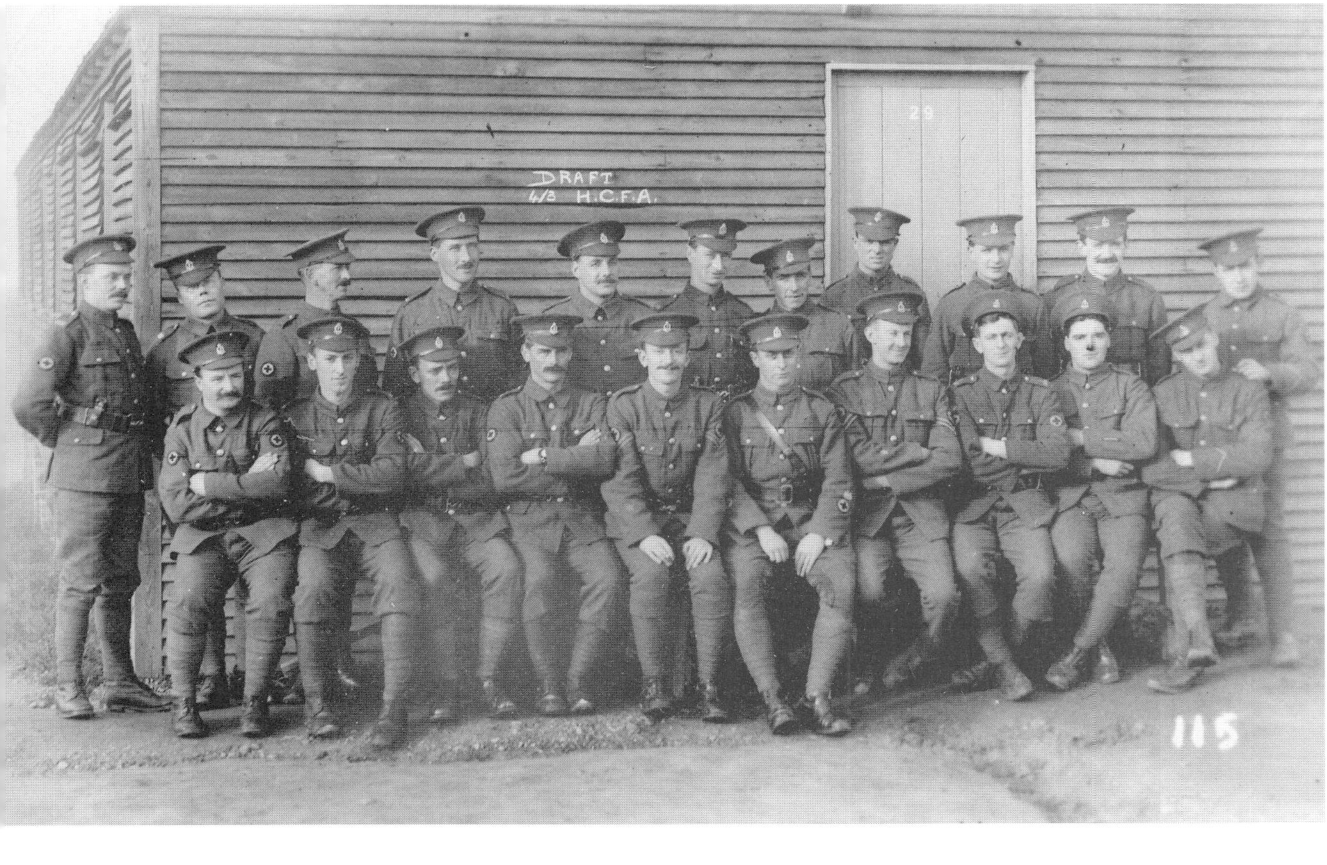

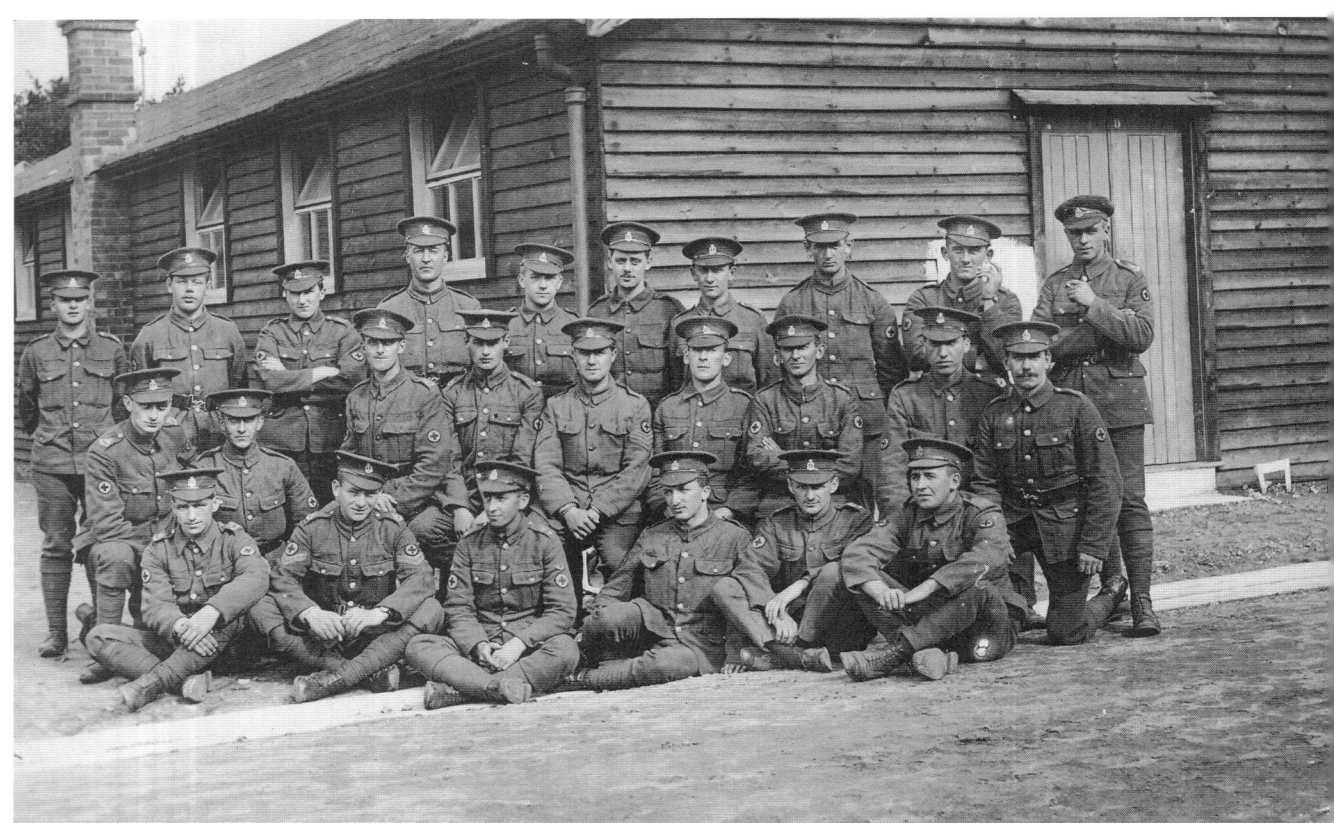

The reverse of the photograph was signed on 21 August 1916 by 1217/386048 Sergeant John Brown Ash, RAMC. The photo was sent from Farnham, Surrey, to 1025/386029 Warrant Officer Class 1 Andrew Nixon Vinycomb, RAMC. Both soldiers would serve overseas after the photo was taken, with the 2/1st Northumbrian Field Ambulance in Salonika.

John Brown Ash was born in Walker, Newcastle upon Tyne. In 1911, aged 20, he was working as a barman in a hotel managed by his father. He enlisted in February 1912 in the 1st Northumbrian Field Ambulance at Newcastle upon Tyne. Later in 1915 he married Elizabeth Nichols at Tynemouth. Prior to the First World War he worked at the Armstrong Whitworth Naval Yard, Walker-on-Tyne, as an Ambulance Room Attendant. Serving in Salonika from September 1916, with the 2/1st Northumbrian Field Ambulance, he was transferred to a hospital in Malta during November 1916 suffering from dysentery and malaria. On 3 January 1917 he was transferred from Malta, to the UK on the Hospital Ship, *Neuralia*. After recovery, from spring 1917, Sergeant Ash served with No. 8 Company RAMC, in the UK. During 1919 he was awarded the Territorial Efficiency Medal. He was discharged with a Silver War Badge, due to illness contracted on active service, on 4 July 1919, aged 29. He died on 15 December 1929 at Walker.

Andrew Nixon Vinycomb was born in Jesmond, Newcastle upon Tyne. He enlisted in the 1st Northumbrian Field Ambulance on 20 July 1910, aged 25 years and 9 months. He lived at 15 Holly Avenue, Jesmond and worked as a clerk in an insurance office. Prior to the First World War he attended a number of training camps, including one at Haltwhistle from 18–25 June 1911 and Scarborough from 22–30 June 1912. He was promoted corporal on 1 February 1912 and sergeant on 1 October 1914. During the First World War he served with the 2/1st Northumbrian Field Ambulance in Salonika from September 1916. On 31 March 1920 he was discharged from the Territorial Force. He died on 23 March 1965 at High Heaton, Newcastle upon Tyne.

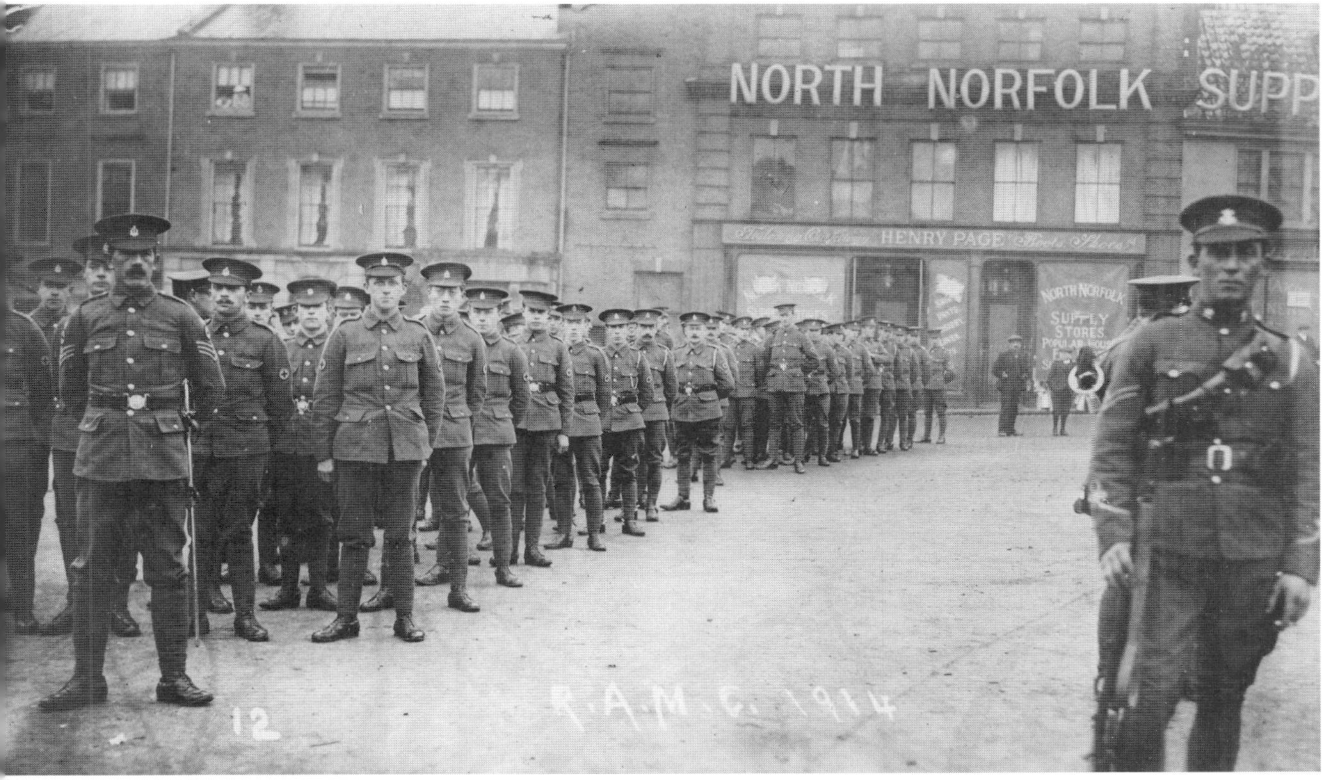

RAMC personnel at a church parade, Aylsham, Norfolk, 1914.

A group of RAMC recruits at Aldershot, wearing a variety of uniforms.

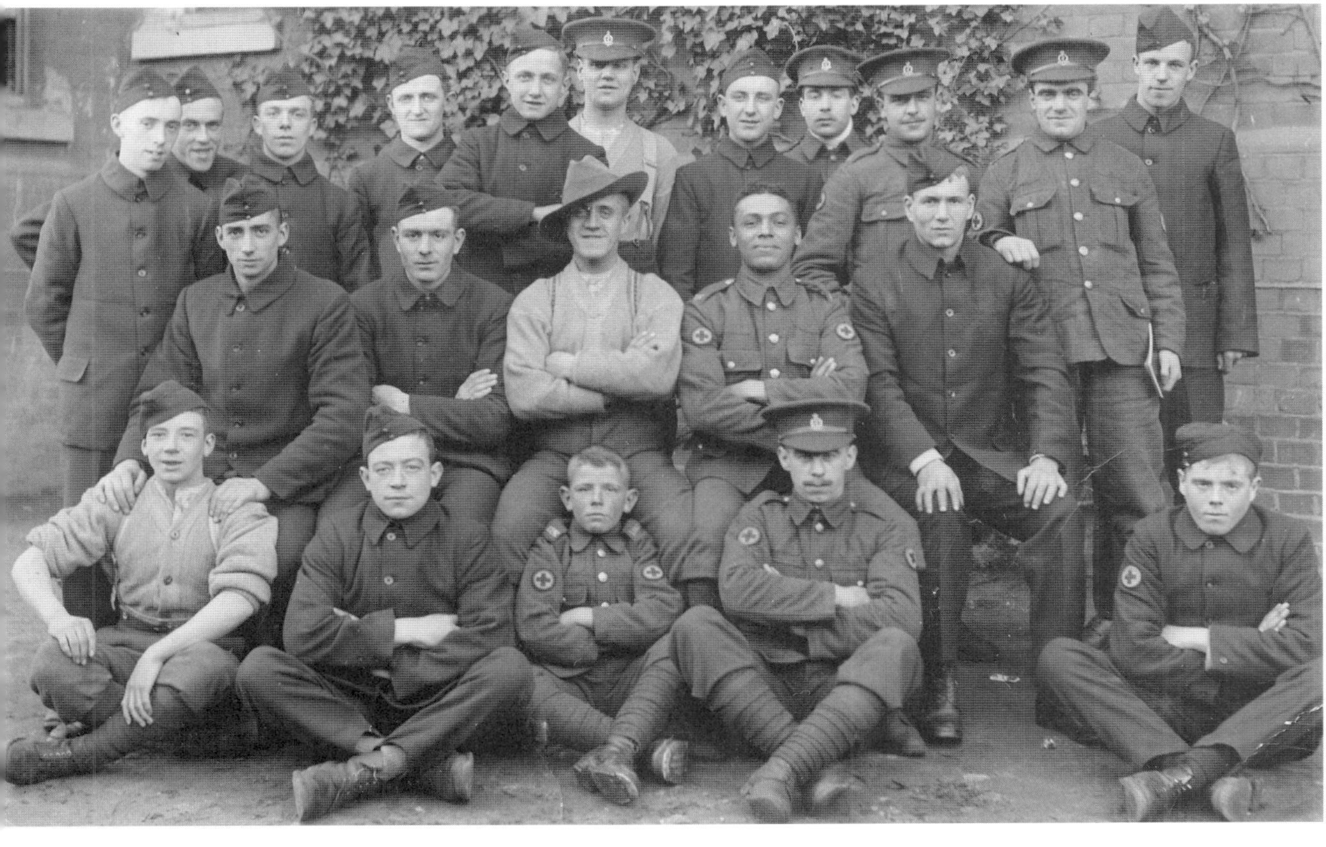

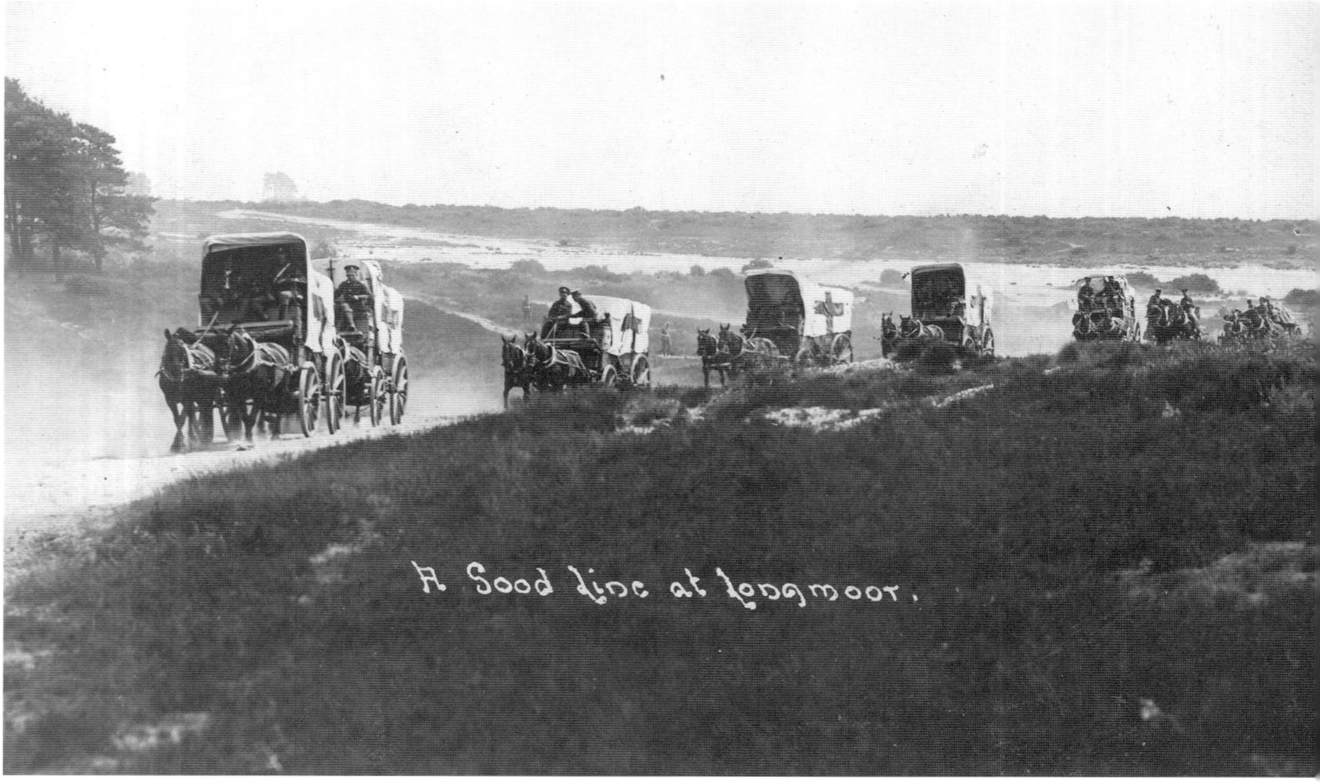

RAMC horse drawn ambulances, Longmoor Military Camp, Hampshire.

RAMC personnel with motor ambulances and the unit mascot.

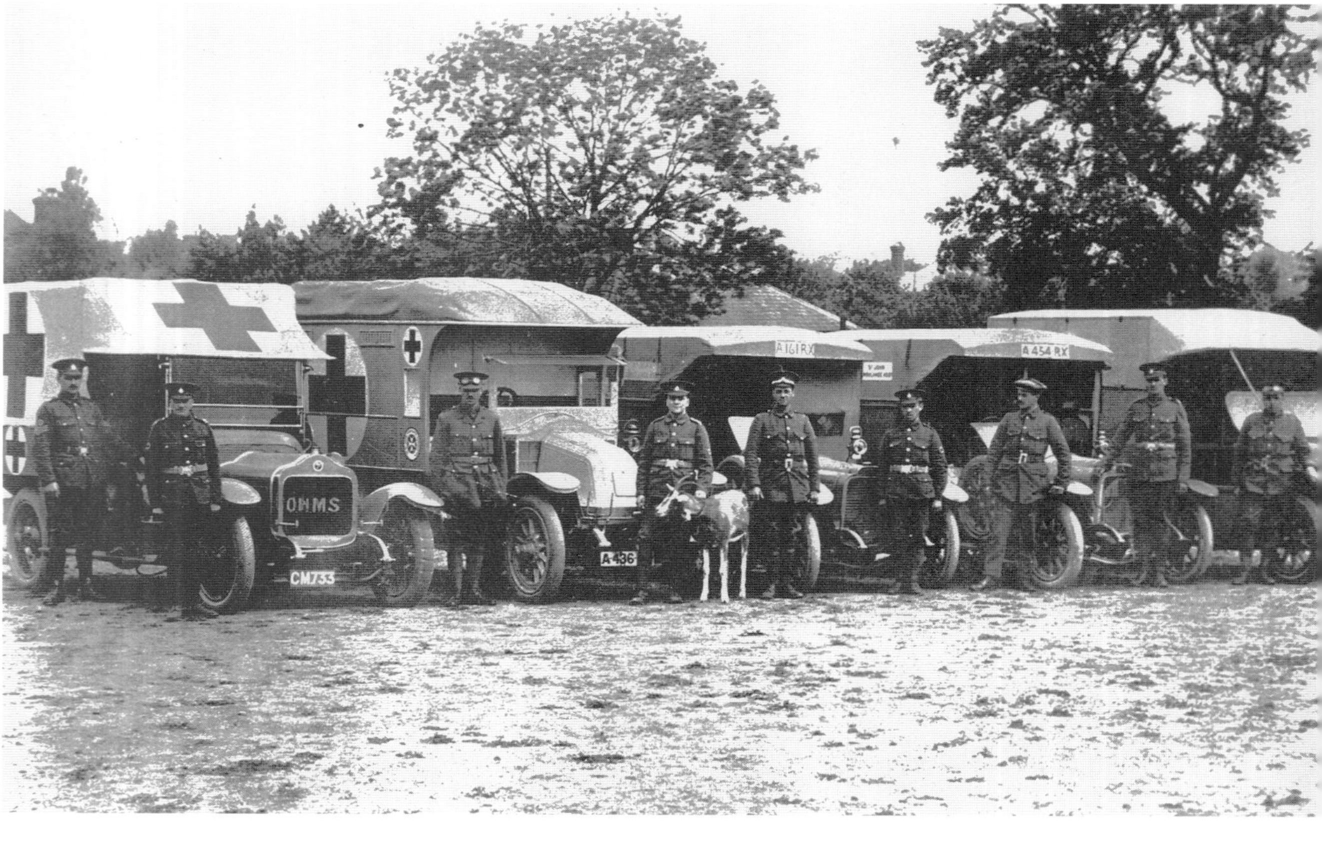

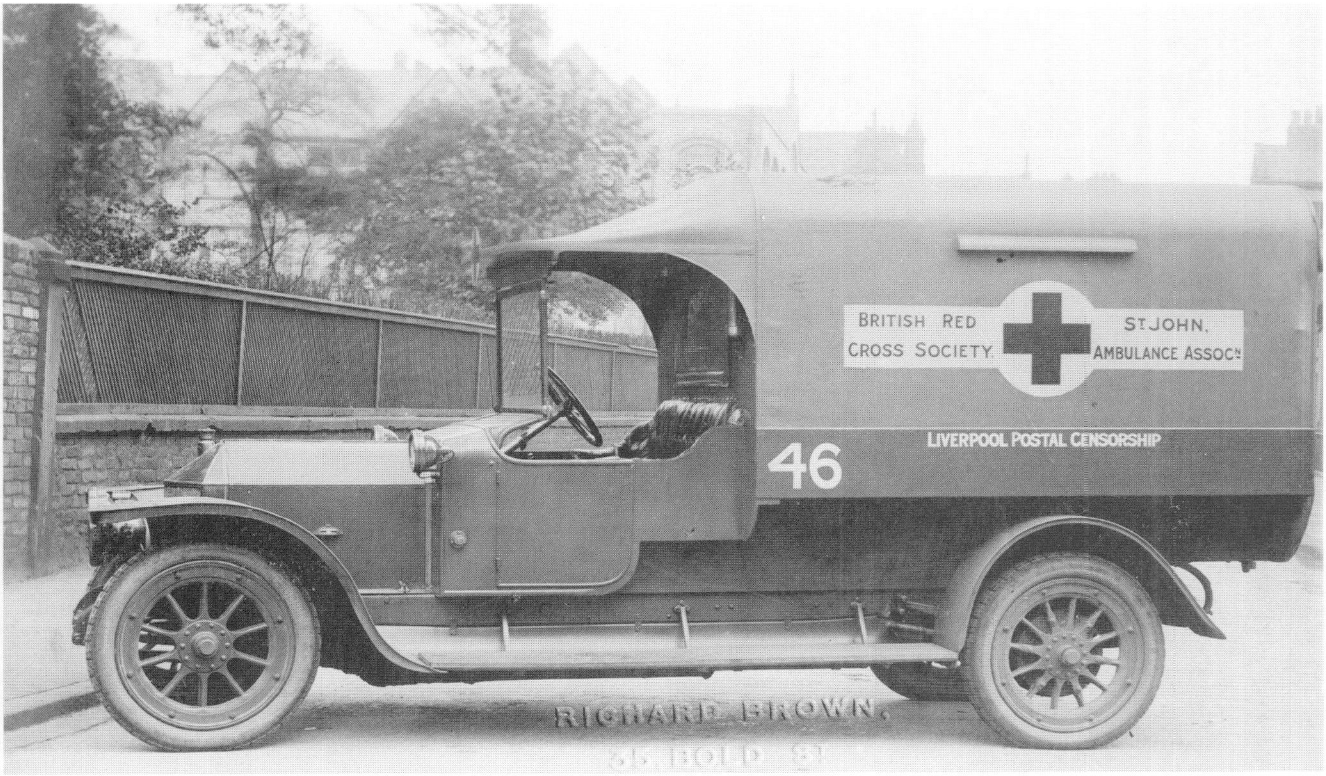

A British Red Cross Society ambulance, photographed in Liverpool. (*Mr Andrew Read*)

Casualties being received by a RAMC sergeant at a London hospital.

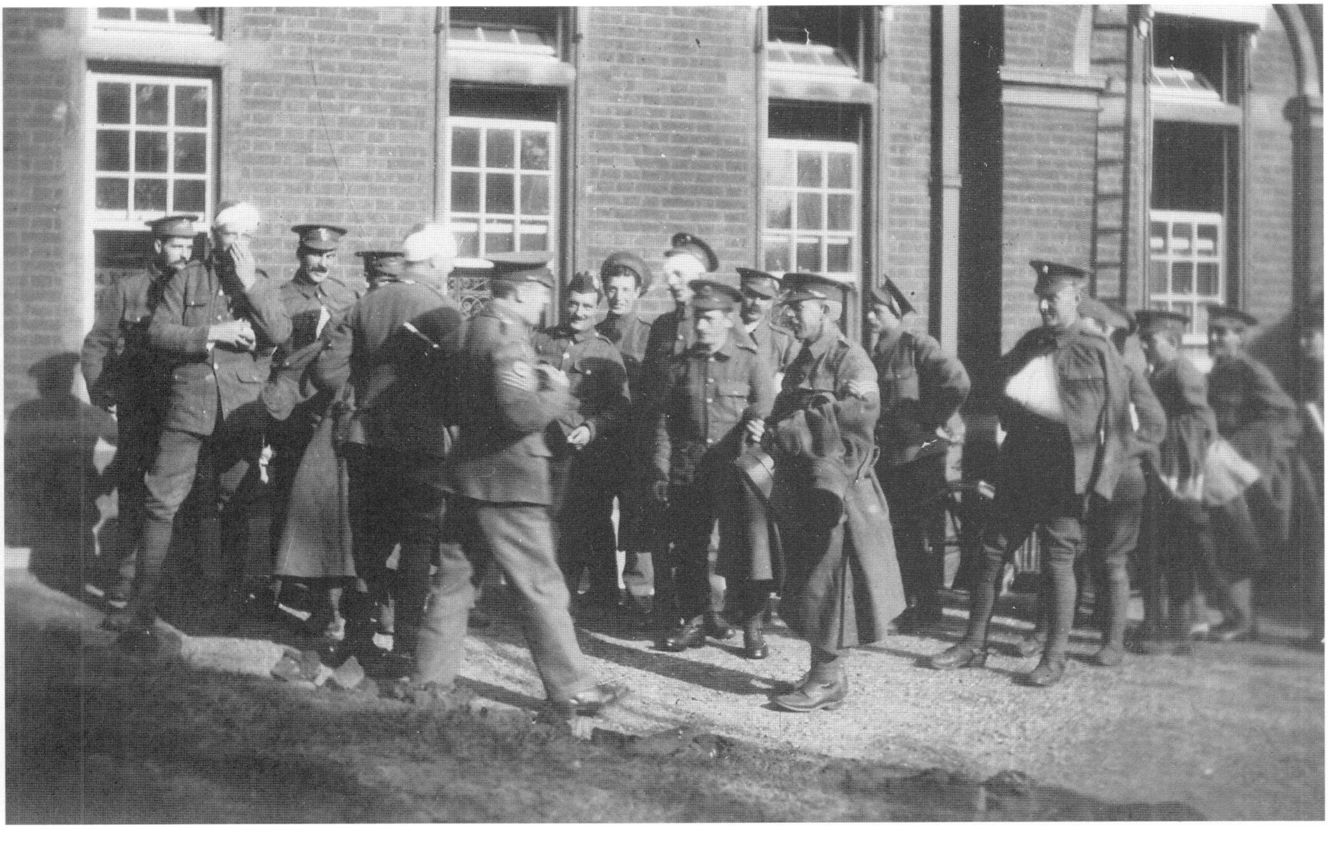

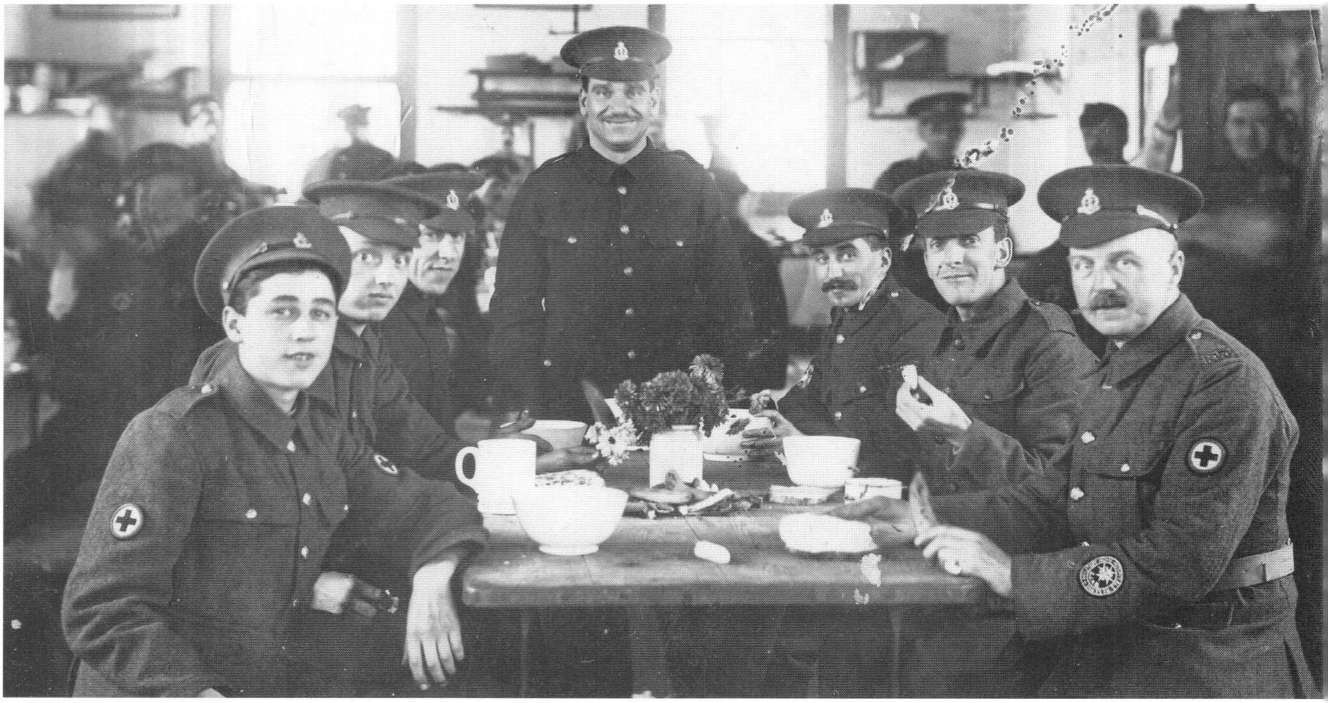

RAMC personnel having a meal break. The private seated on the right wears a St John Ambulance Brigade badge of the Home Hospital Reserve on his uniform cuff.

Two nurses serving with the Queen Alexandra's Imperial Military Nursing Service Reserve – a nursing sister and a staff nurse – with RAMC personnel. The nursing sister (seated left) wears a Princess Christian's Army Nursing Service Reserve badge.

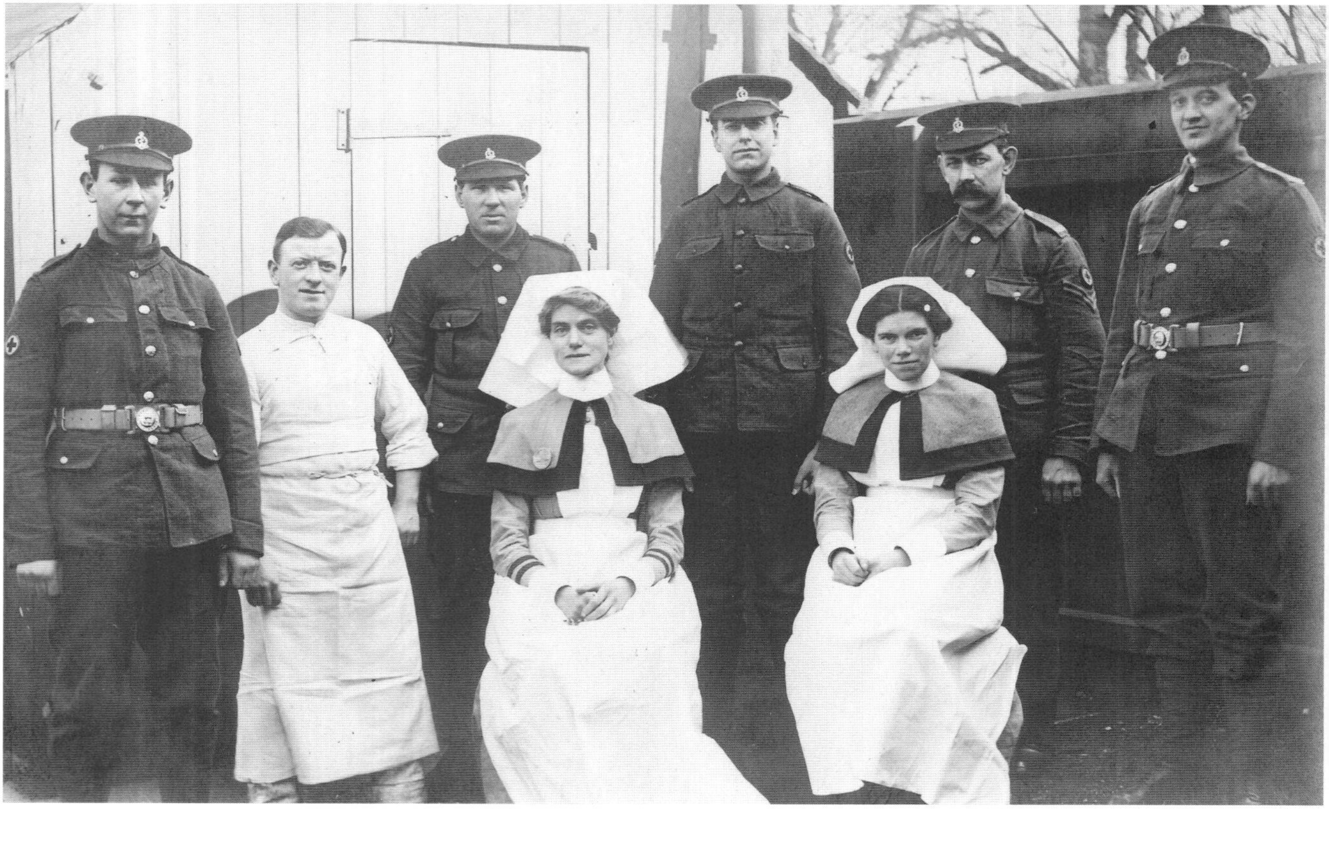

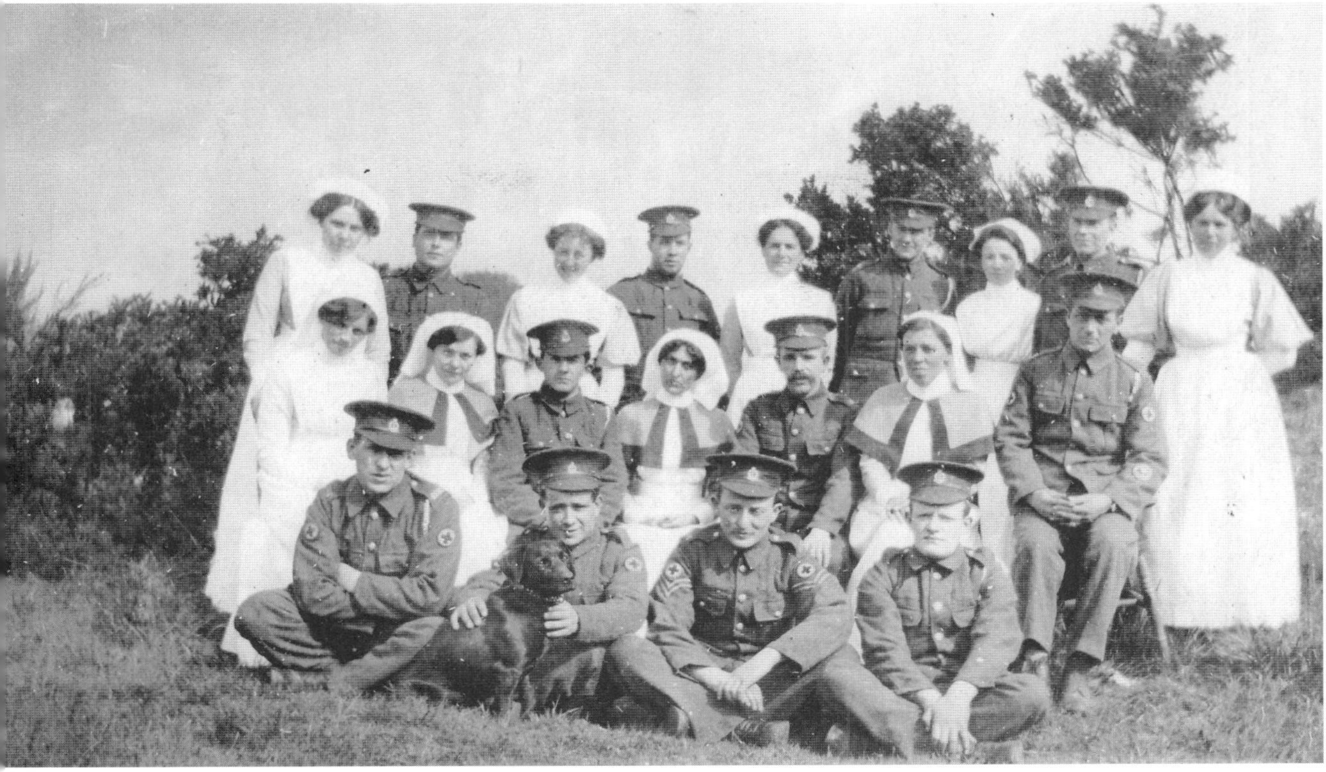

Queen Alexandra's Imperial Military Nursing Service Reserve Nurses and RAMC personnel at Walmersley, Greater Manchester.

RAMC personnel and Voluntary Aid Detachment nurses.

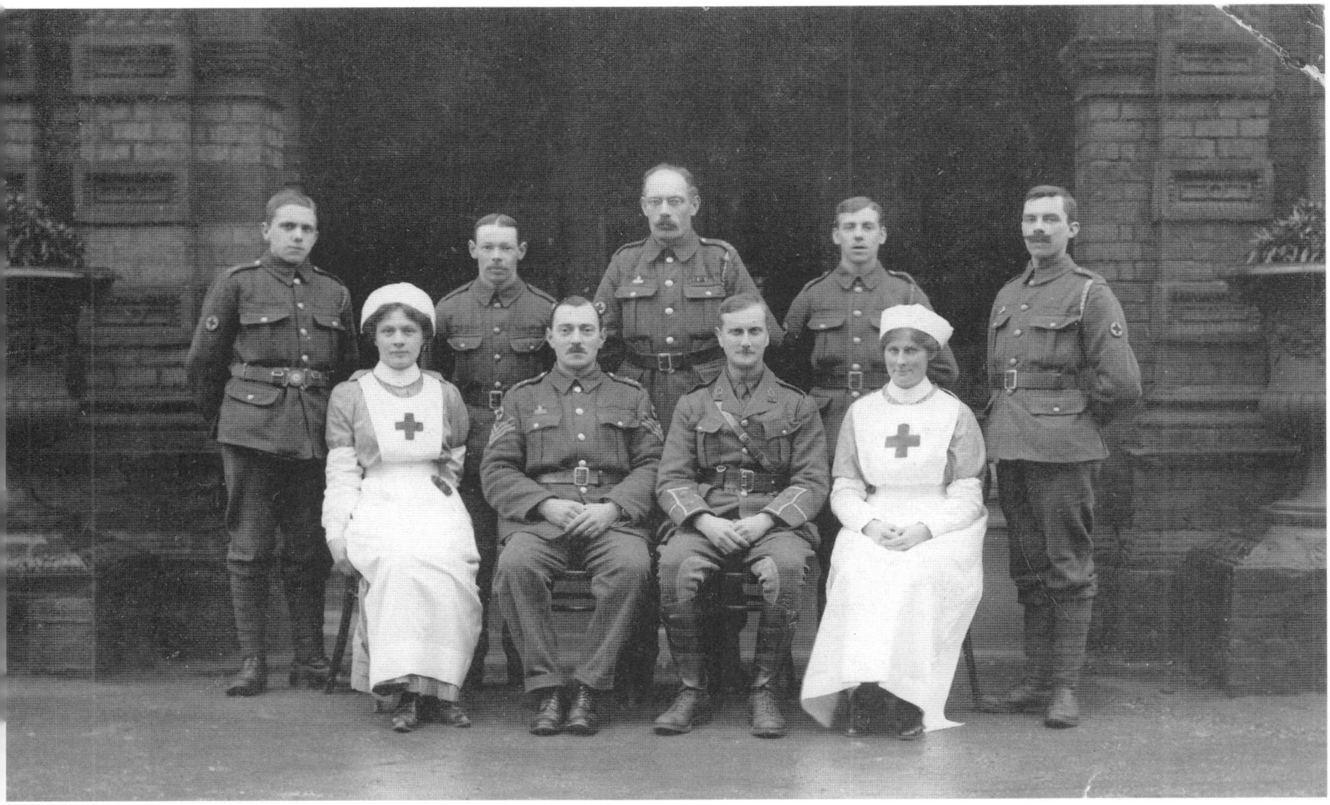

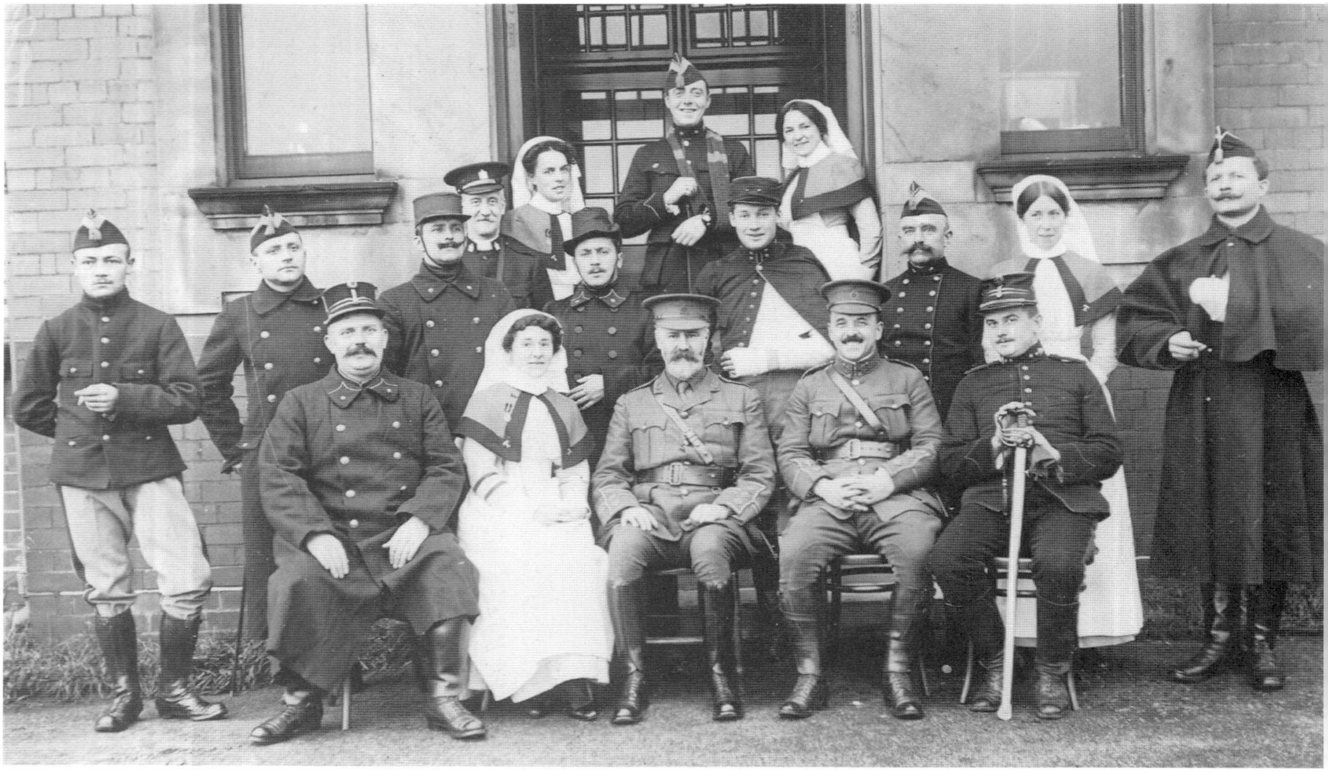

Nurses of the Territorial Force Nursing Service, RAMC officers and wounded Belgian soldiers, at a UK military hospital.

Personnel of 2nd Northern General Hospital, RAMC Territorial Force. The 2nd Northern General Hospital was located in the teacher training college at Beckett's Park, Leeds, during the First World War. The hospital had around 1,800 beds.

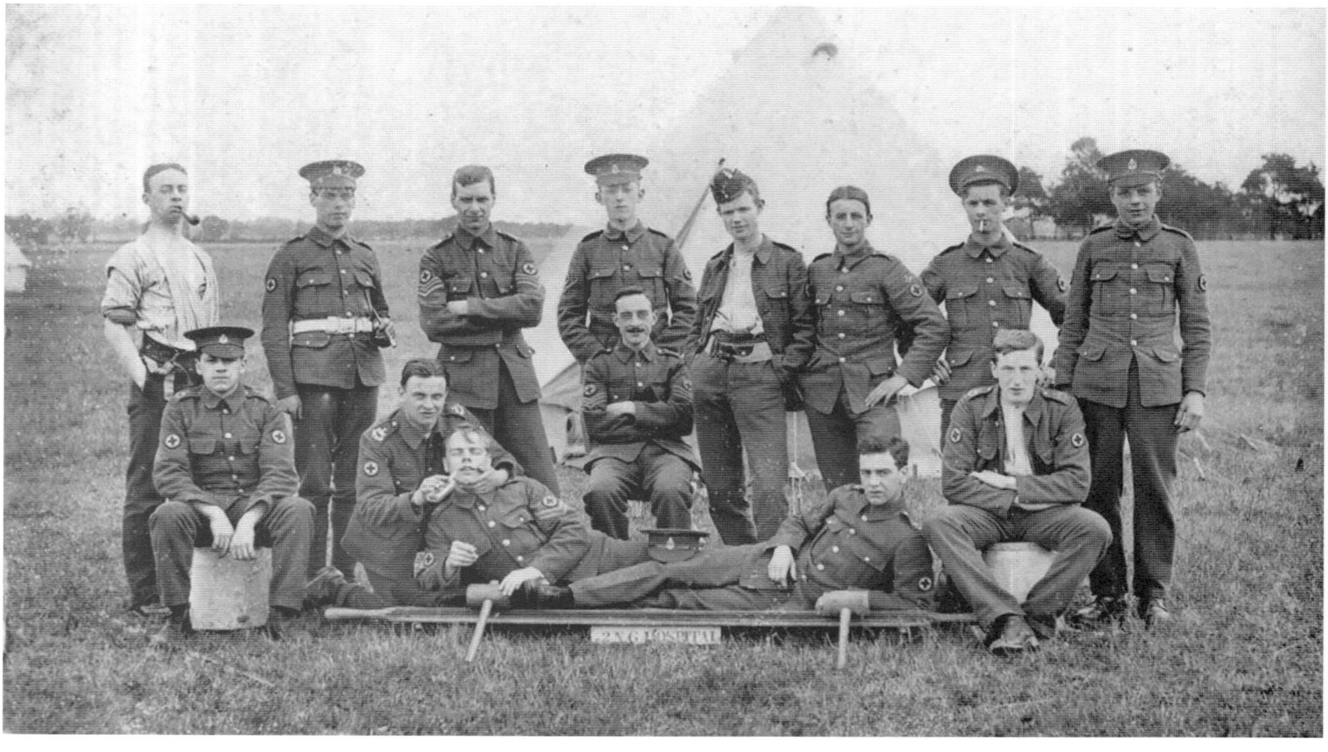

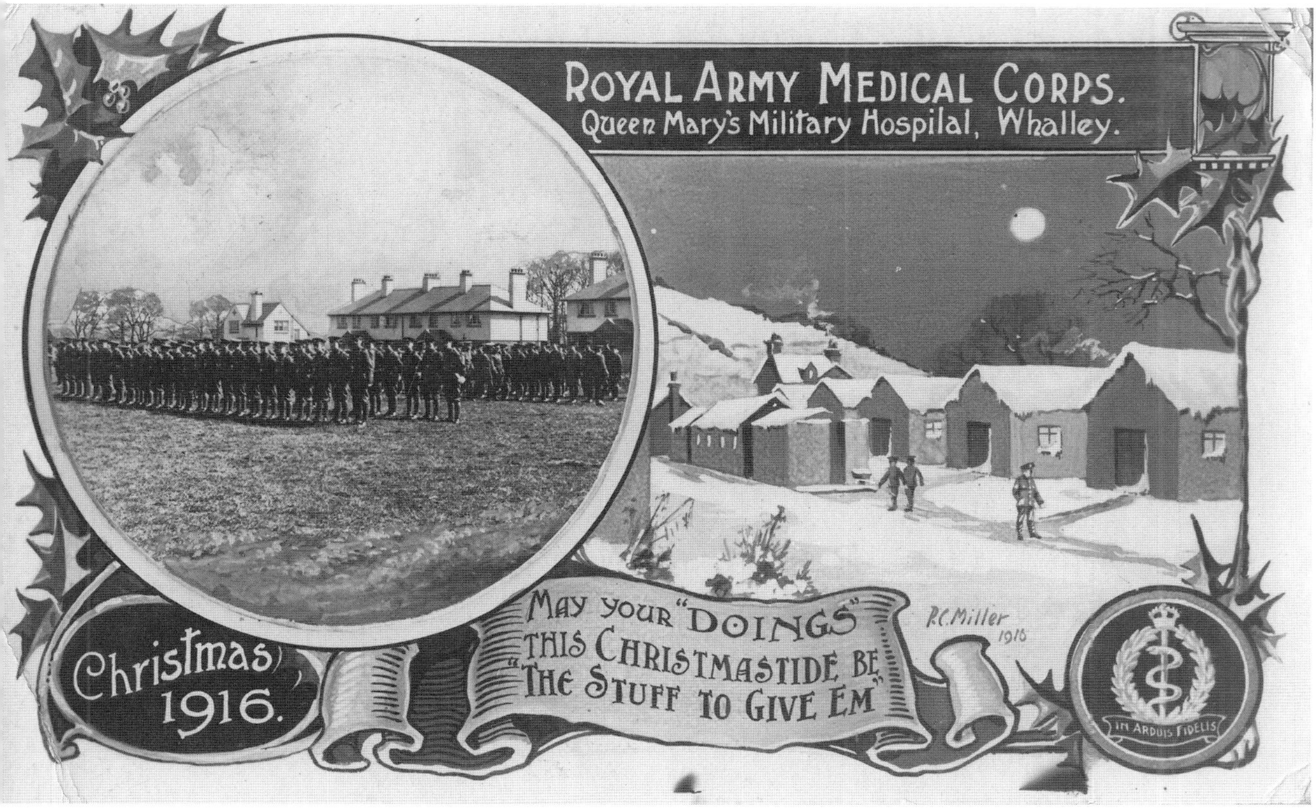

ROYAL ARMY MEDICAL CORPS.
Queen Mary's Military Hospital, Whalley.

Christmas 1916.

May your "DOINGS" this Christmastide be "The Stuff to Give 'Em"

P.C.Miller 1916

IN ARDUIS FIDELIS

Queen Mary's Military Hospital, Whalley, Lancashire. This Christmas card was produced for the hospital in 1916. During the war the 2,000 bed hospital was located in the county asylum at Whalley, remaining there until June 1920.

A RAMC Territorial Force officer seated on hospital mattresses, with a lady serving with the British Red Cross Society. They appear to be outside a workshop.

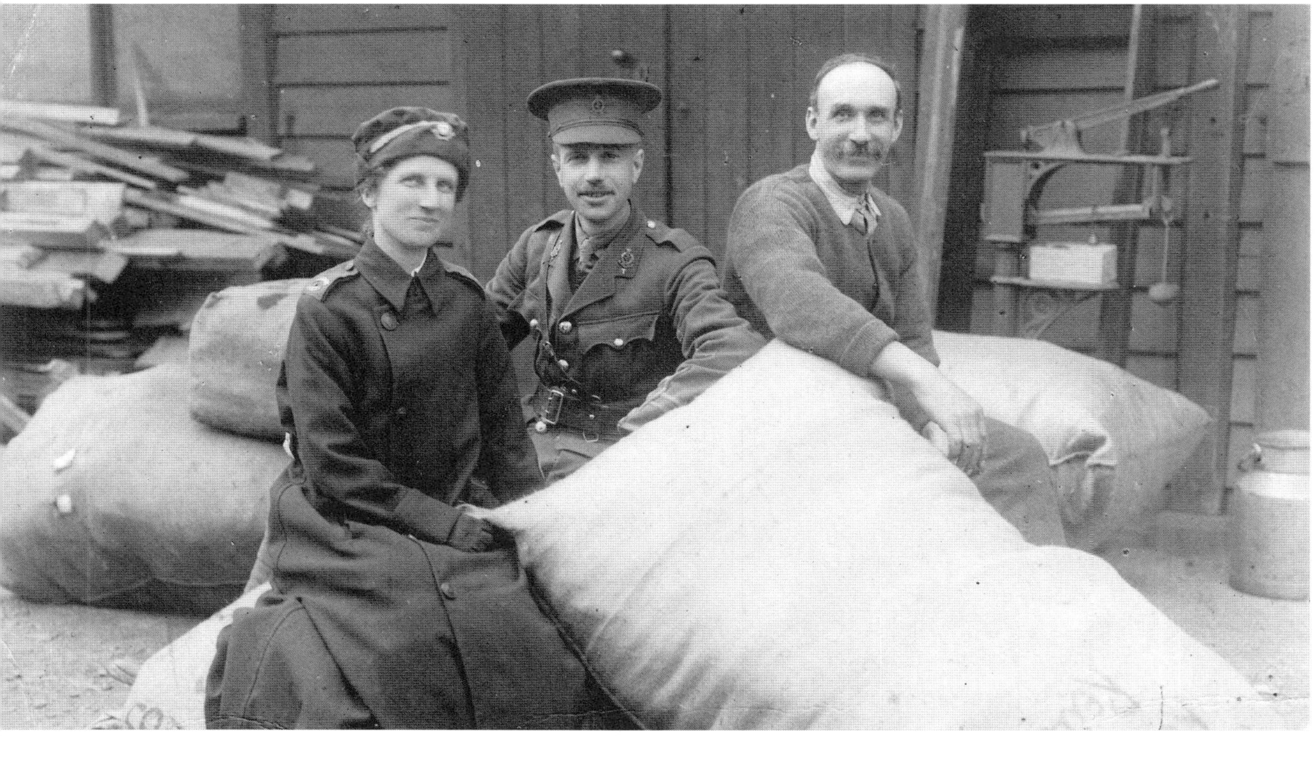

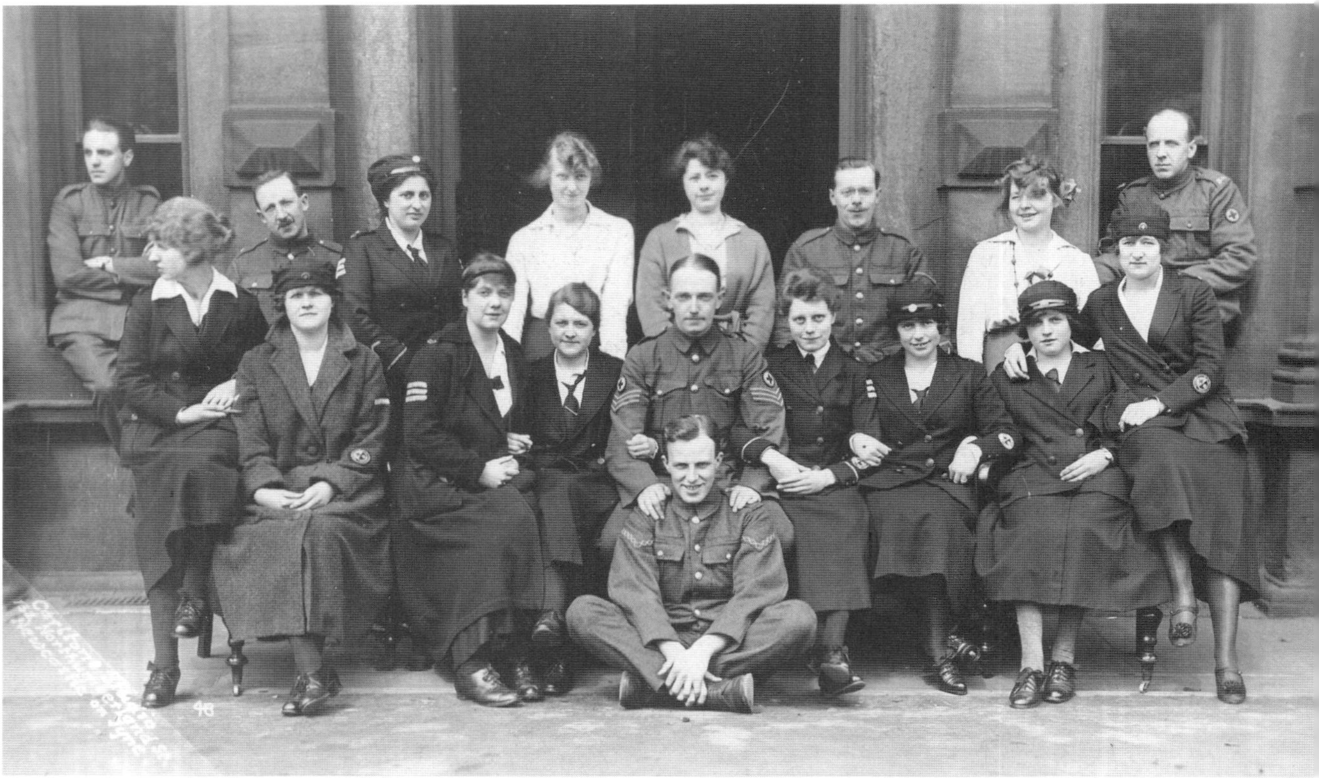

RAMC personnel and ladies serving with the British Red Cross Society. The photograph was taken in Newcastle upon Tyne.

Lewisham Military Hospital during the First World War.

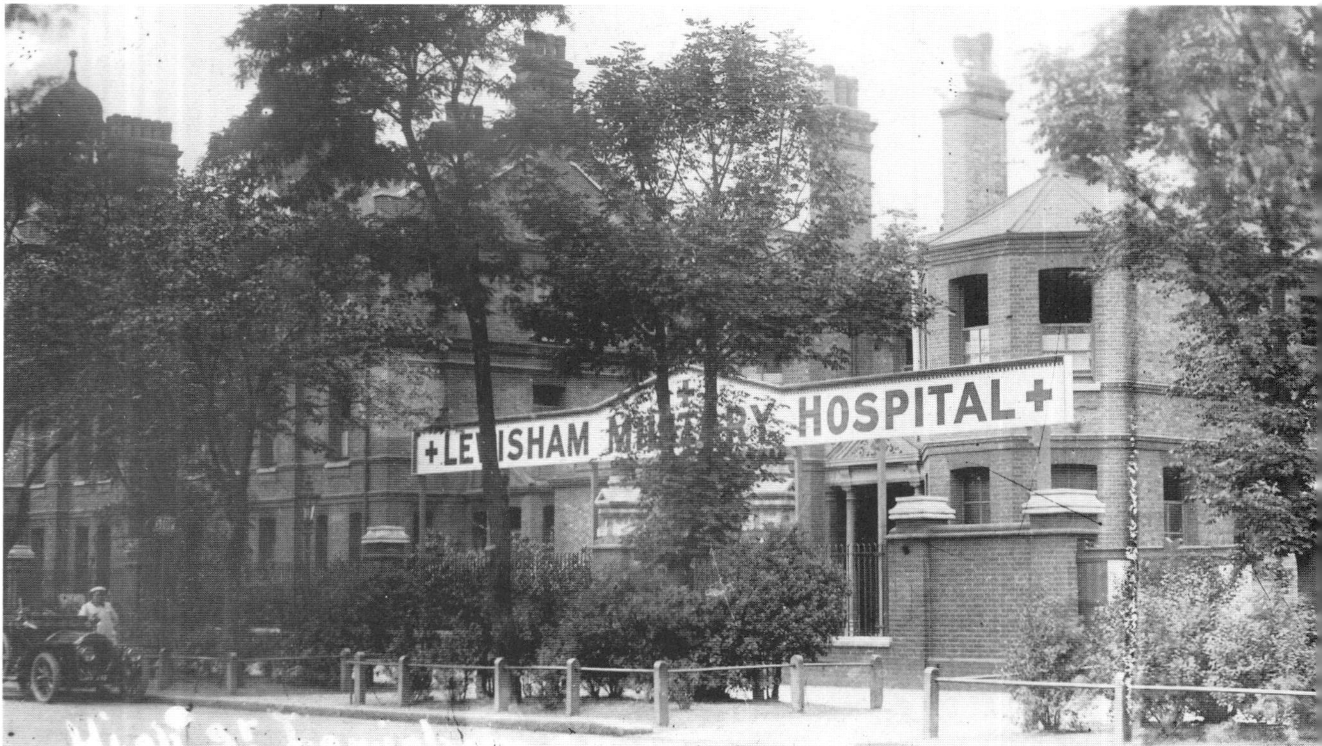

An operation at Lewisham Military Hospital, 1918. Managed by the RAMC, military hospitals were predominately staffed by RAMC personnel and the military nursing services. They were supported by voluntary workers from a number of organisations, including the British Red Cross and local Voluntary Aid Detachments.

During the First World War the Royal Pavilion, Brighton, was converted into a hospital for wounded soldiers. From 1914 to 1916 it was used for Indian Army soldiers who had been wounded on the Western Front. In late 1915 the Indian Army was redeployed to the Middle East and most Indian Army soldiers were withdrawn from Europe. Consequently the hospital closed in January 1916. In April 1916, however, the Royal Pavilion reopened as a hospital for British Army troops who had lost limbs during the conflict. The Pavilion Hospital helped with their rehabilitation, and from 1916 to 1920 over 6,000 patients were treated.

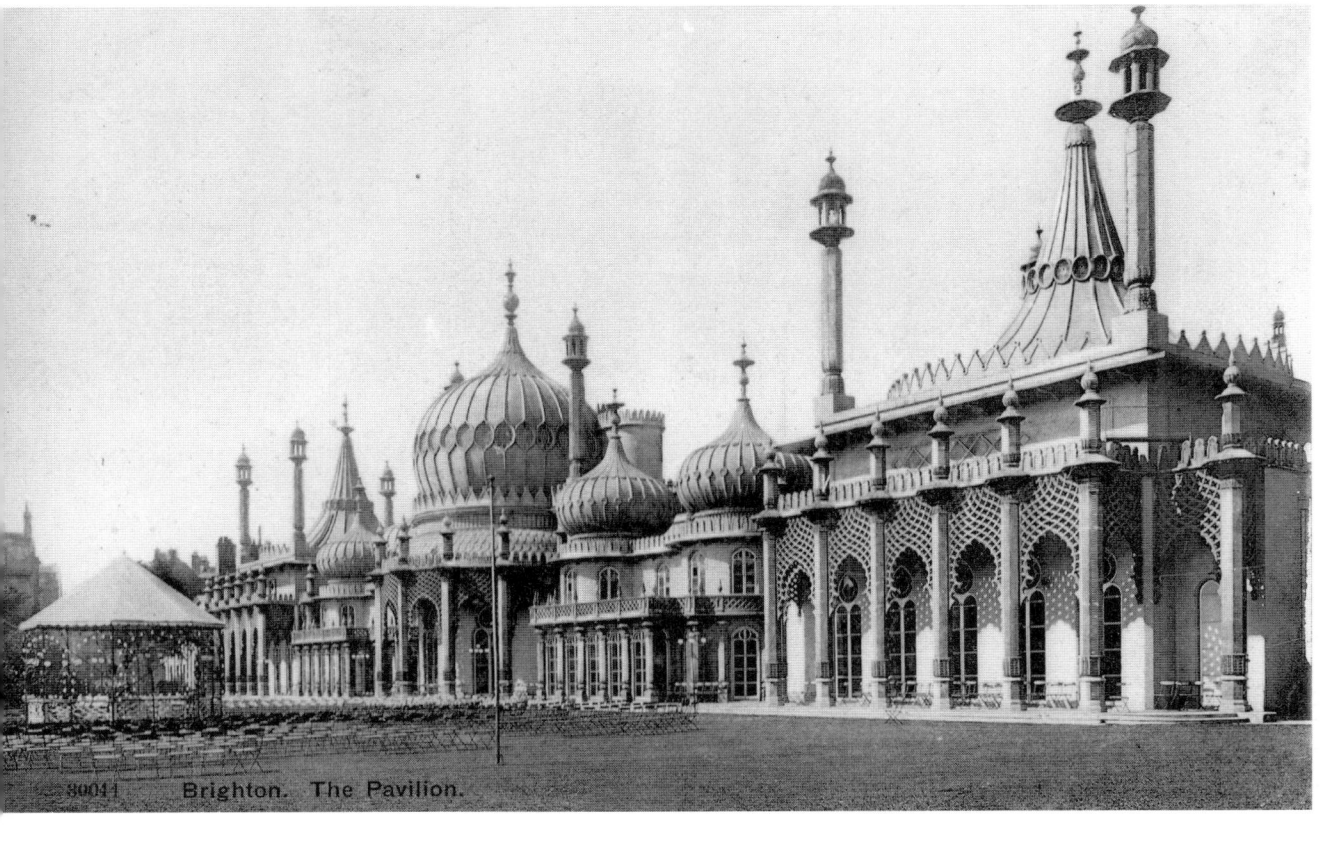

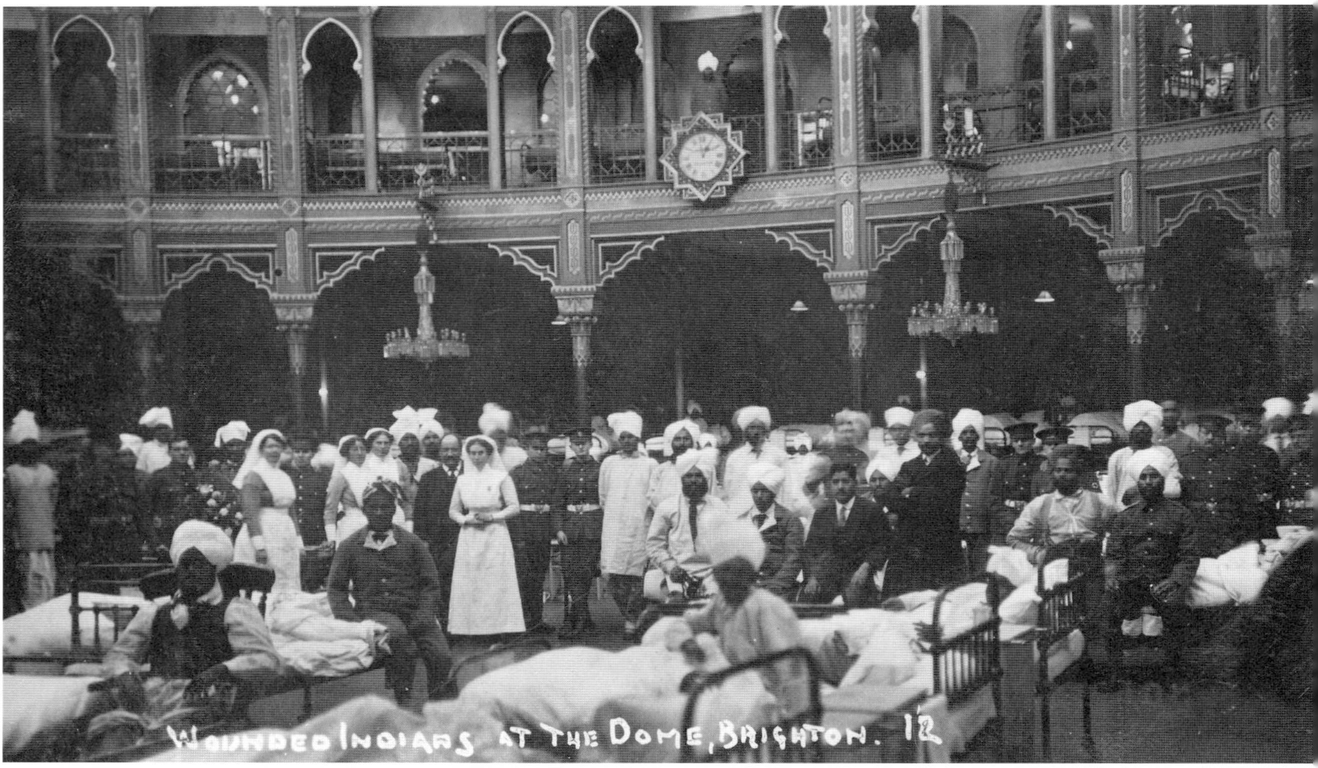

Wounded Indian Army soldiers with RAMC personnel and nurses at the Royal Pavilion, Brighton, 1915.

The Royal Pavilion, Brighton, when in use as a military hospital for British Army troops who had lost limbs during the First World War. A message on the reverse of the photo reads – 'What do you think of this for a hospital ward – over 160 beds in it and it looks a treat.'

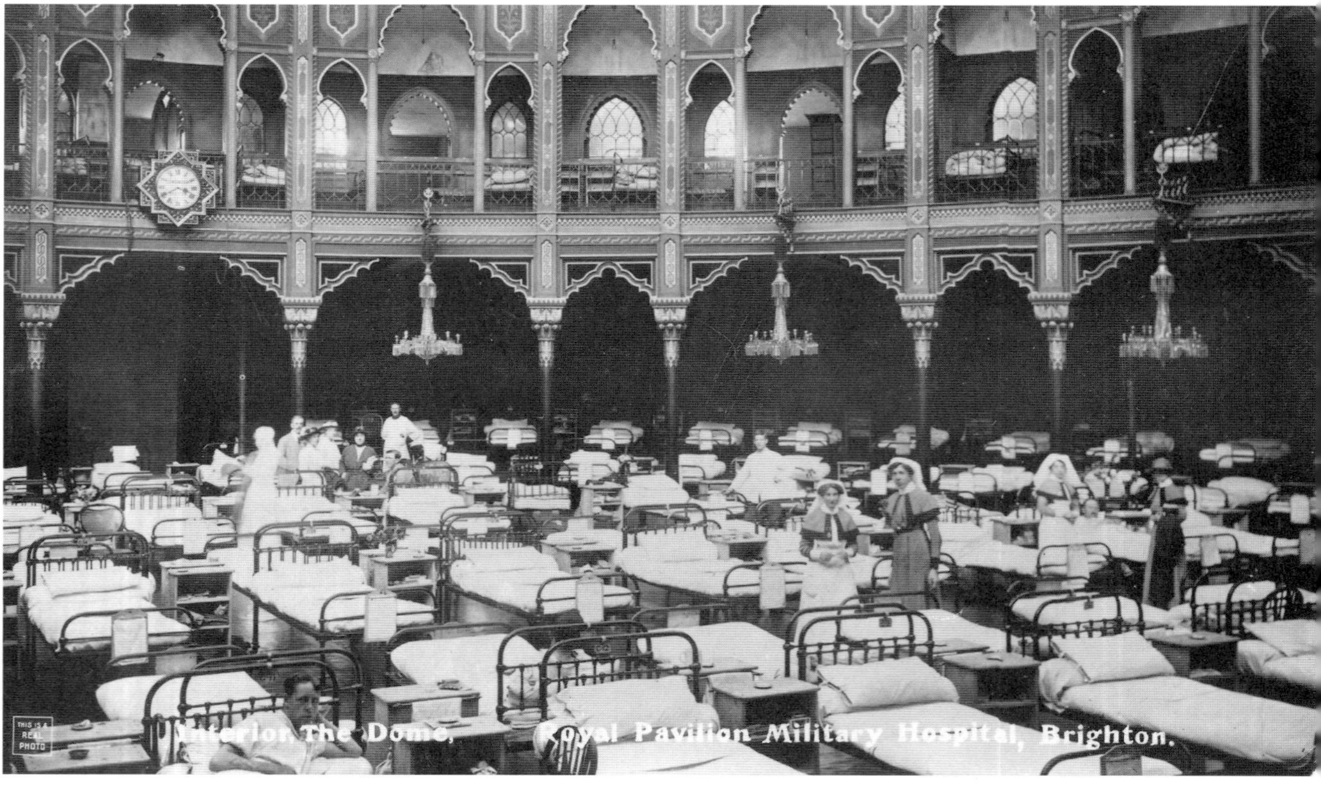

Cover of the *Pavilion Blues* magazine, October 1916. The magazine, produced by RAMC personnel and patients at the Royal Pavilion Military Hospital, Brighton, was bought and sold locally.

Royal Army Medical Corps catering staff at the Royal Pavilion Military Hospital, Brighton. The photo was included in the *Pavilion Blues* magazine. An accompanying article, entitled 'A word on the Men Behind the Scenes', noted thanks and appreciation for 'the R.A.M.C men, who toil behind the scenes, morning, noon and night by serving up tasty meals'. The article went on to note that 'though they do not get the opportunity for the honours of war, we should like them to know we appreciate very much their efforts on our behalf to serve King and Country. We reproduce their photos; and wish them all that is best in life and a happy future.'

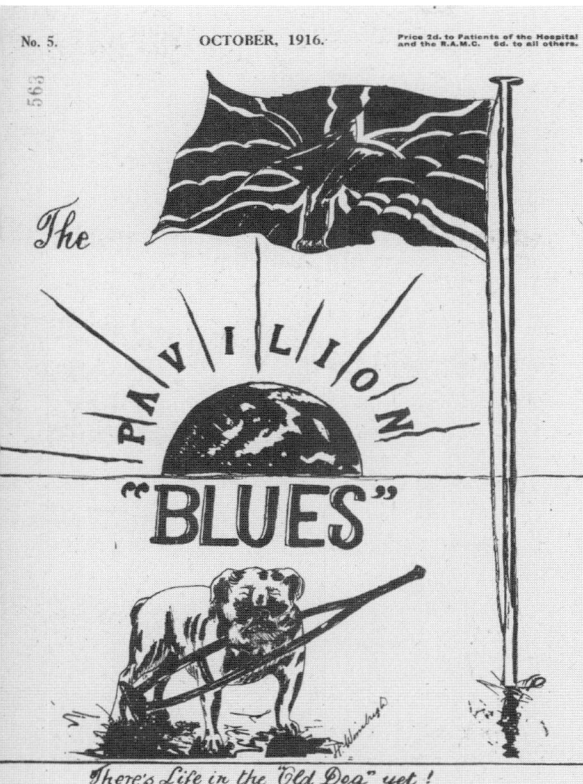

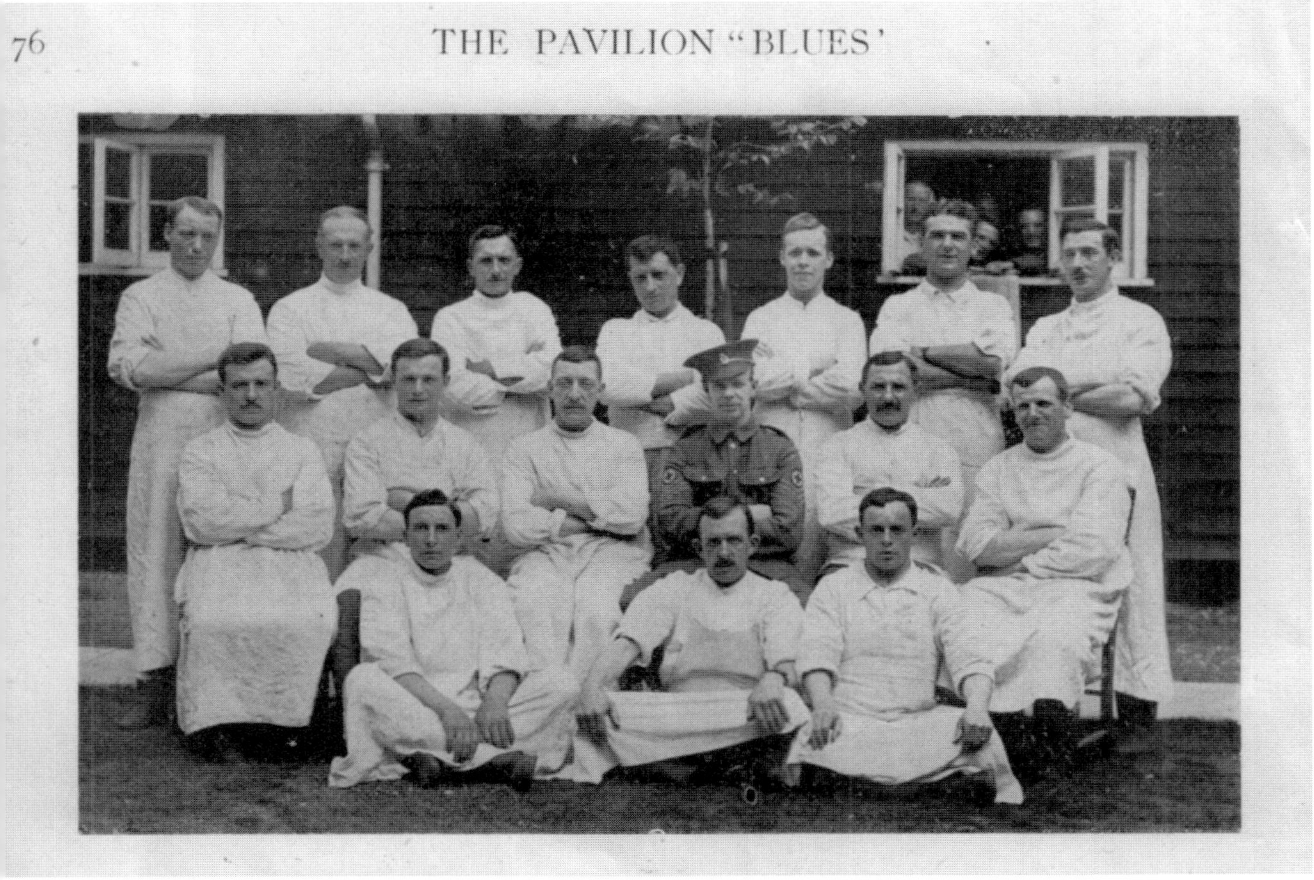

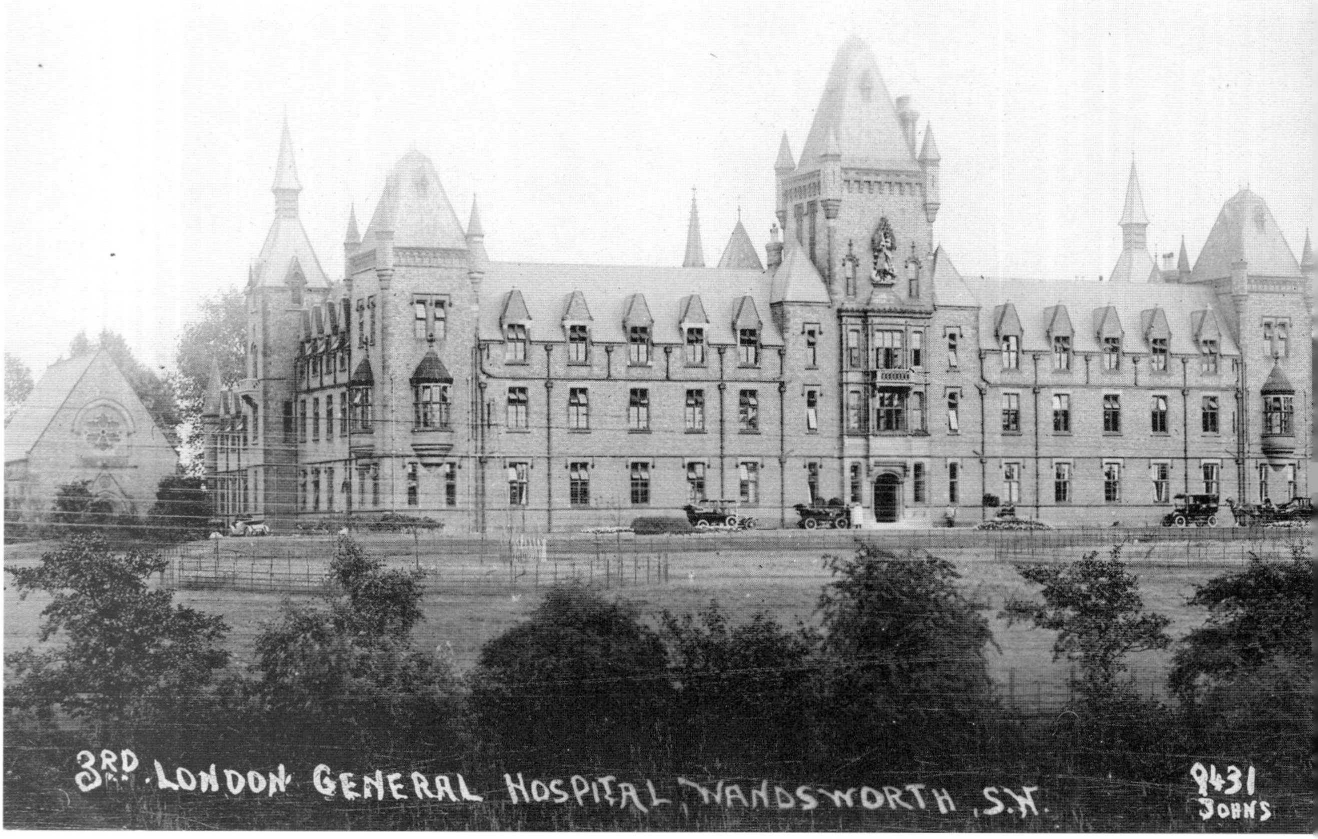
3RD. LONDON GENERAL HOSPITAL, WANDSWORTH, S.W.
9431
JOHNS

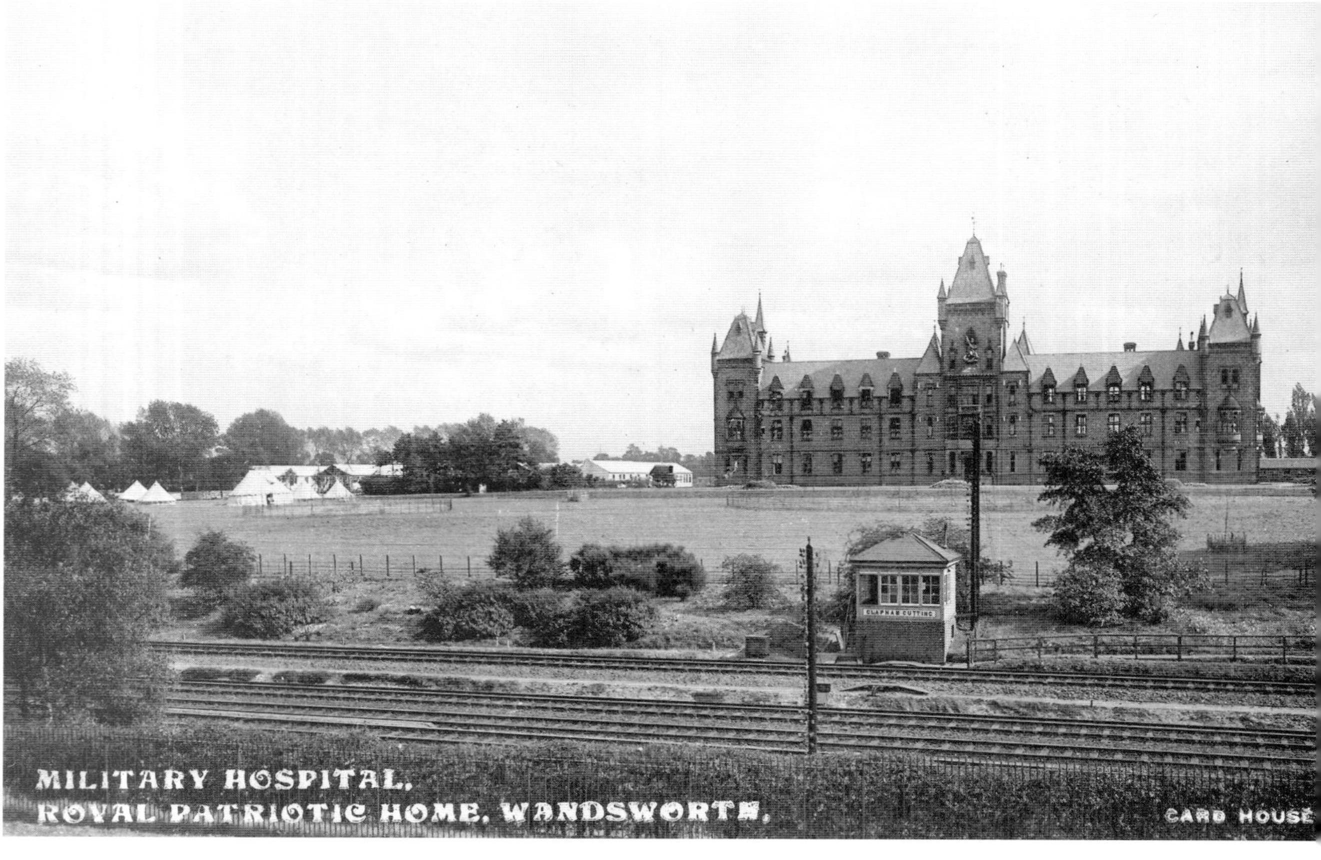

CLAPHAM CUTTING
MILITARY HOSPITAL.
ROYAL PATRIOTIC HOME. WANDSWORTH.
CARD HOUSE

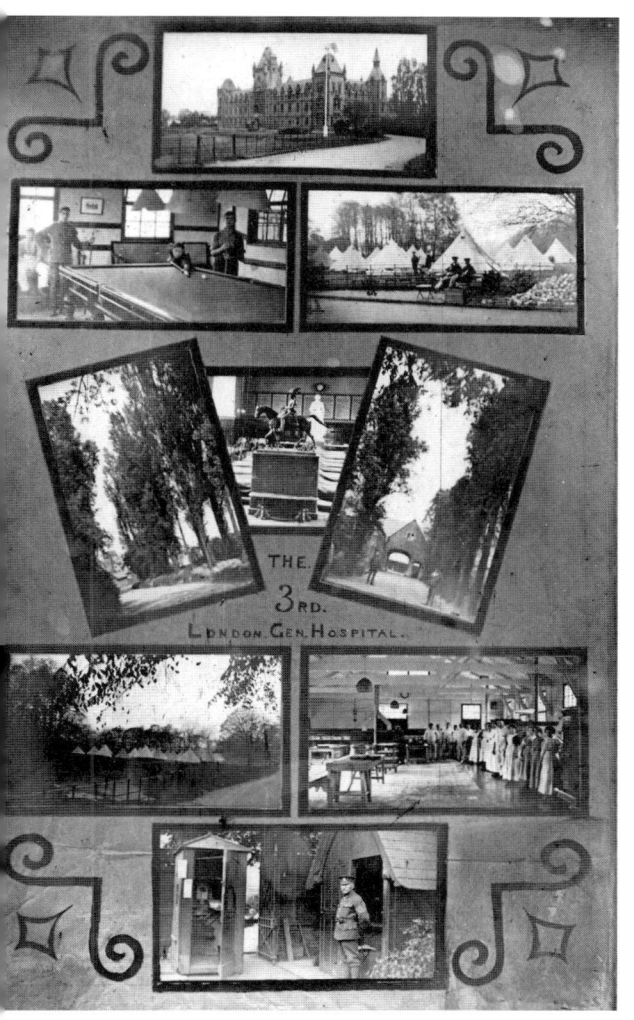 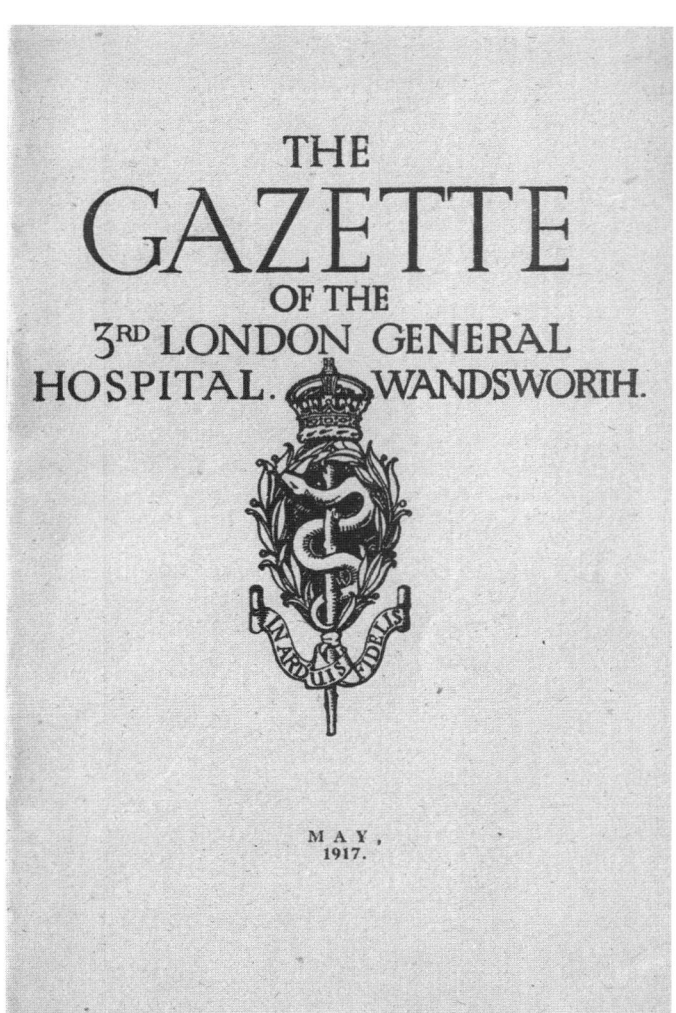

(**Above, left**) A collage postcard made of photographs taken at the 3rd London General Hospital, RAMC (TF). The photos show a variety of aspects around the hospital including tented accommodation, the surrounding gardens, the laundry and patients playing snooker.

(**Above right**) Front cover of the May 1917 edition of the *Gazette* of the 3rd London General Hospital, RAMC Territorial Force. Editions of the *Gazette* were produced regularly, with hospital patients and personnel contributing material to the magazine. Proceeds from its sale supported hospital fundraising.

(**Opposite page**) The 3rd London General Hospital, RAMC (TF) which was located at the Royal Victoria Patriotic School in Wandsworth. The lower photograph shows additional tented accommodation to the left of the hospital.

(**Right**) The *Gazette* included a range of cartoons and graphics drawn by hospital patients and staff.

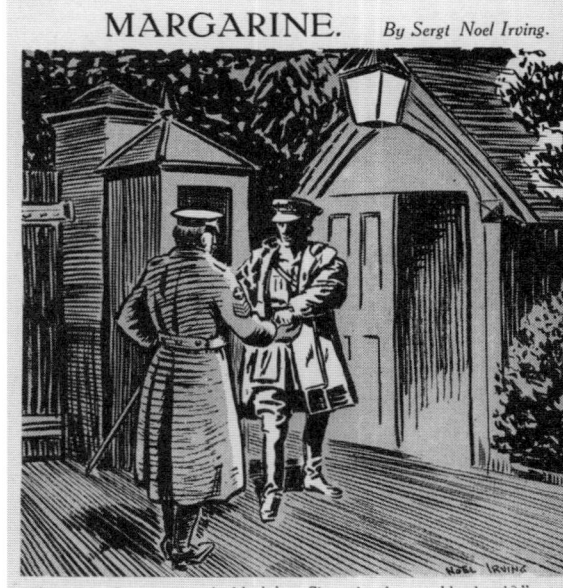

(**Below, left**) Editions of the 3rd London General Hospital *Gazette* also included a range of photographs taken around the hospital of patients and staff. In these photographs, taken at the front of the hospital, a number of Australian patients can be identified wearing slouch hats.

(**Below, right**) Patients and staff enjoy a boxing exhibition at the 3rd London General Hospital.

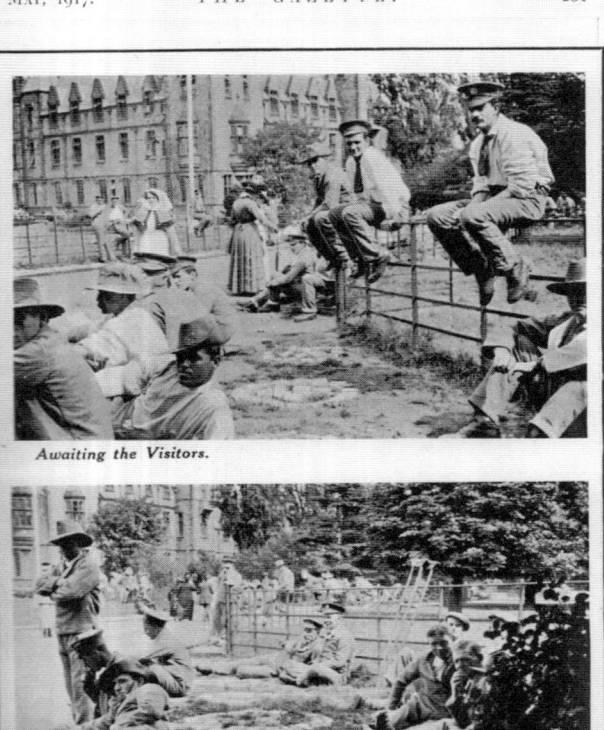

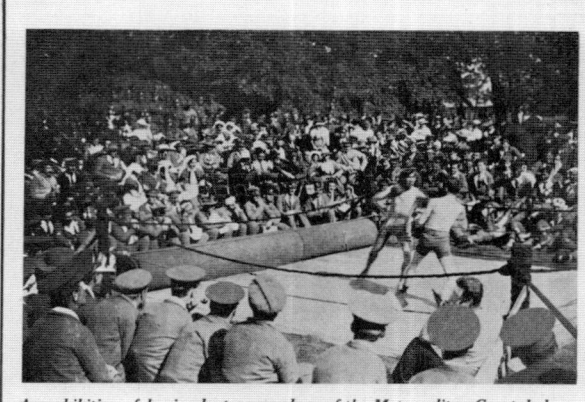

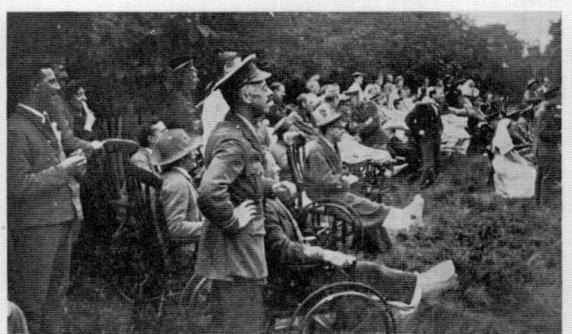

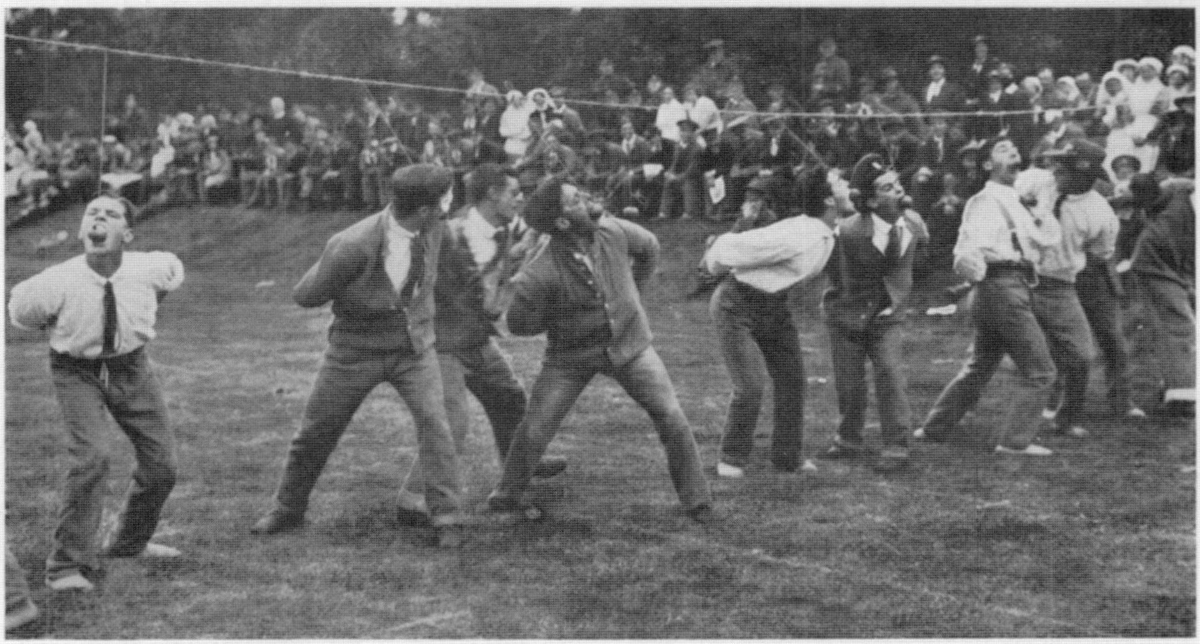

Mr. Howard William's Sports Meeting for the Wounded.   I. The Suspended Apple Event.   *"Gazette" Photograph.*

A range of activities were organised for patients at military hospitals; this was photographed at the 3rd London General Hospital.

RAMC personnel of the 3rd London General Hospital contributed material to the *Gazette*.

OUR CONTRIBUTORS.

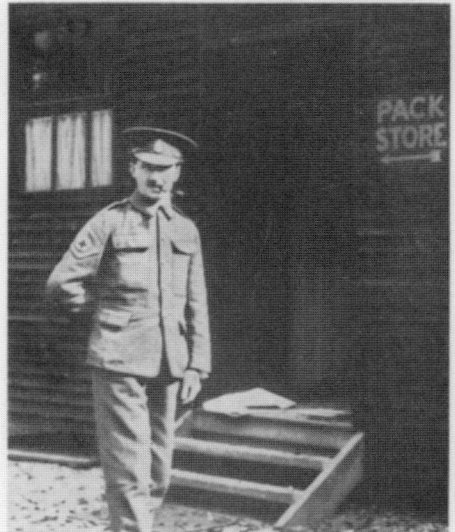

Cpl. W. R. S. STOTT.

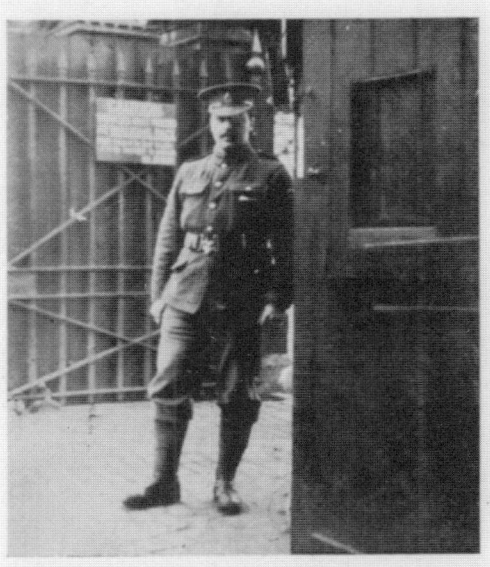

Pte. R. B. OGLE.

"Gazette" Photographs.

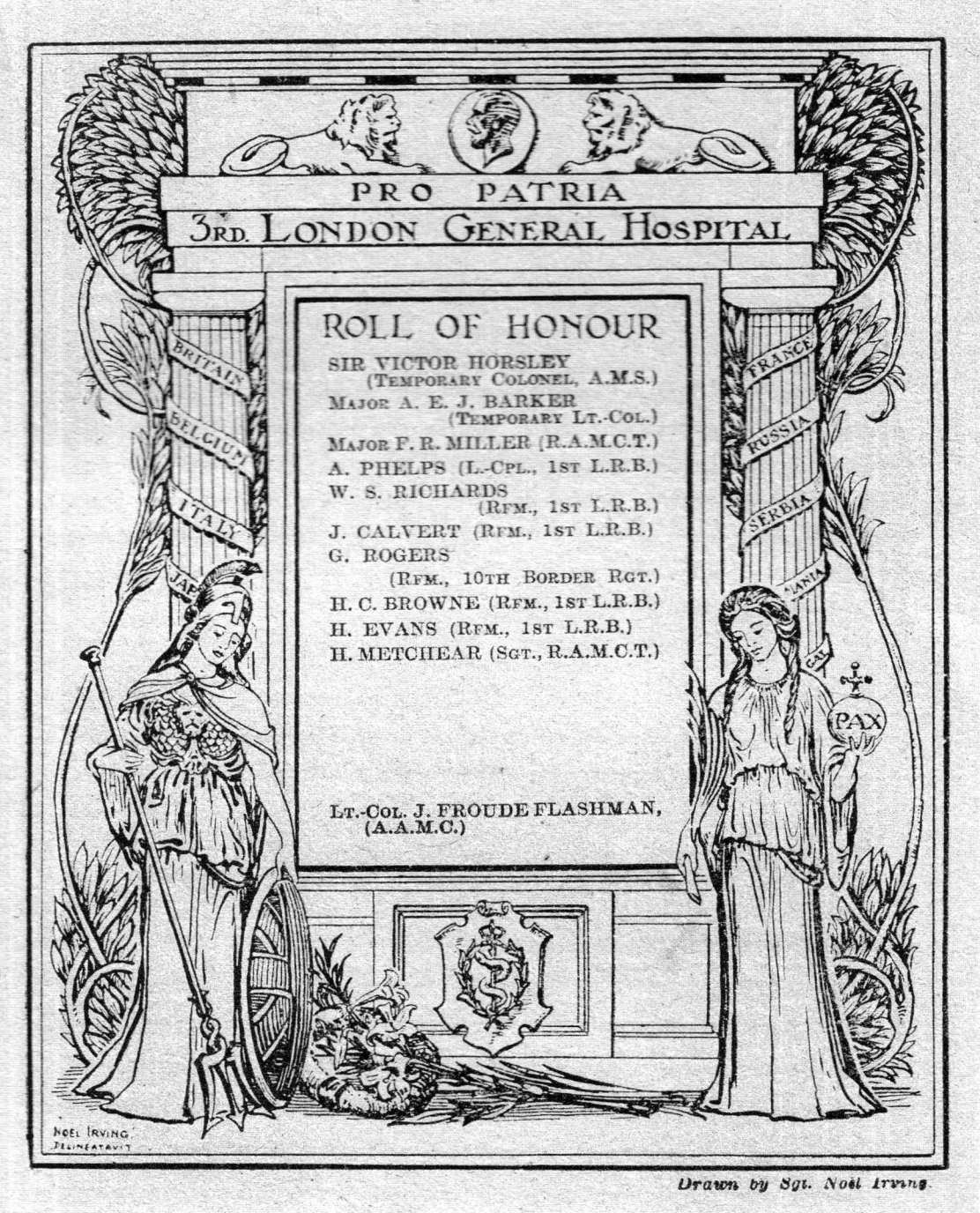

In the May 1917 edition of the *Gazette* a Roll of Honour was printed, including the names of patients and staff who had died at the hospital. Included in the Roll of Honour is 1696 Sergeant George Henry Metchear, 3rd London General Hospital, RAMC (TF), who died of nephritis on 12 November 1916, age 49. He was the son of George Henry and Sarah Metchear, of Portsmouth and the husband of Louisa Mary Metchear, of 105, Grosvenor Park, Camberwell, London. He is buried in Wandsworth (Earlsfield) Cemetery.

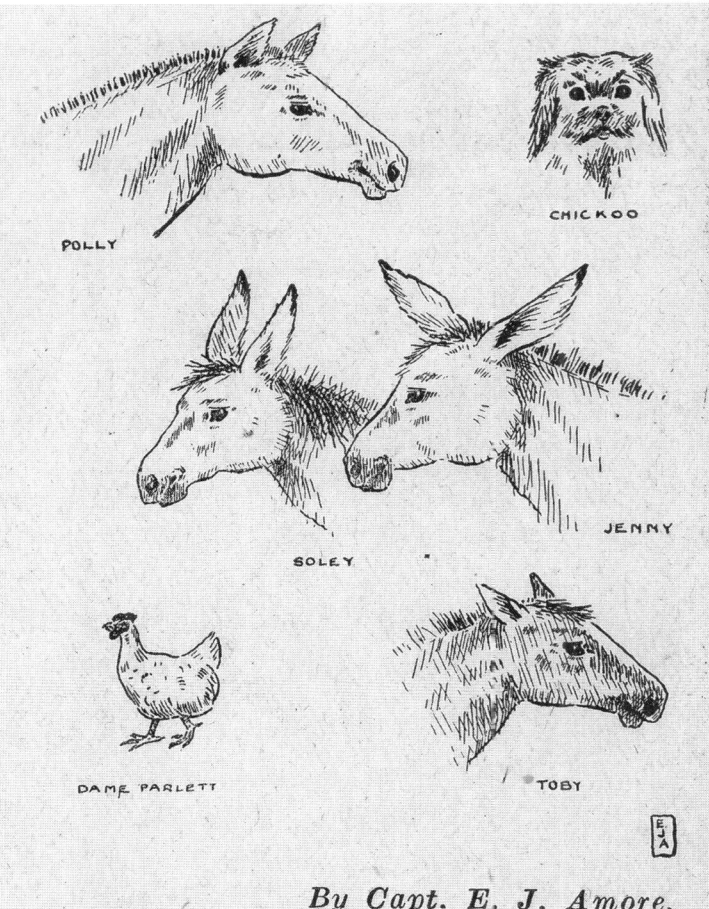

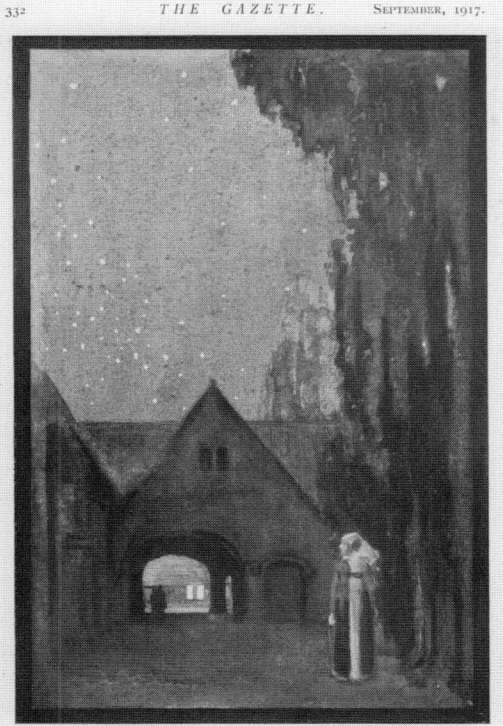

The September 1917 edition of the 3rd London General Hospital *Gazette* included a painting of the hospital courtyard and a nurse. It also had drawings of animals kept at the 3rd London General Hospital.

The September 1917 edition of the *Gazette* contained photos of sports events which had taken place at the hospital during the summer.

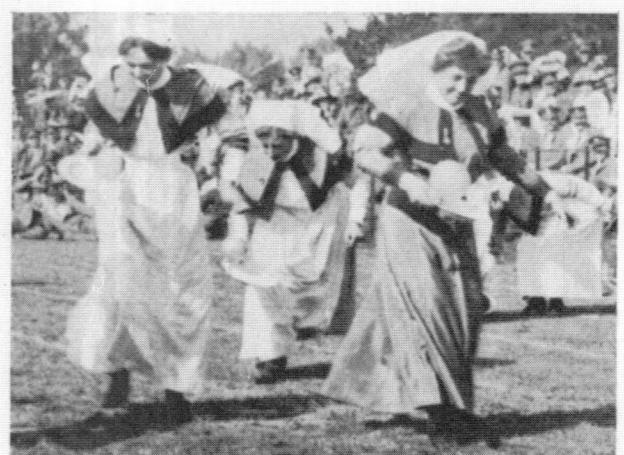
"Gazette" Photograph.
THE MATRON COMPETES.

Three photographs showing nursing staff and patients of the 3rd London General Hospital taking part in sporting events, included in the September 1917 *Gazette*.

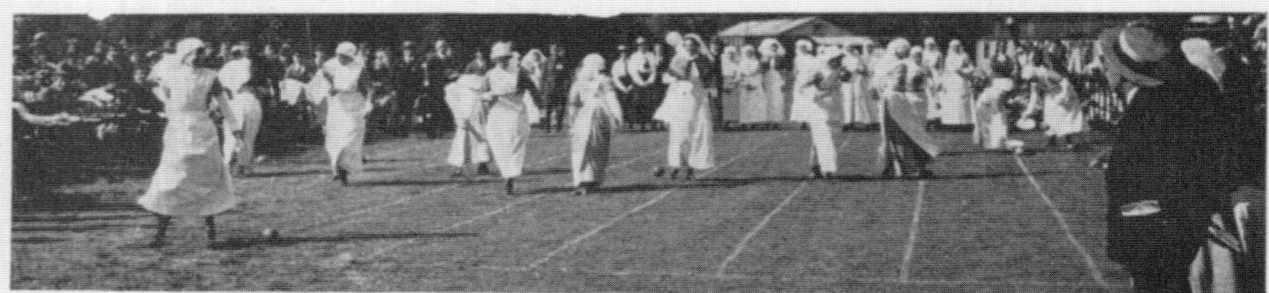
THE BALLOON RACE.   *"Gazette" Photograph.*

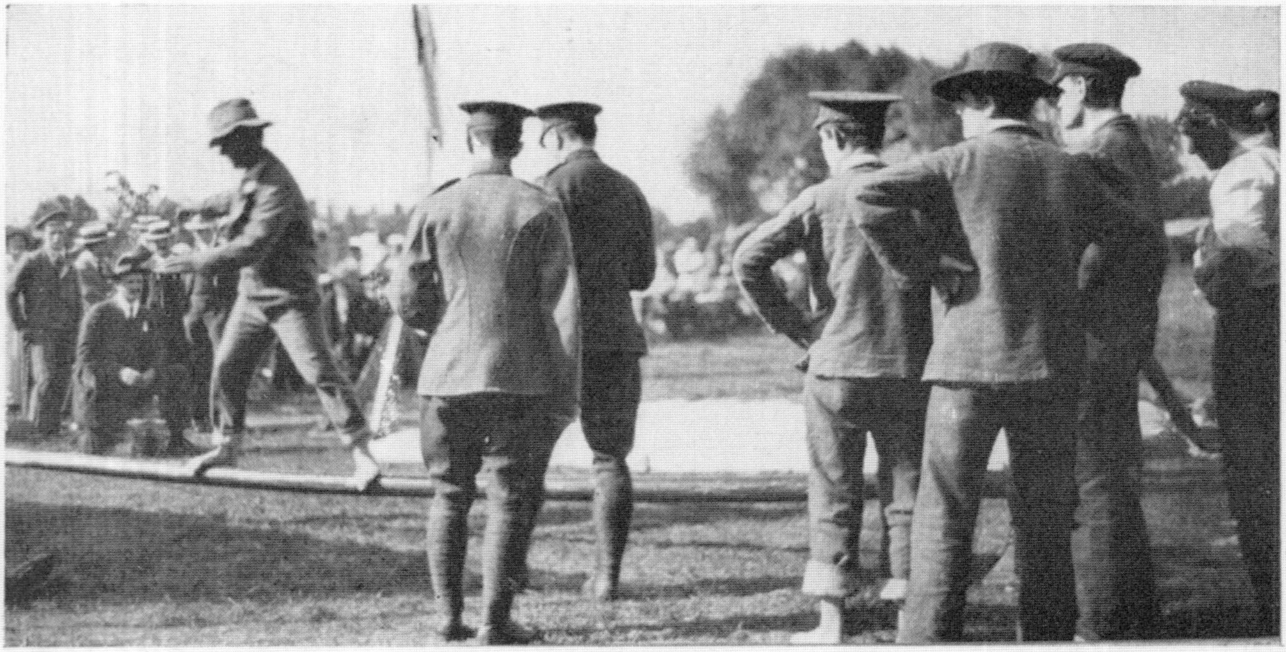

WALKING THE GREASY POLE.   *"Gazette" Photograph.*

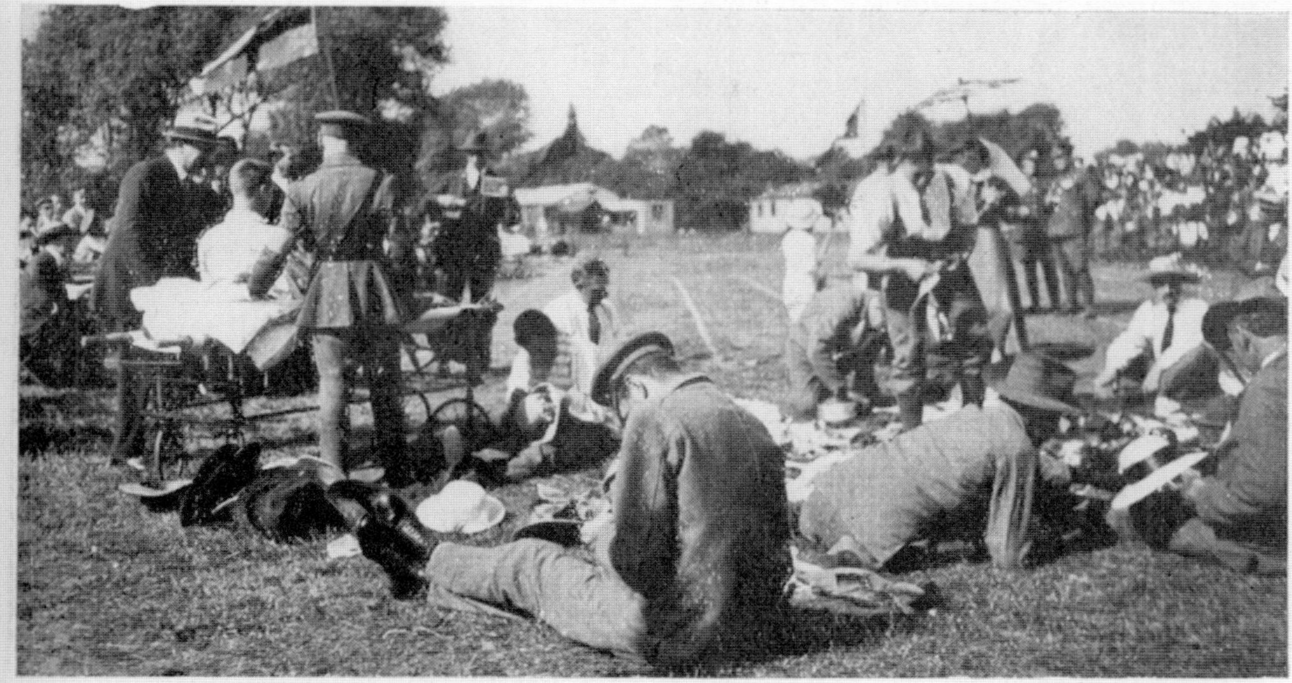

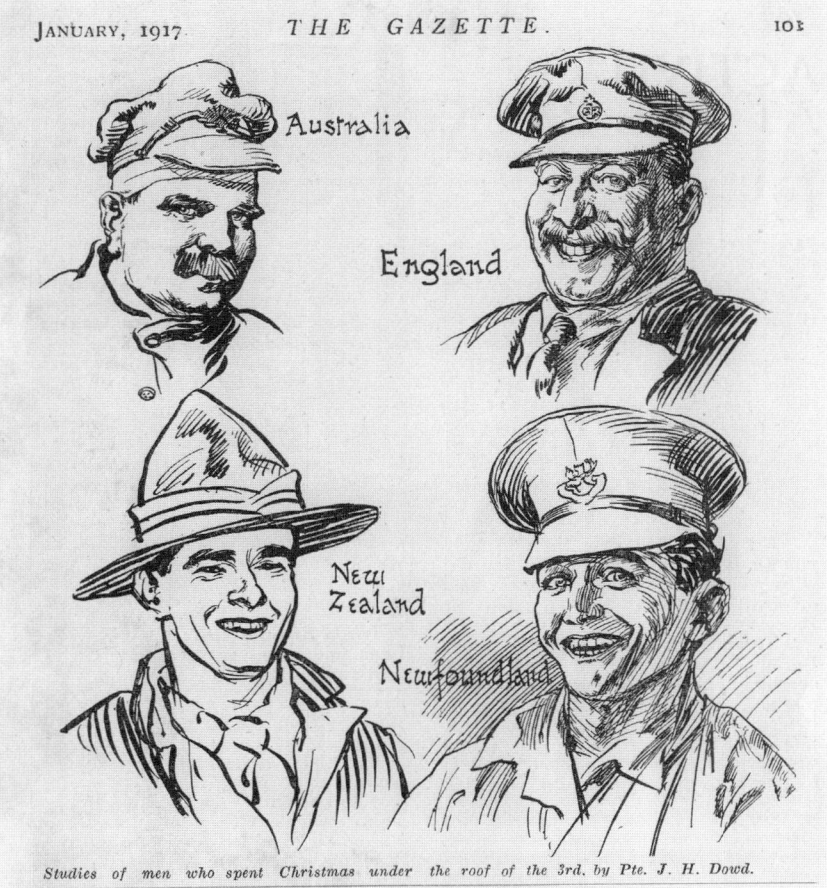

HAT TRIMMING COMPETITION. *"Gazette" Photograph.*

Here patients are taking part in a hat trimming competition, another photo from the September 1917 *Gazette*.

JANUARY, 1917. THE GAZETTE. 103

Studies of men who spent Christmas under the roof of the 3rd, by Pte. J. H. Dowd.

The January 1917 edition of the *Gazette* included sketches of patients.

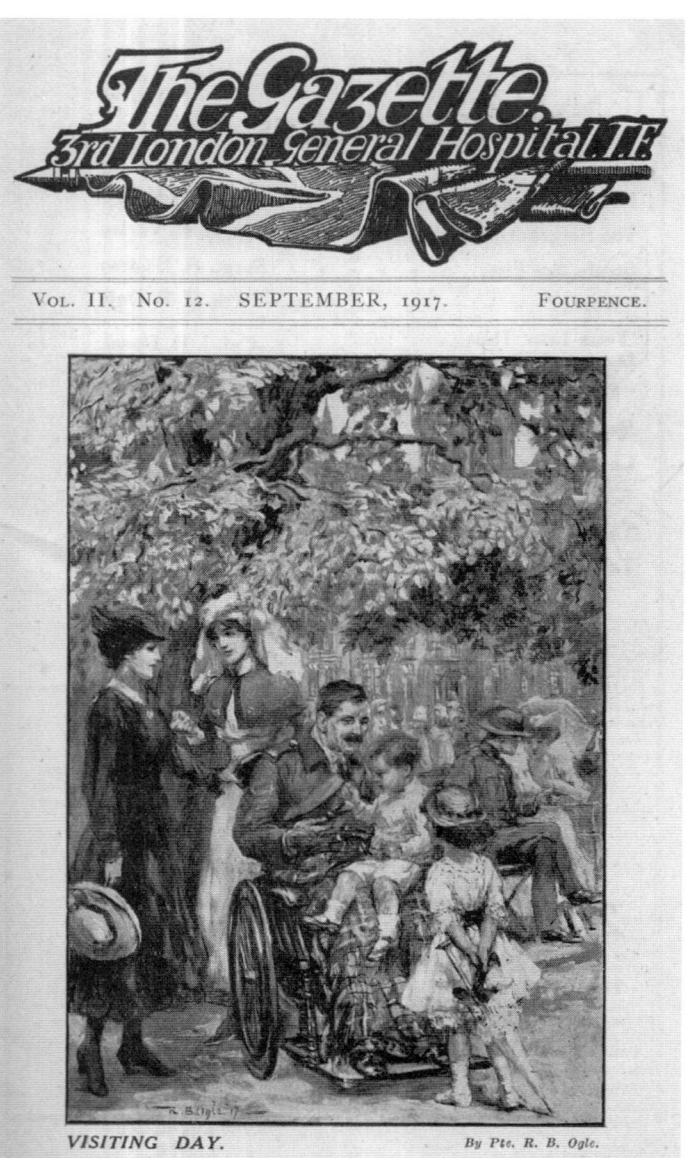
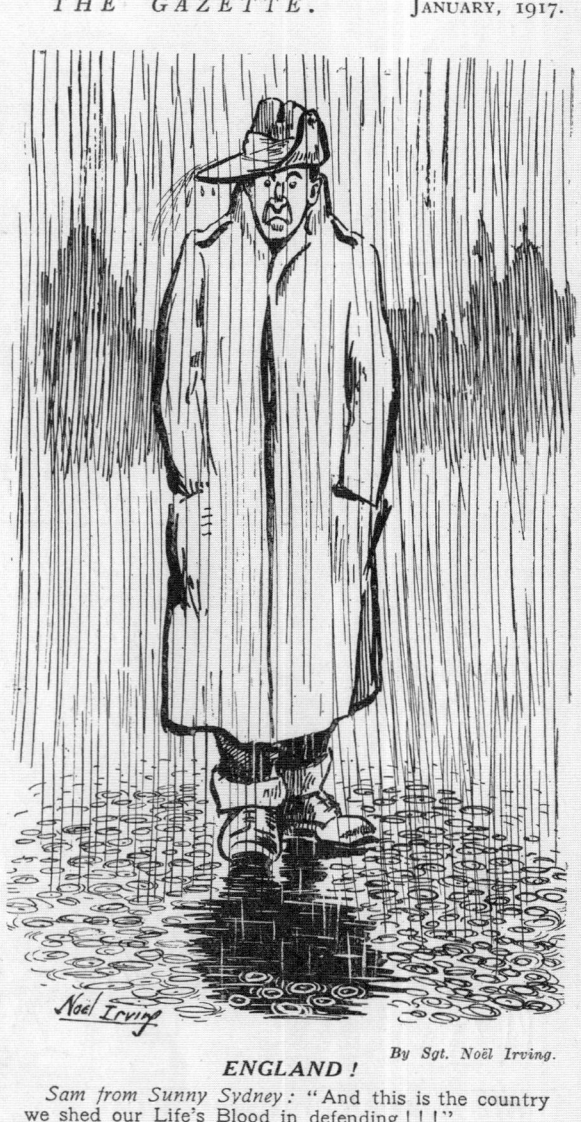

(**Left**) The September 1917 edition of the 3rd London General Hospital *Gazette* included a painting of a visiting day at the hospital.

(**Right**) This comic sketch of an Australian patient was drawn for the January 1917 edition of the 3rd London General Hospital *Gazette*.

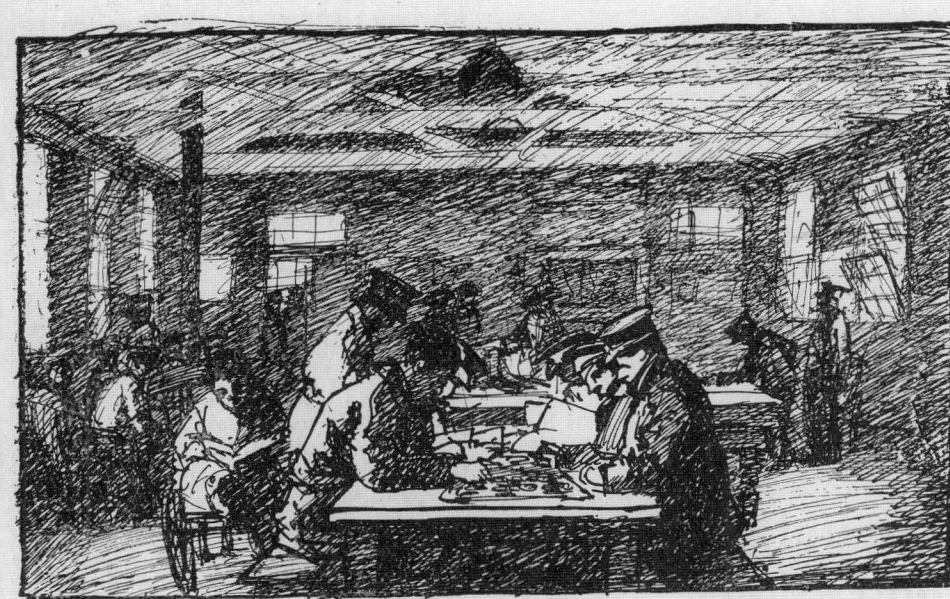

A sketch of the recreation room of the 3rd London General Hospital.

THE NEW RECREATION ROOM. *By L.-Cpl. J. H. Lobley.*

Two of the animals kept at the hospital that were featured in cartoons.

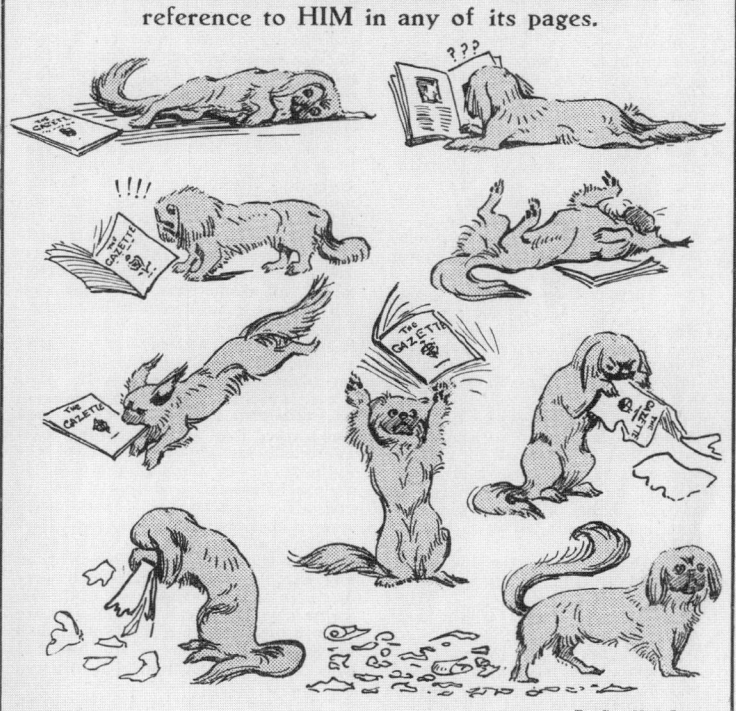

CHICKOO finds a "GAZETTE" which contains no reference to HIM in any of its pages.

By Sgt. Noël Irving.

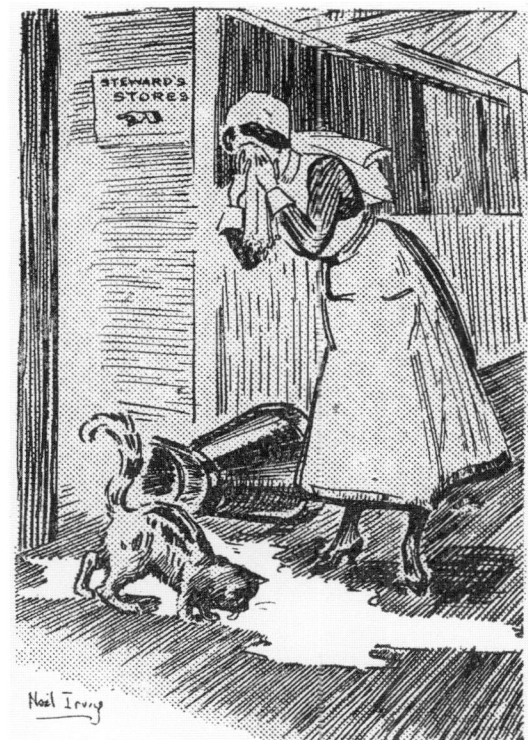

By Sgt. Noël Irving.

Night Sister's Cat: I'm bothered if I can understand why Humans cry over spilt milk. I'm sure I don't.

WINTER AT THE 3rd L.G.H.

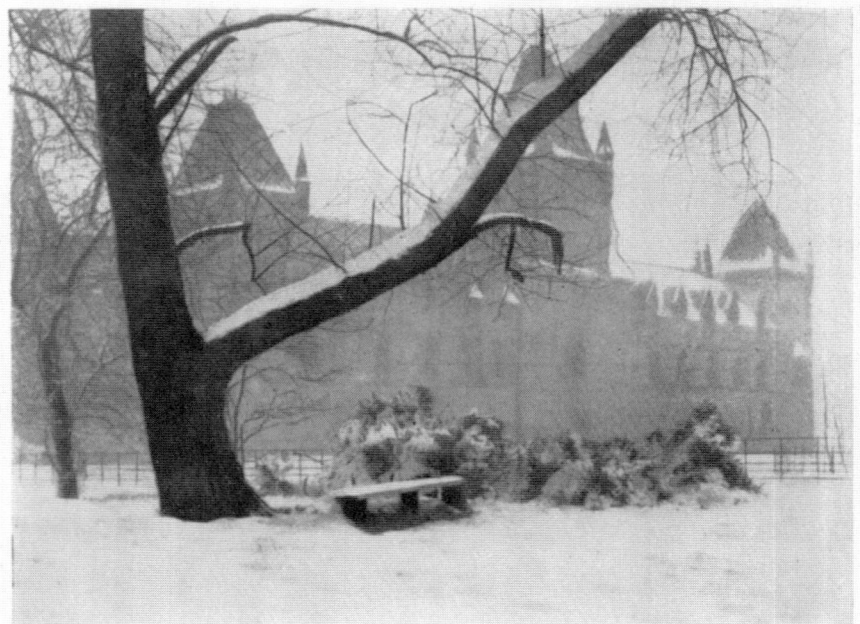

Morning.

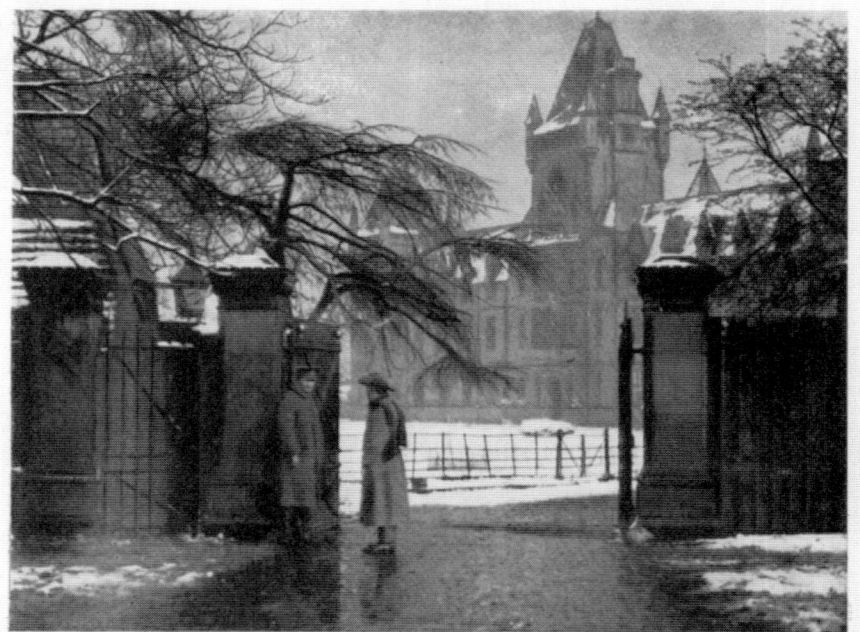

Evening.　　　　　　　　　　　　　　　　*"Gazette" Photographs.*

Photographs of the 3rd London General Hospital taken during winter.

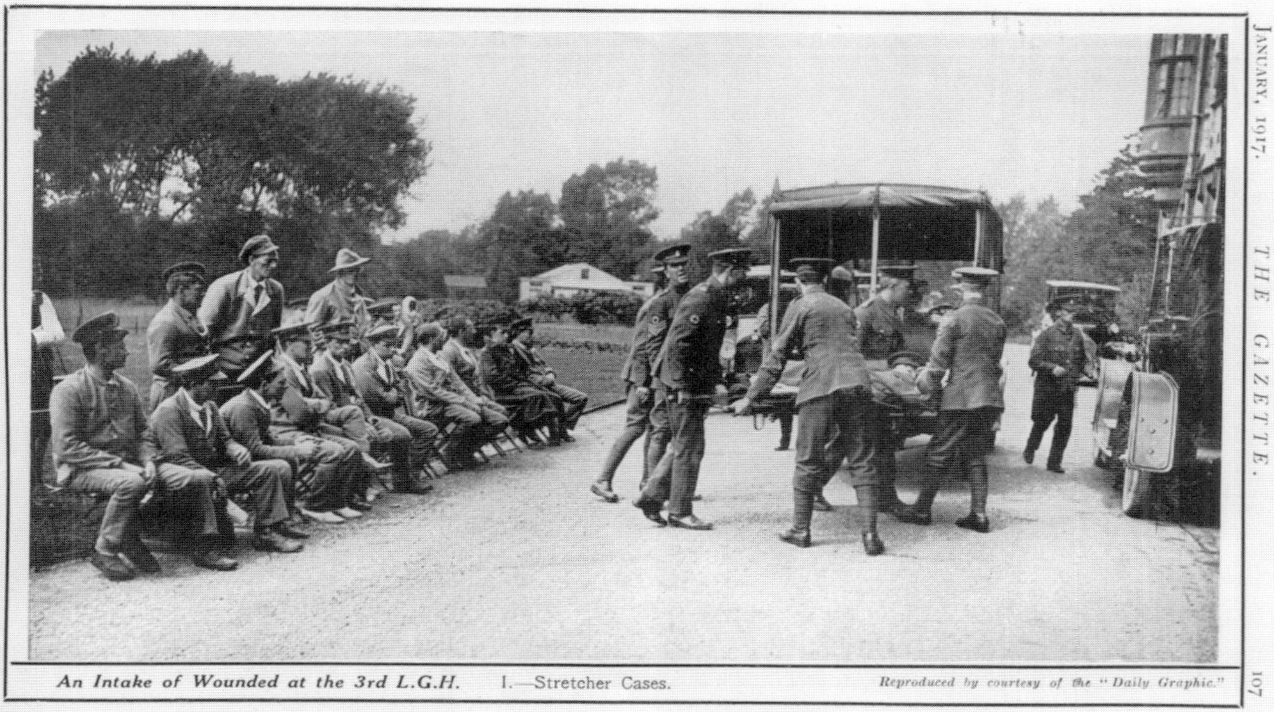

An Intake of Wounded at the 3rd L.G.H.   I.—Stretcher Cases.   Reproduced by courtesy of the "Daily Graphic."

A more sombre note – patients watching the arrival of wounded at the 3rd London General Hospital.

Voluntary Aid Detachment nurses with patients outside Sussex No. 1 Hut. Following the outbreak of war in August 1914, the British Red Cross and the Order of St John worked together, forming the Joint War Committee. The Joint War Committee organised Voluntary Aid Detachments; their work was vital in the treatment of sick and wounded military personnel in the UK and overseas.

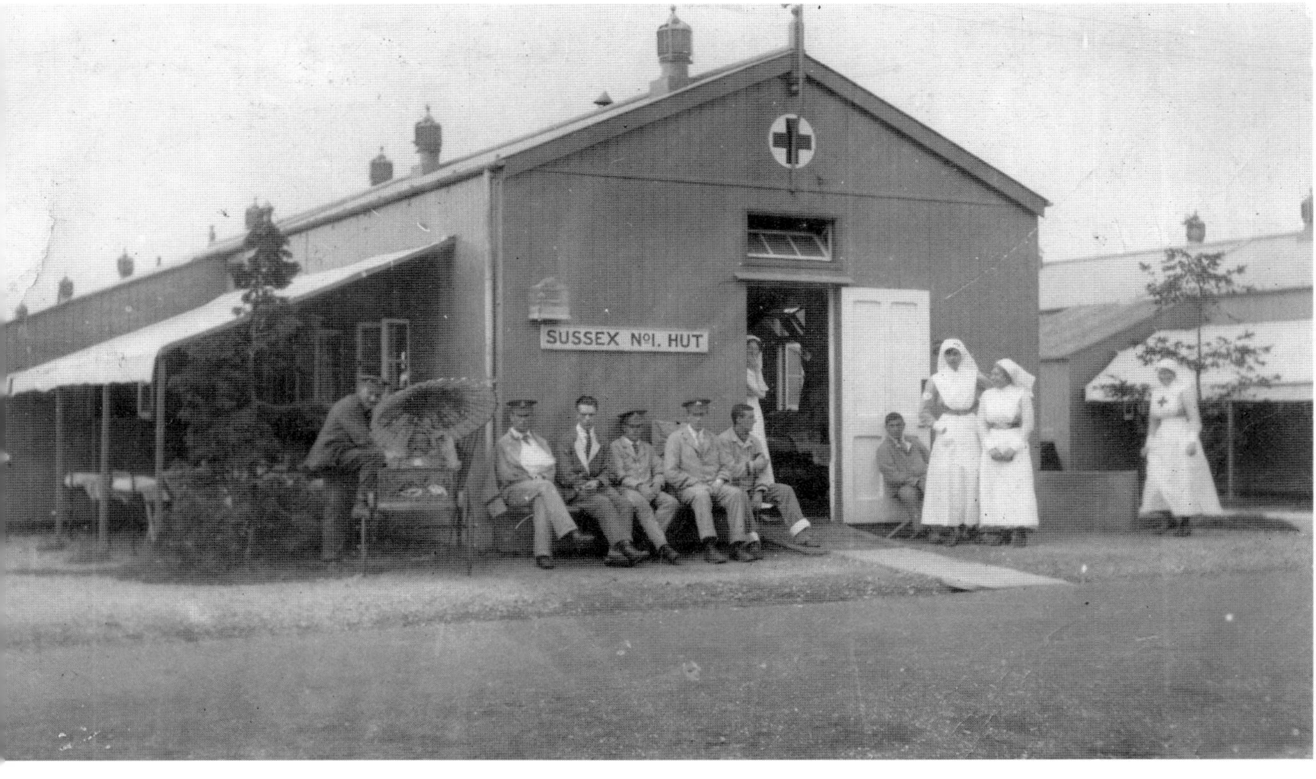

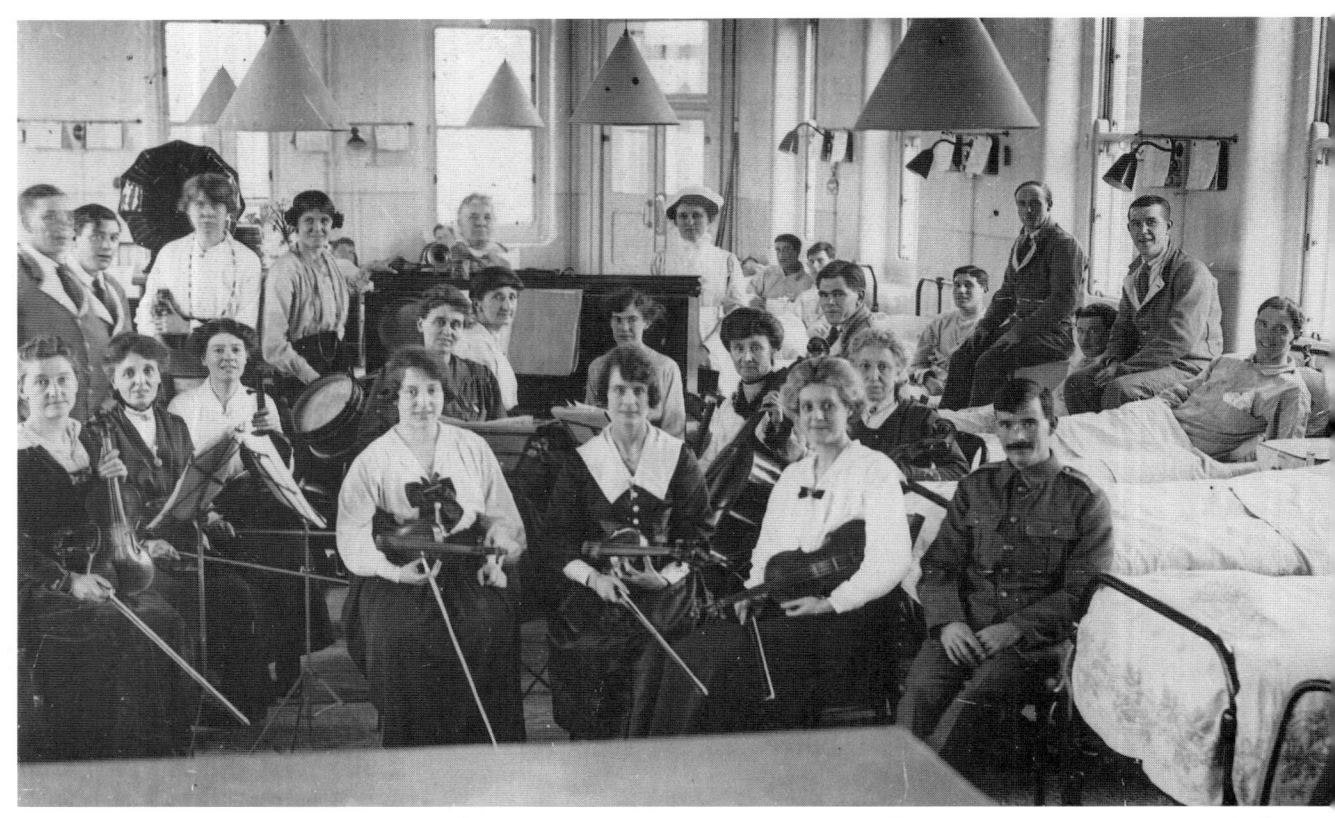

Musical entertainment for patients at St Andrew's Hospital, Dollis Hill, London. The hospital had around seventy beds and formed part of the 2nd London General Hospital, RAMC (TF). During the war over 2,000 patients were treated there. The reverse of the photo, written by a member of the orchestra, describes the musical performance.

Dear Molly,

This is the little ragtime orchestra I belong to; we had it taken at St Andrews Hospital Dollis Hill on the 400th performance. It was put in the Daily Graphic, rather amusing is it not? I hope you recognise me, it really is quite a good photo. You might write to me soon I have not heard from you for ages. I saw Skinny about a fortnight ago, she is working in London now.

Well good bye for to-day

Best love from Fanny

Love to Joan & Brenda

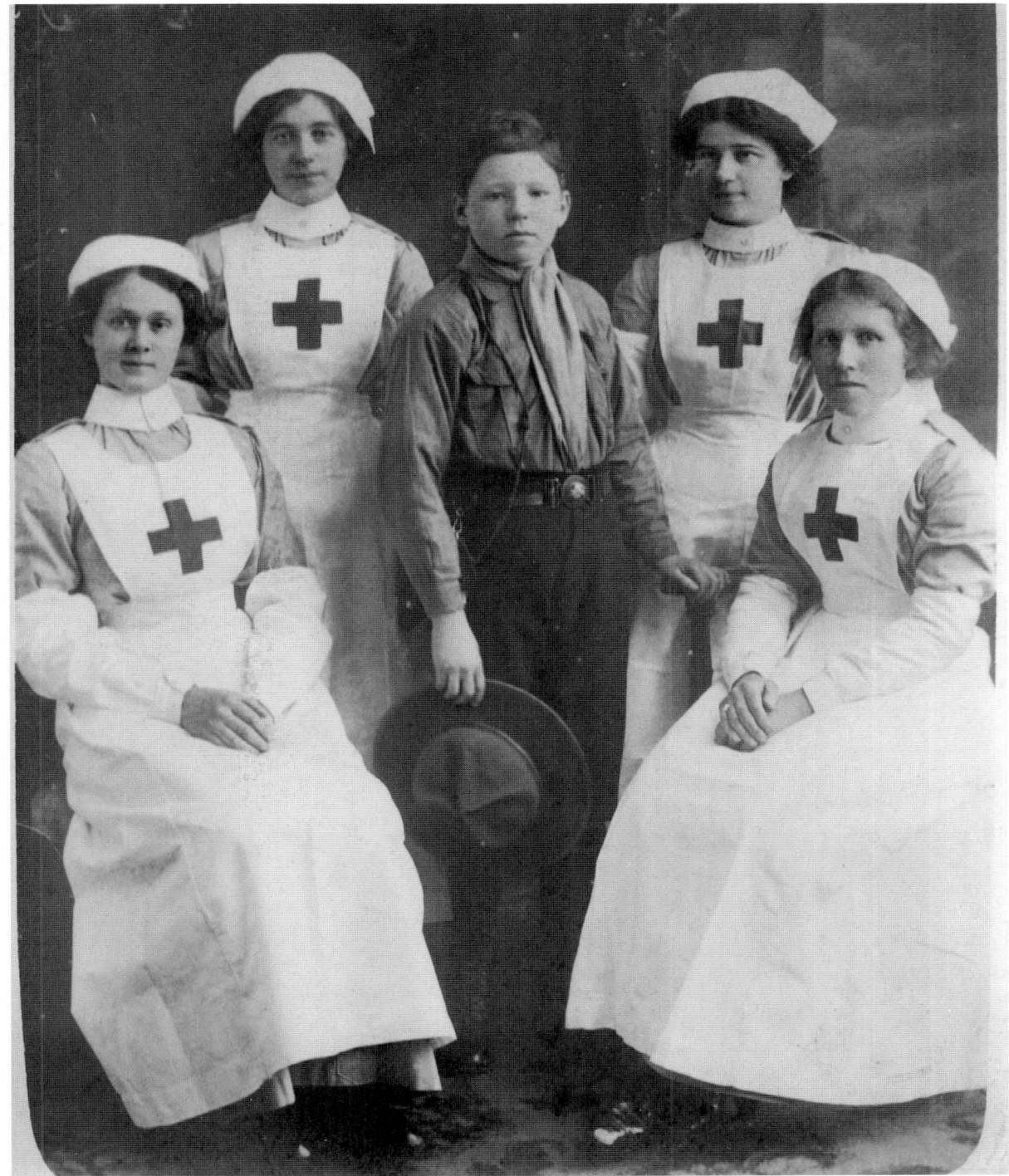

VAD nurses photographed in Dumfries, Dumfriesshire. A Scout, who would have served as a messenger, is also pictured. In October 1914, the Dunbar Terrace Red Cross Auxiliary Hospital was established in Dumfries. When the Hospital closed in February 1919, a total of 1,069 wounded soldiers had been treated since 1914

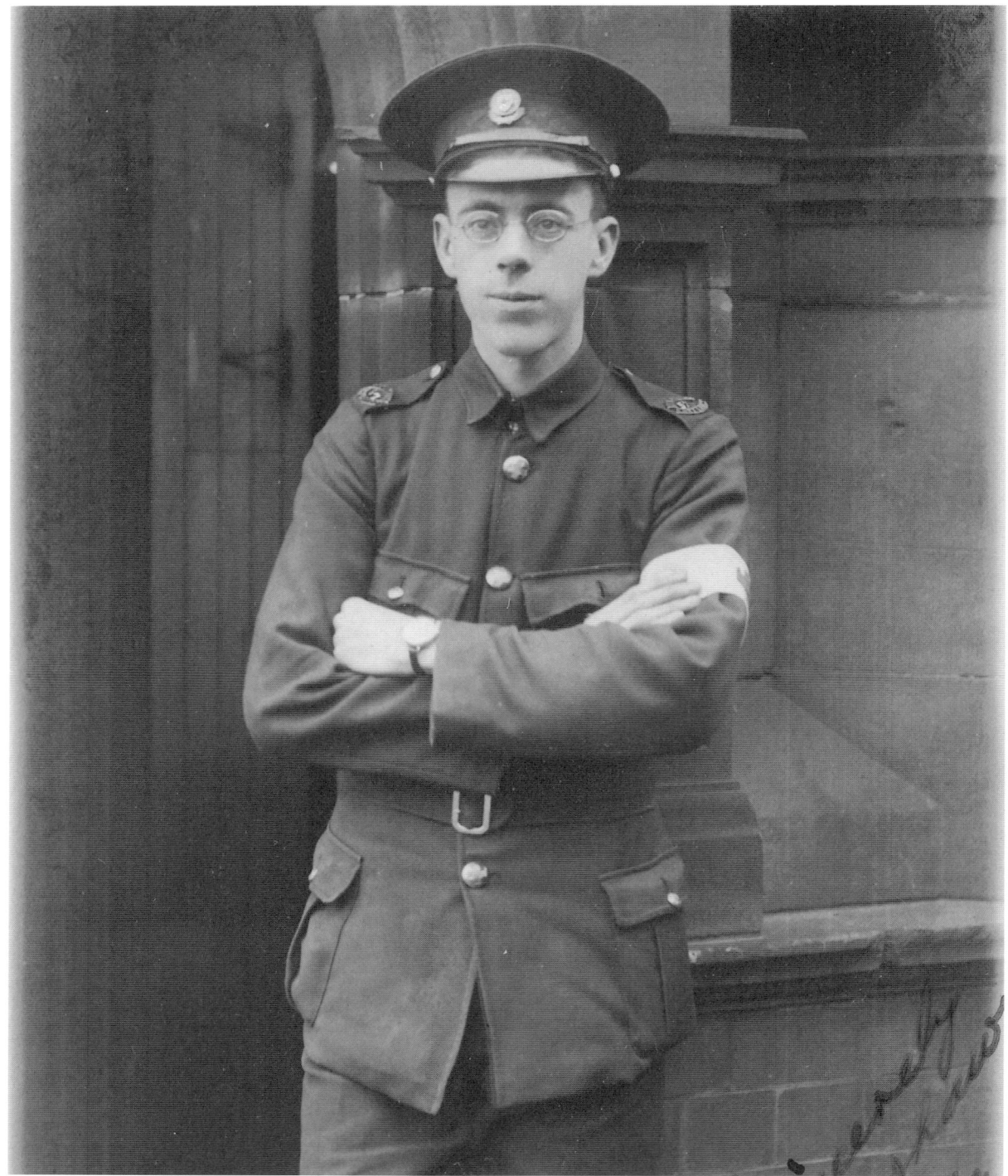

Fred Renshaw lived at 168 Oswald Road, Chorlton, Manchester. He served with No. 57 Detachment, East Lancashire Brigade, British Red Cross Society. From October 1914, he worked as a Hospital Orderly and a member of the Train Party, transferring casualties from Hospital Trains arriving in Manchester to local hospitals. He was still serving in May 1919.

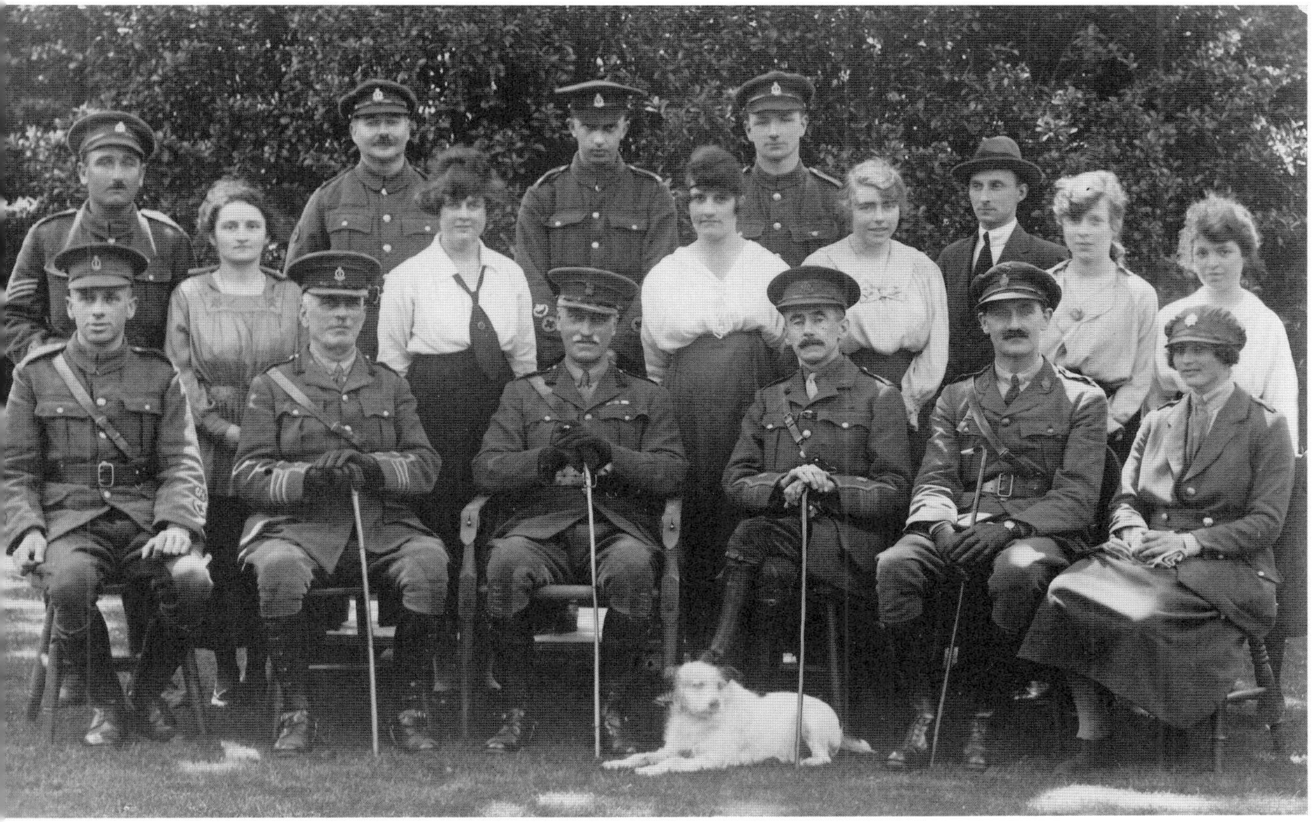

Clerkesses, officers, warrant officers and sergeants serving at a Royal Army Medical Corps hospital. Sitting on the right is a Women's Army Auxiliary Corps officer.

The Pipe Band of the Lowland Field Ambulance, RAMC. The photograph was taken whilst the unit was stationed at Chelmsford, Essex. On the reverse is written 'Our Band (with officers). Royal Stewart tartan'.

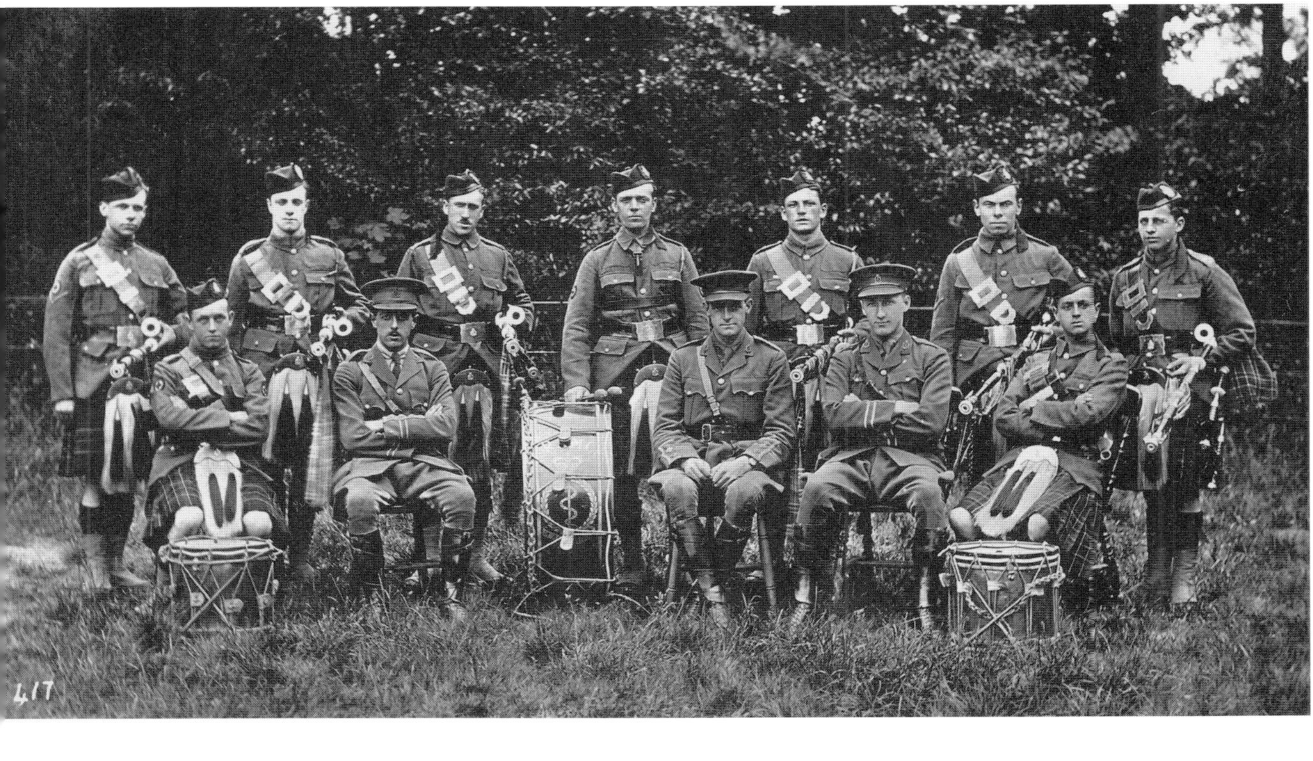

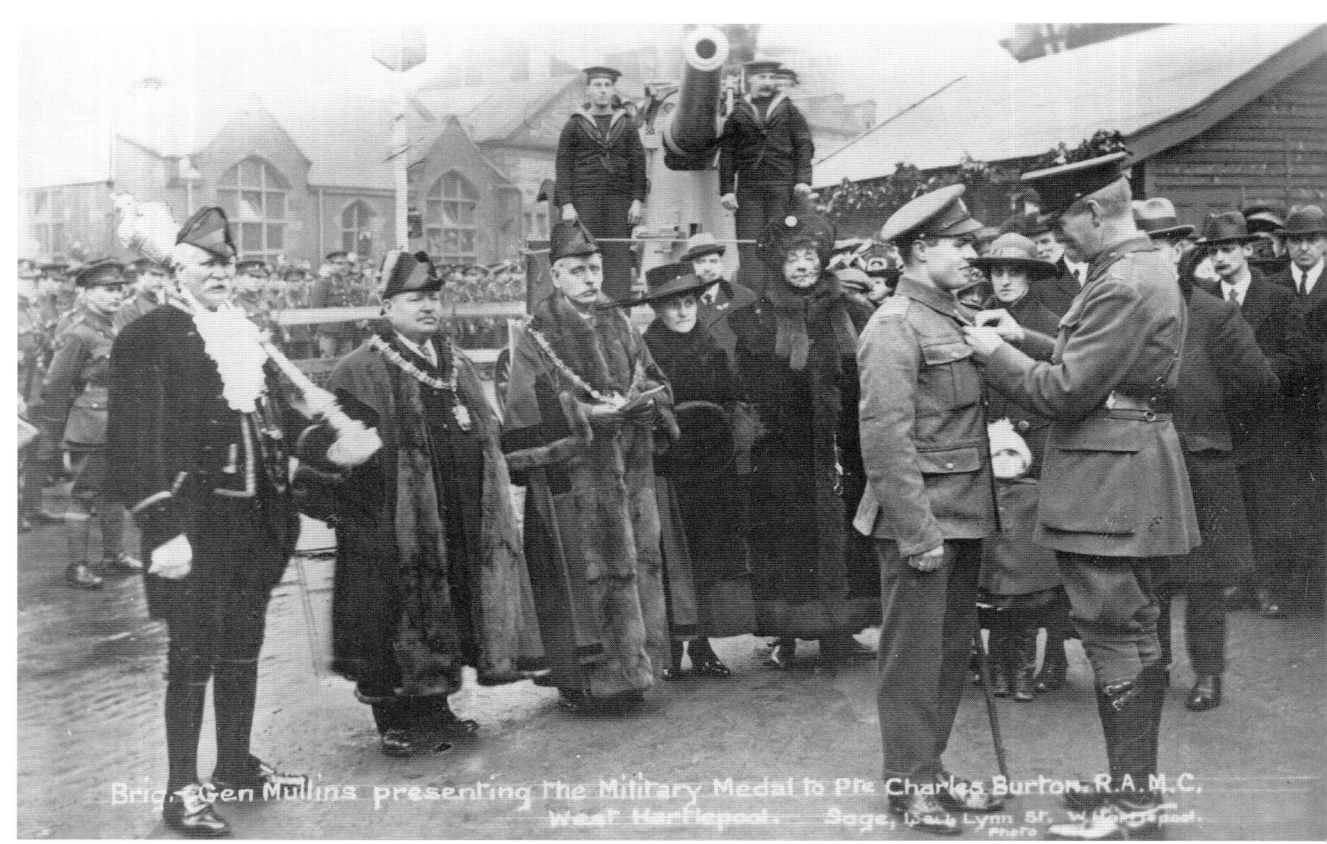

32055 Pte Charles Burton RAMC, being presented with the MM by Brig Gen Mullins at West Hartlepool. The award of the Military Medal to Pte Burton was announced in the *London Gazette*, 28 January 1918. *(Mr Andrew Read)*

Chapter Three

France and Belgium

The First World War resulted in casualties on a scale never before experienced in warfare. Advances in technology resulted in injuries caused by a range of new weaponry including poison gas, aerial bombing and flamethrowers. The size of the armies, the intensity of the combat and the power of modern armaments meant the number of casualties proved challenging for the medical services of all combatants, including the RAMC. At many times on the Western Front the medical services experienced great strain. The *Medical Services General History – Official Medical History of the War* records that between 1 July and 30 November 1916, the number of wounded admitted to field ambulance units of the Fourth, Fifth and Third Armies was 316,073.

On many occasions casualty clearing stations were overwhelmed; in the early days of the Battle of the Somme the 29th CCS at Gézaincourt admitted 5,346 casualties in a twenty-four hour period, from 6.00am on 2 July to 6.00am on 3 July 1916. During twelve weeks of the German Army offensives of 1918 more than 335,000 sick and wounded were treated and evacuated from the front line to the base area by British medical services.

The medical services had to respond to casualties suffering from the effects of new weapons; on one such occasion, on the night of 12/13 July 1917 in the Ypres area, the first mustard gas attack occurred and 1,800 cases were admitted to casualty clearing stations on the following day.

To address the scale and complexity of the casualties a number of innovative solutions were needed. One such innovation, suggested in early 1915 and developed by British medical services, was the use of barges for the evacuation of seriously wounded soldiers on the Western Front. Three Ambulance Barge Flotillas were established and during 1915 they brought severely wounded patients directly to hospitals at St Omer, reducing the suffering caused to serious cases by road or rail transport. Two further flotillas, Nos 4 and 5, were added to the fleet, establishing a total of twenty-four ambulance barges. The barges operated on the canals between Calais, the northern battle areas and the Somme. Each barge had space for thirty-one beds and also had a kitchen, dispensary, storeroom, toilets and accommodation for a medical officer, two nurses, eight RAMC personnel and three crew of the Inland

Water Transport, Royal Engineers. Electricity was provided by generators and skylights provided ventilation. Initially a tug towed only one barge, but subsequently two ambulance barges were towed by a tug. In July 1915 it was decided to transfer several ambulance barges to the River Somme. By spring 1916 twelve ambulance barges were located there. During the 1916 Somme battles patients were taken on board at Corbie and transported to Abbeville or Amiens. The barges moved back to the northern canals in June–July 1917.

In July and August 1917, when the British Army was operating on the Belgian coast, ambulance barges operated on the Dunkerque–Furnes Canal and moved casualties to St Omer. In 1918 when large numbers of wounded soldiers needed to be evacuated during the Battle of the Lys, several barges were adapted to accommodate sixty non-critical cases. The ambulance barges only operated in daylight and on the northern canals moved patients to Arques, St Omer or Calais. The average travel time by barge from Béthune to St Omer was ten and a half hours and from St Omer to Calais, eleven hours. Ambulance barges on the Western Front carried around 70,000 cases from 1915 to 1918. Although this was a relatively small proportion of the casualties, ambulance barges played an important role in the evacuation of patients suffering from injuries such as fractured thighs, head trauma and chest wounds.

Photographs were taken of individuals and units prior to service on the Western Front, with some unit photos taken shortly after the enlistment of personnel, before the issue of uniforms. Many photos taken at medical facilities show the vital role played by military nursing services and voluntary medical personnel overseas. Photos were taken to send home and also illustrate the challenges faced, with personnel wearing a range of clothing to reduce the risks of service including gas masks and goatskin tunics. The RAMC suffered many casualties whilst treating the sick and wounded and photographs of RAMC casualties are a poignant reminder of the sacrifices made by medical personnel.

(**Opposite, above**) Volunteers on enlistment in A Section, 49th Field Ambulance RAMC. The 49th Field Ambulance served with the 37th Division in the Second New Army from the summer of 1915. Around 30,000 personnel of the 37th Division were killed, wounded and missing on the Western Front.

(**Opposite, below**) A Section, 2nd West Riding Field Ambulance RAMC (TF). This unit served with the 49th (West Riding) Division which was raised in West Riding of Yorkshire and fought on the Western Front from May 1915.

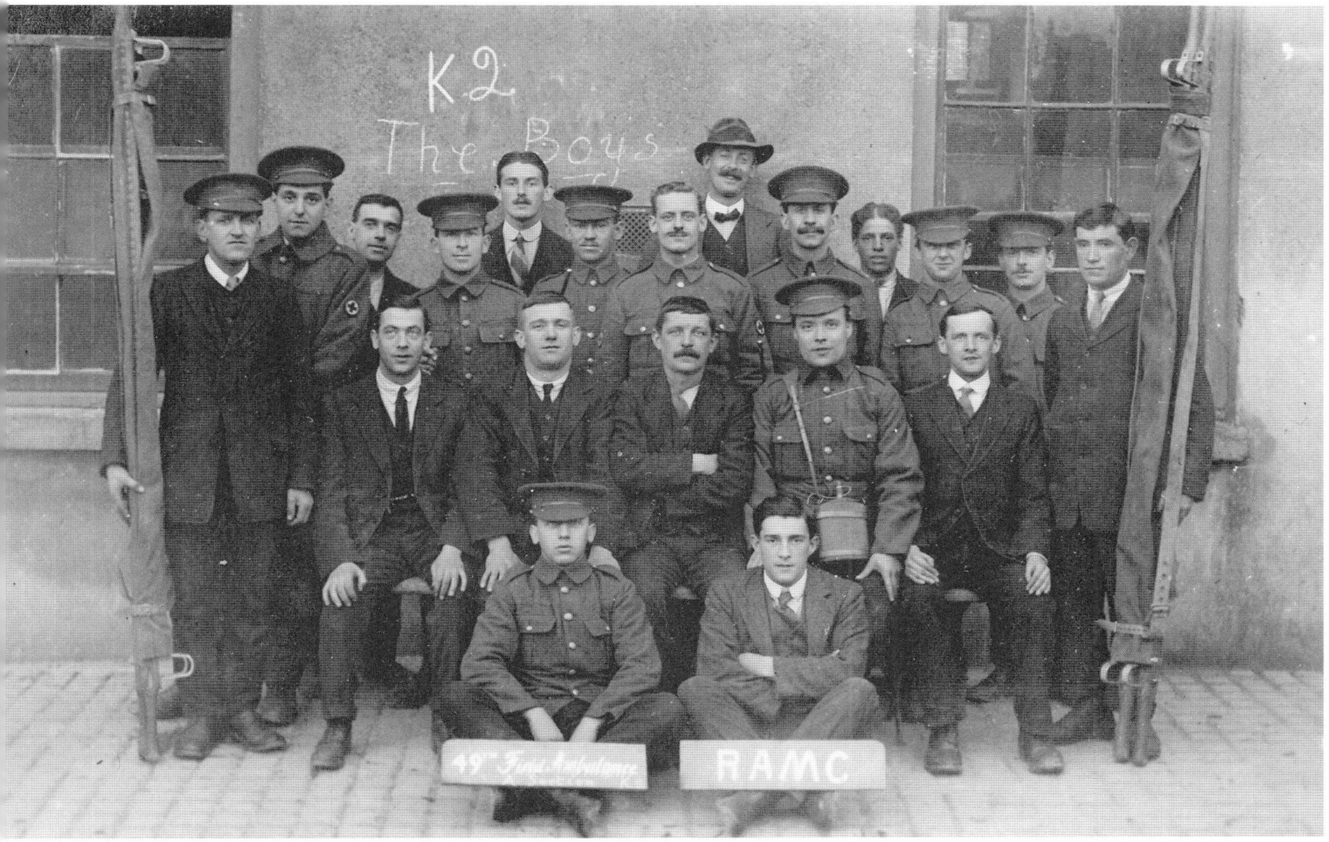

K2
The Boys

49th Field Ambulance   RAMC

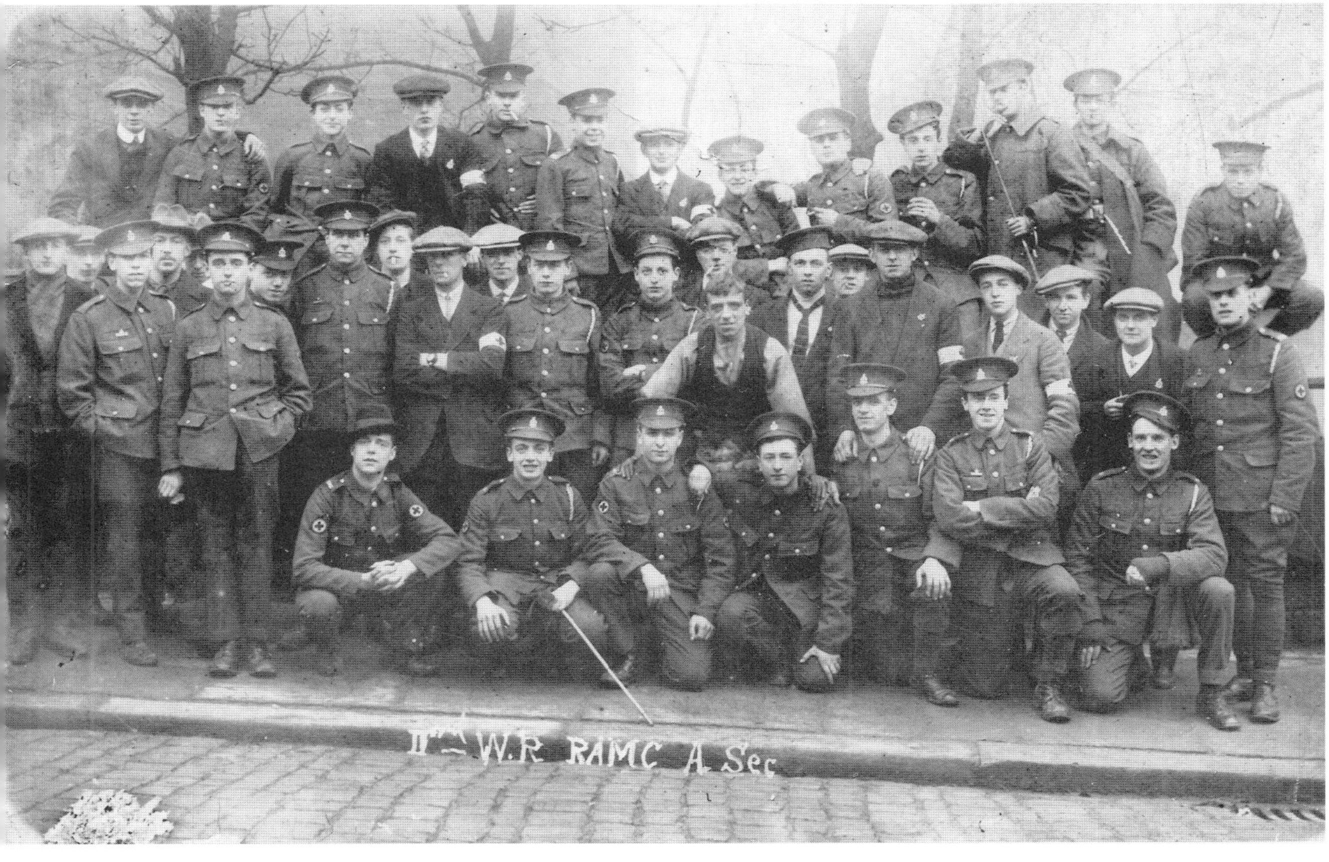

11th W.R. RAMC A Sec

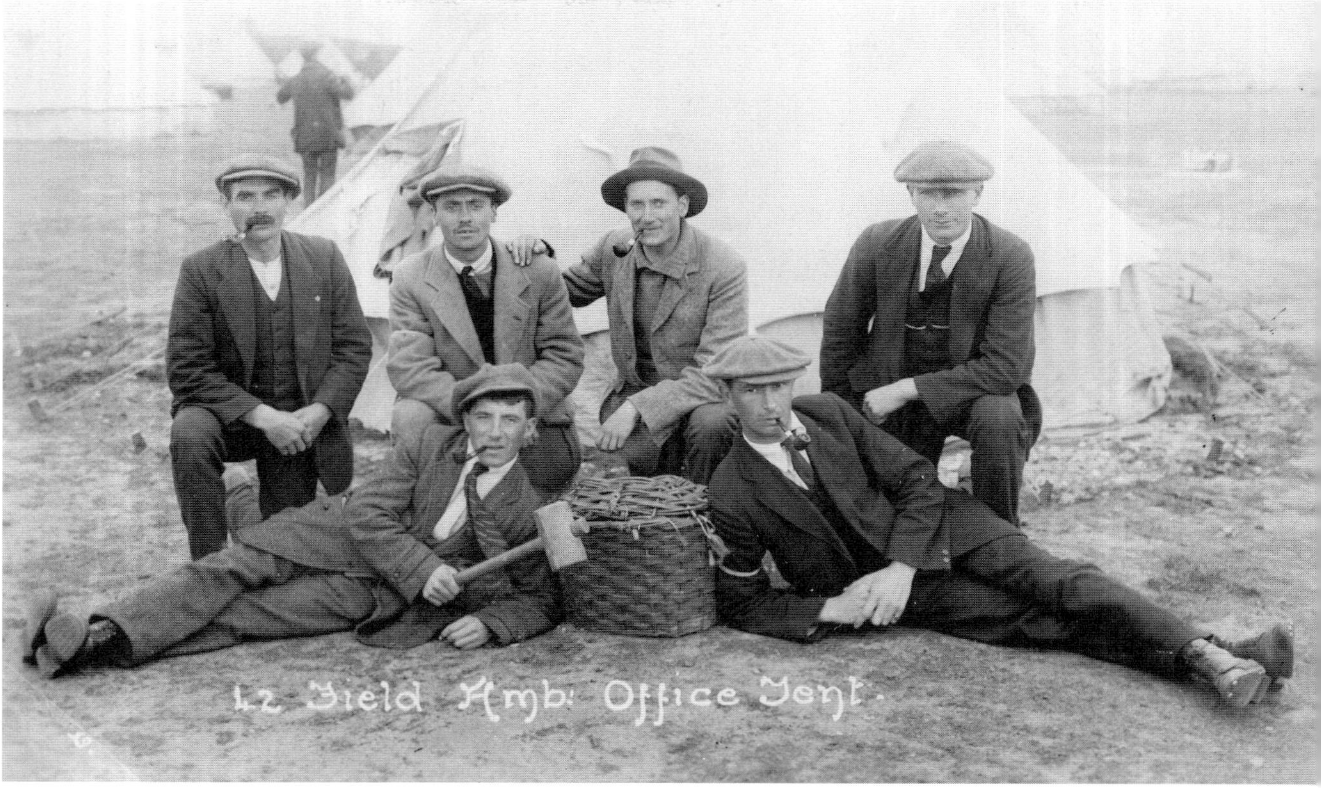

Volunteers on enlistment in the 42nd Field Ambulance RAMC, prior to their issue of uniforms. This unit served with the 14th (Light) Division in the First New Army from the summer of 1915. Around 37,000 personnel were killed, wounded and missing serving with the 14th Division.

Personnel and horse-drawn ambulances of the 17th Field Ambulance, RAMC. This was a regular army unit with the 6th Division on the Western Front from the autumn of 1914.

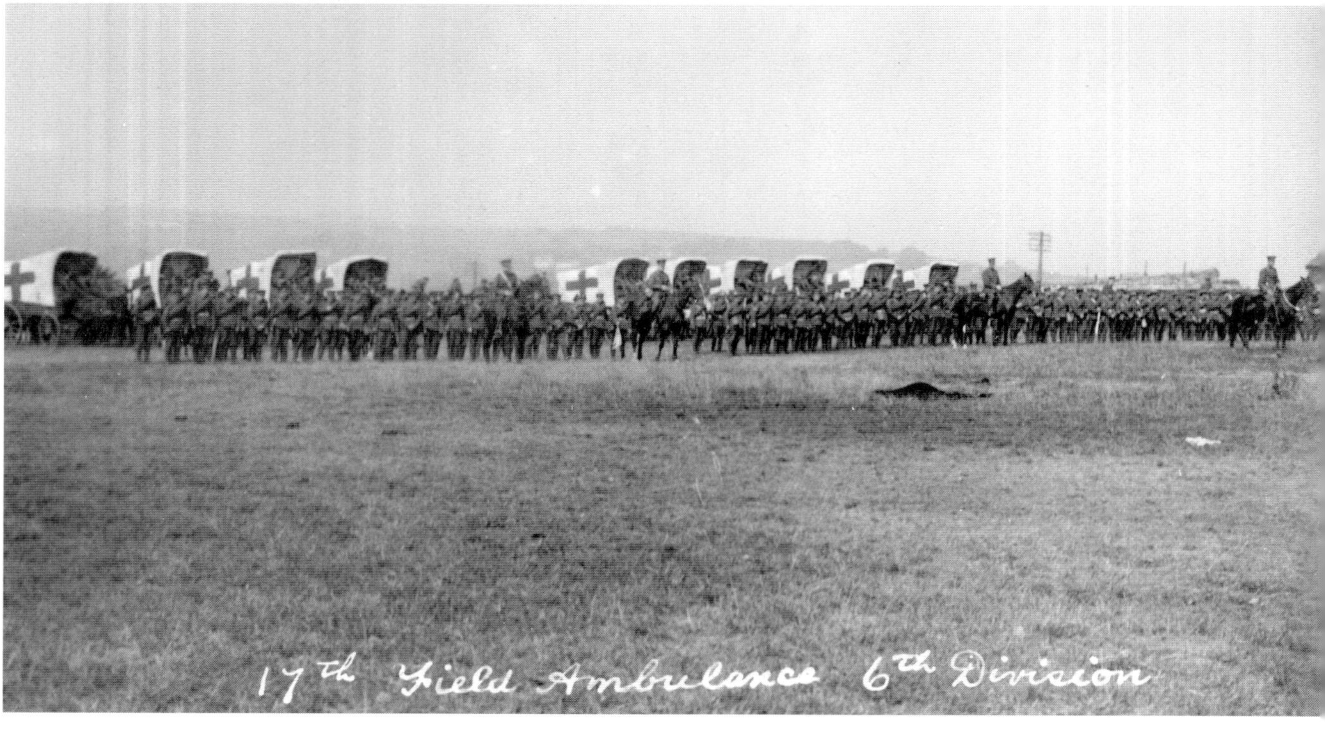

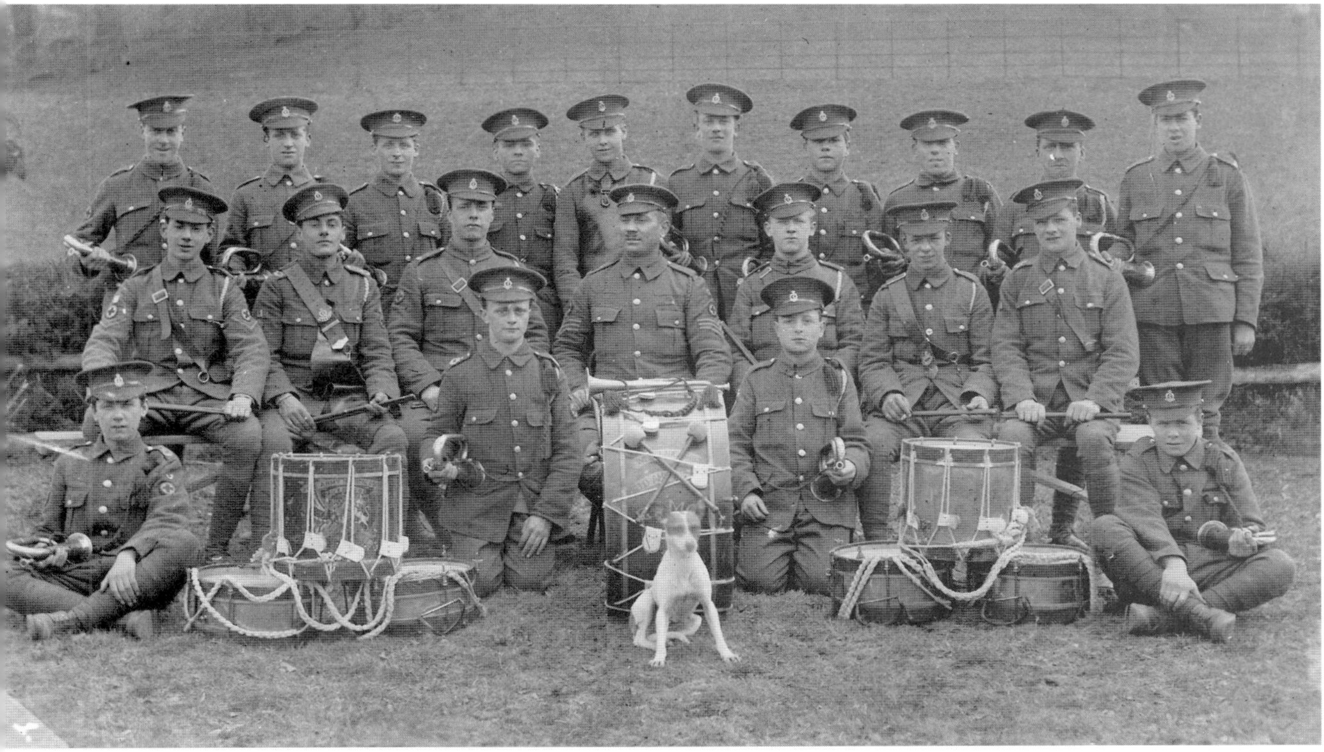

The band of the 1st West Lancashire Field Ambulance, RAMC (TF). The unit was based at Liverpool and during the First World War was renamed the 87th Field Ambulance. It served with the 29th Division, a regular army division, at Gallipoli in 1915 and on the Western Front from early 1916.

Officers of the 2nd West Lancashire Field Ambulance, RAMC (TF). Lieutenant Colonel T. Stevenson, commanding officer, was an oculist who practised in Rodney Street, Liverpool.

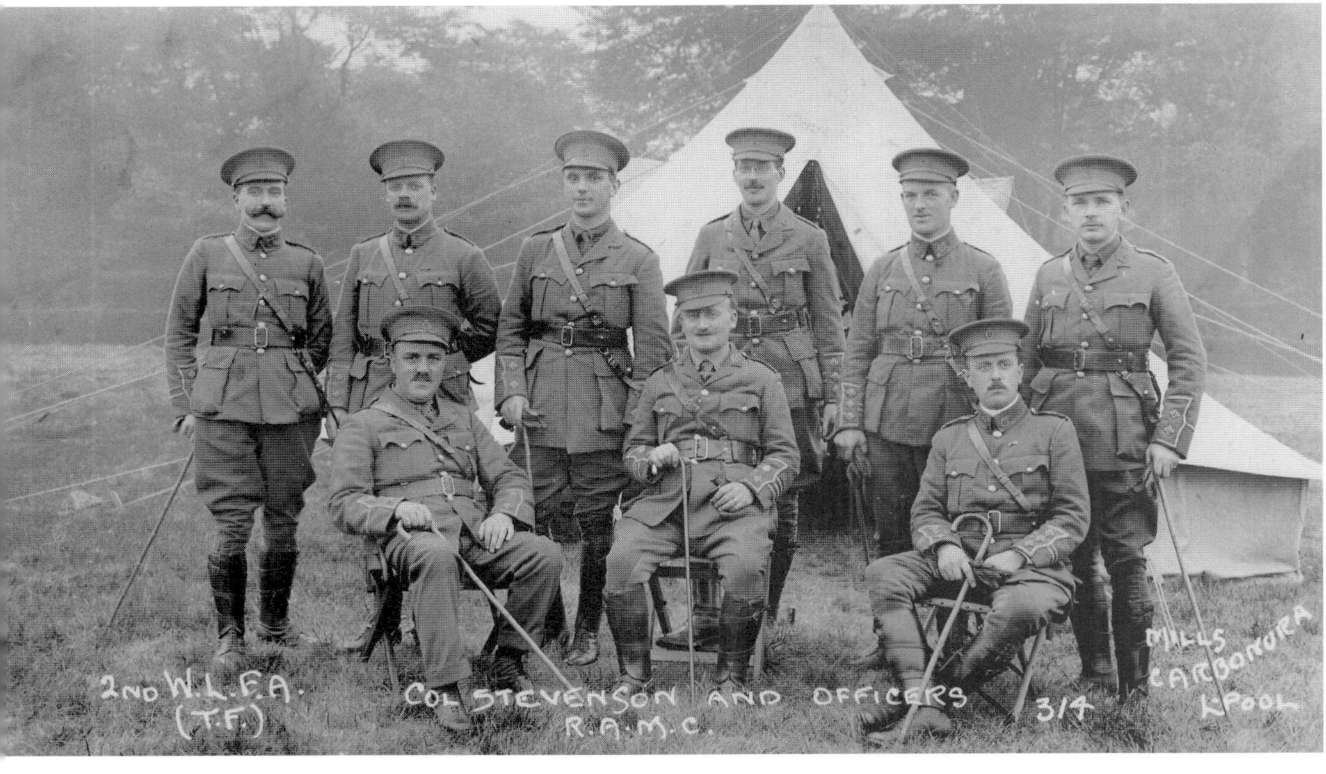

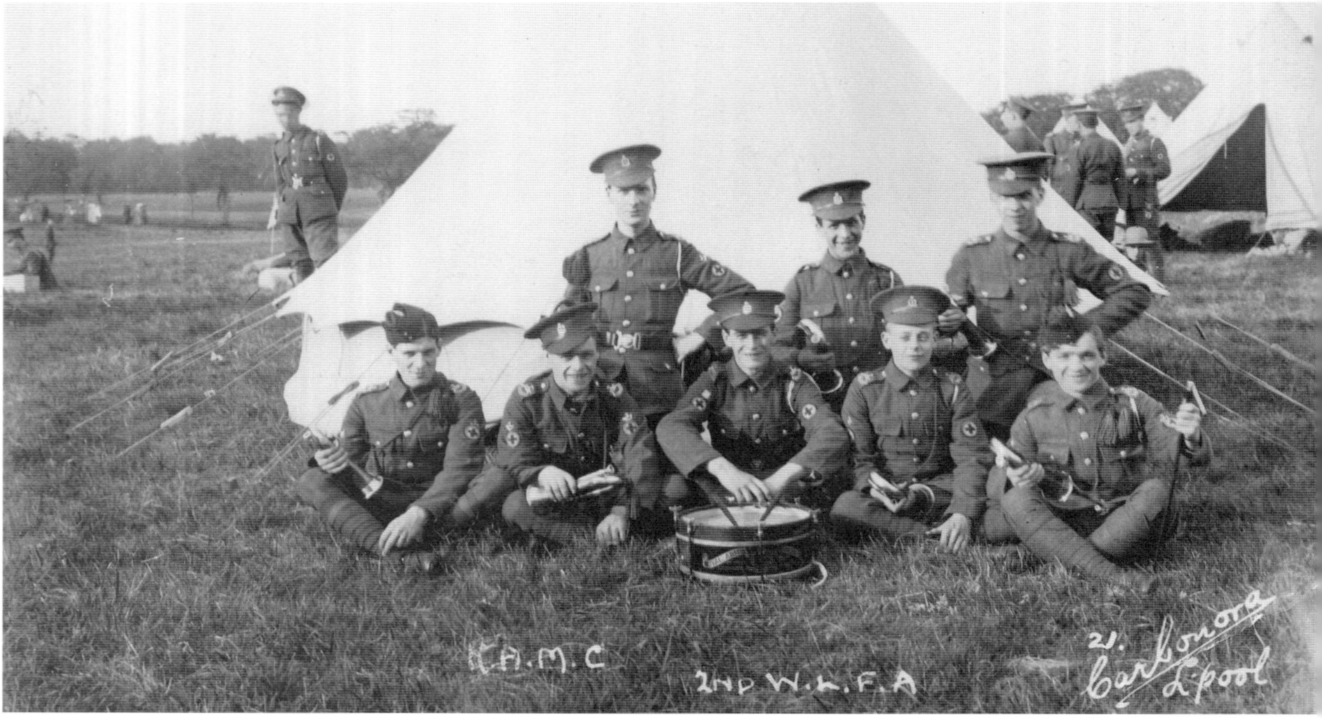

Buglers of the 2nd West Lancashire Field Ambulance, RAMC (TF). The unit was based at Liverpool and during the war was renamed the 98th (County Palatine) Field Ambulance. It served with the 30th Division, a New Army division, on the Western Front from November 1915. Around 35,000 personnel were killed, wounded and missing serving with the 30th Division.

The band of the 3rd South Midland Field Ambulance, RAMC (TF). The unit was based at Bristol. The Field Ambulance served with the 48th (South Midland) Division, on the Western Front from the spring of 1915. In late 1917 the division moved to the Italian Front.

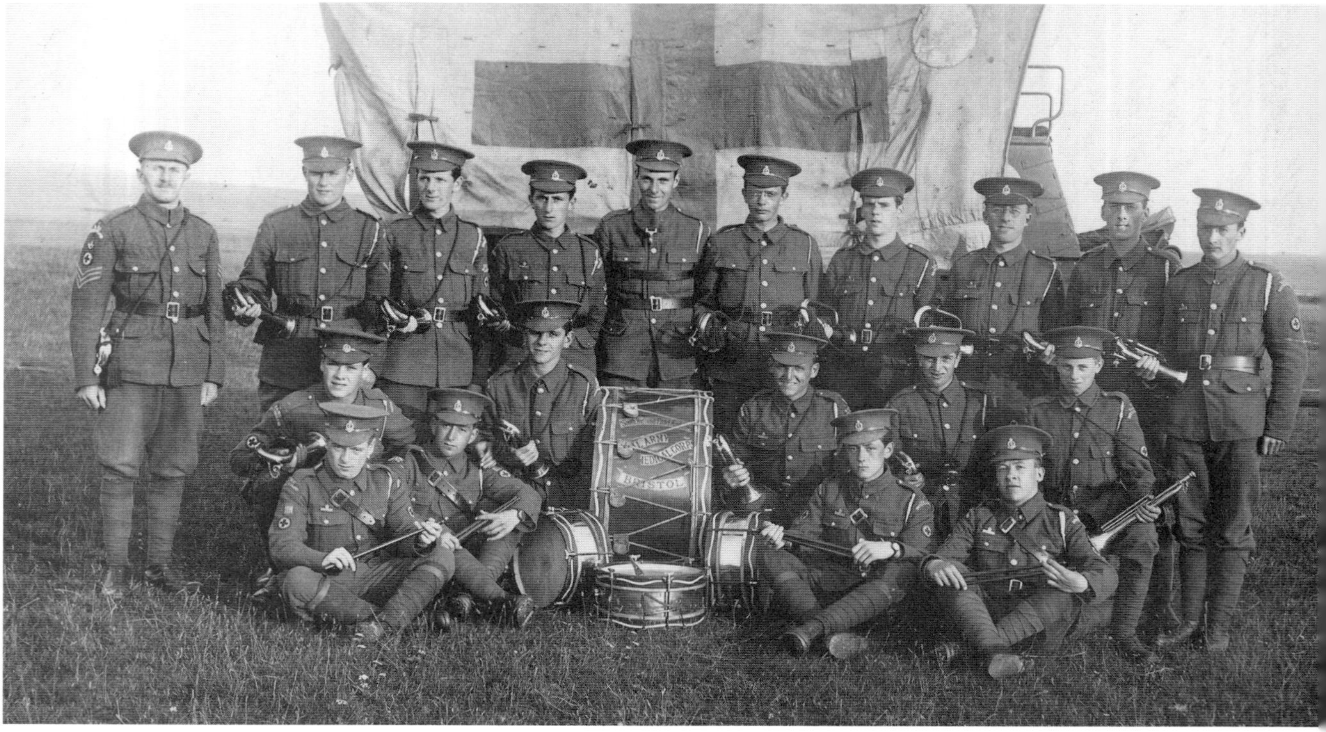

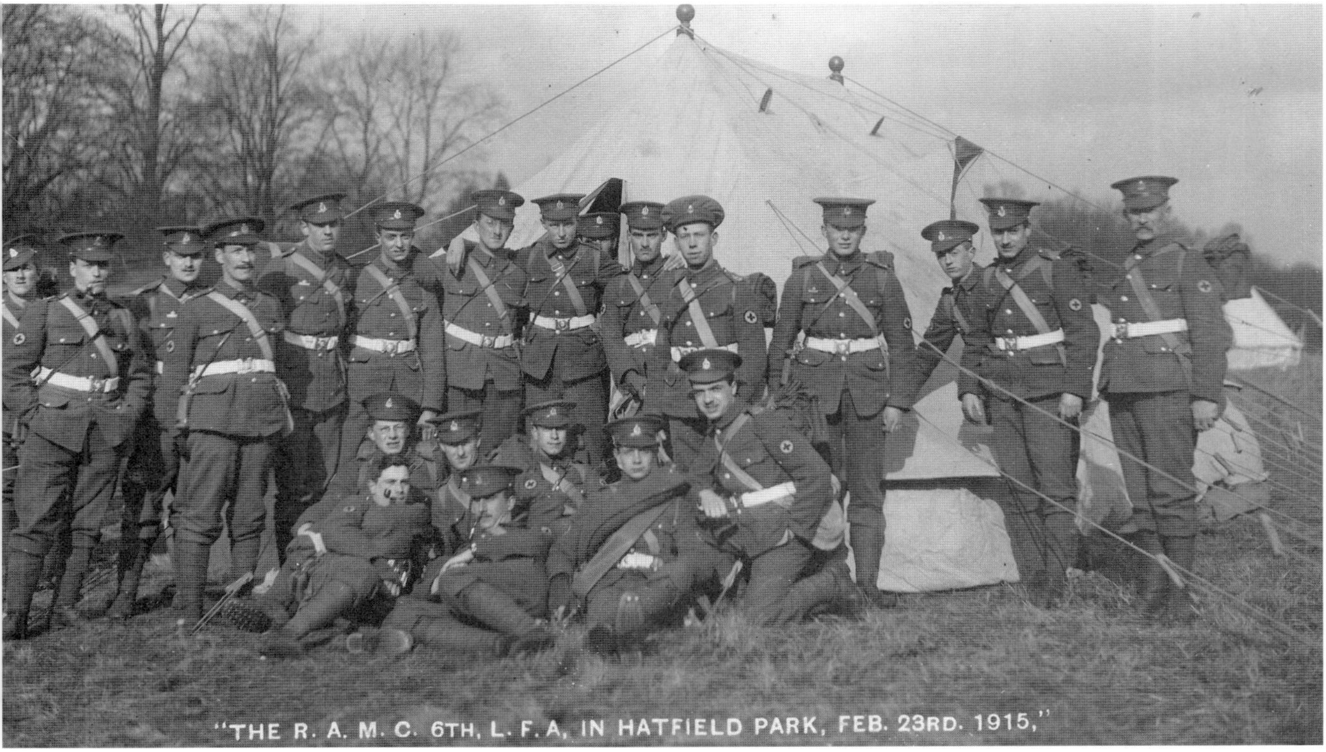

"THE R.A.M.C. 6TH, L.F.A, IN HATFIELD PARK, FEB. 23RD. 1915."

The 6th London Field Ambulance, RAMC (TF) at Hatfield Park, 23 February 1915. This unit served on the Western Front from March 1915 with the 47th (2nd London) Division.

The 130th Field Ambulance RAMC was formed from members of the St John Ambulance Association. The unit served with the 38th (Welsh) Division on the Western Front from December 1915. St John Ambulance Association insignia was worn by personnel on their uniforms.

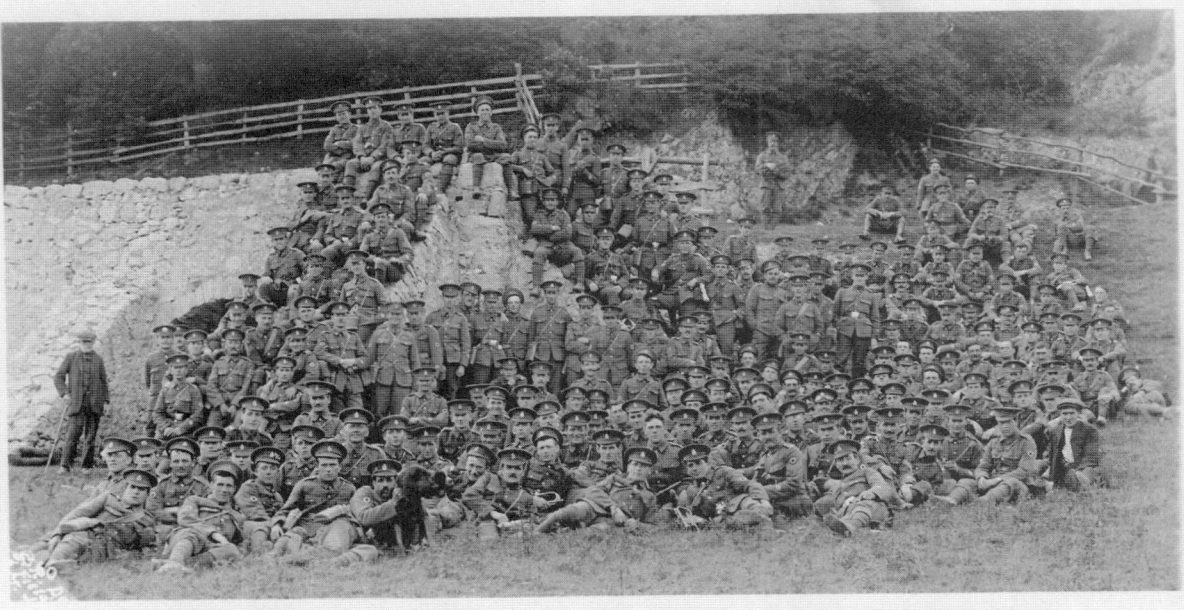

130TH. ST. JOHN. FIELD AMBULANCE R.A.M.C.

TREMEIRCHION ROUTE MARCH JULY 15TH 1915.

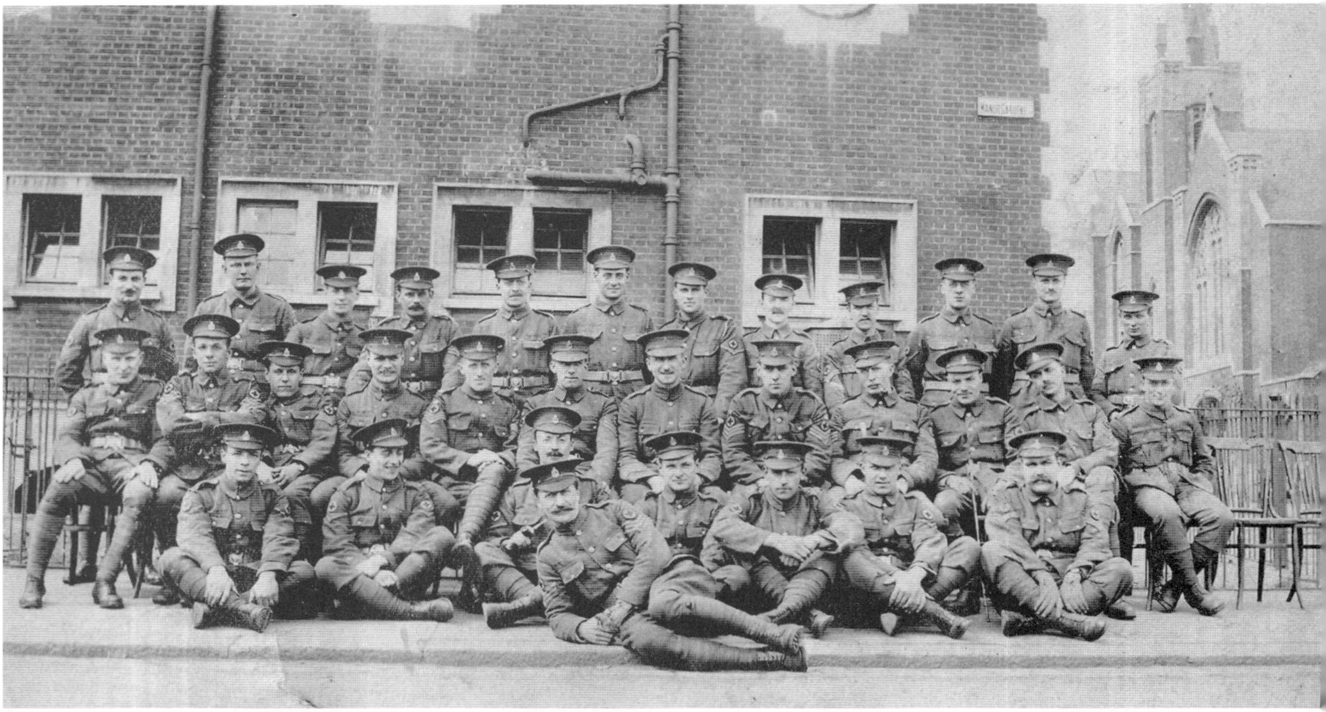

Members of the 41st Sanitary Section, RAMC. The unit served with the 24th Division on the Western Front from the summer of 1915.

Office of the 41st Sanitary Section, RAMC on the Western Front.

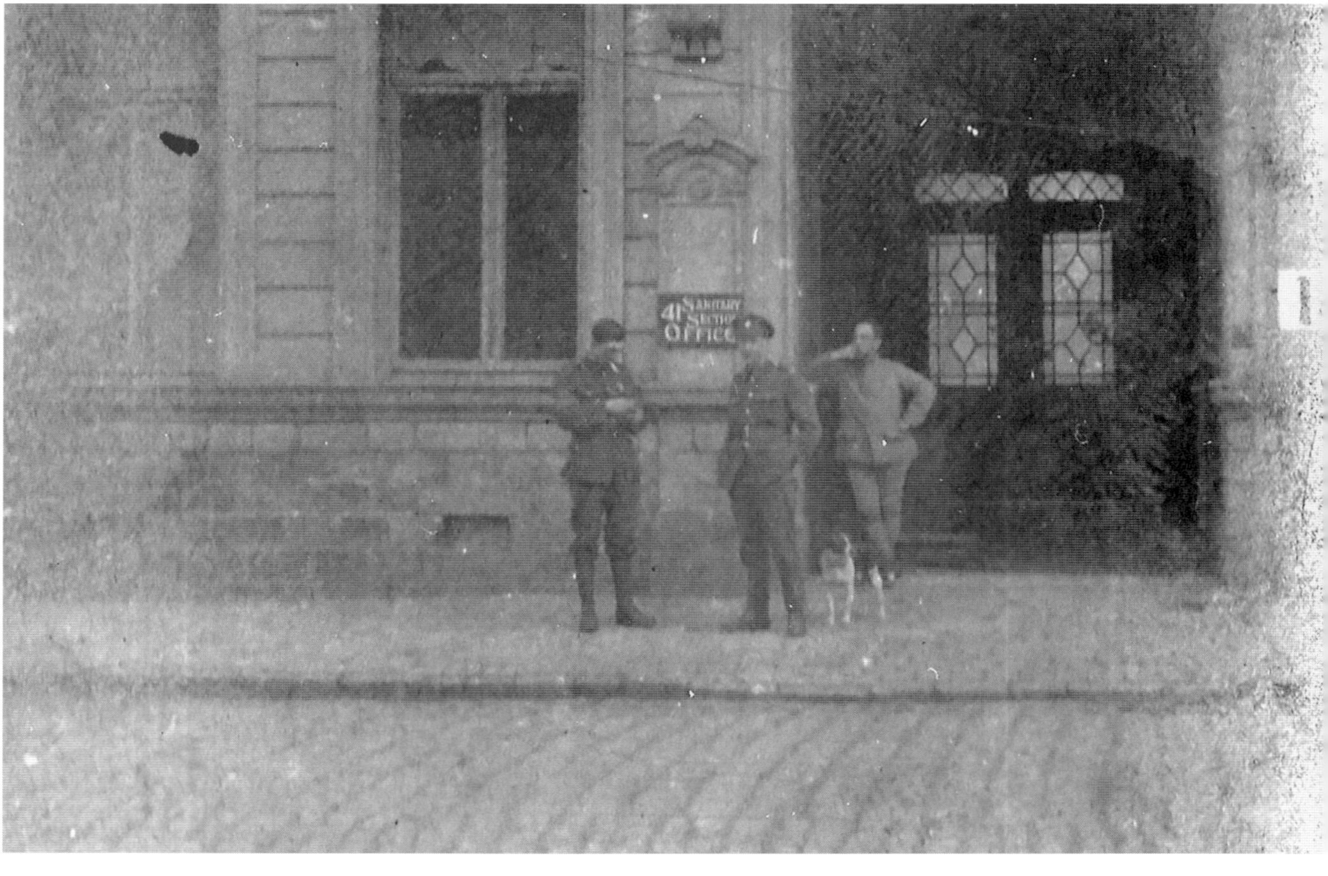

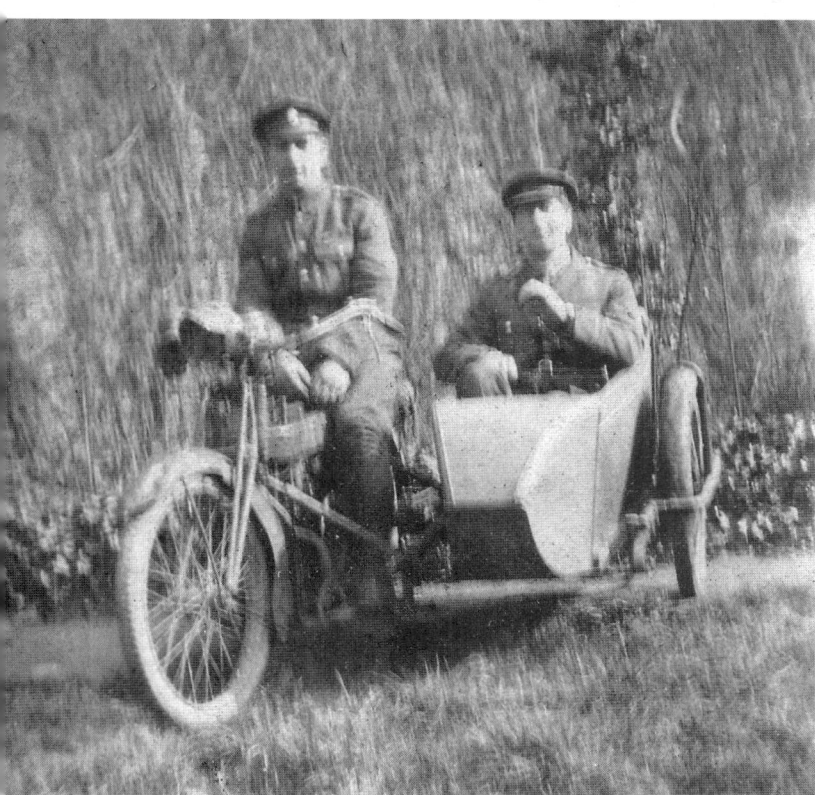

Personnel of the 41st Sanitary Section, RAMC using a motorbike for transportation on the Western Front.

Members of the 41st Sanitary Section, RAMC at Souchez, France.

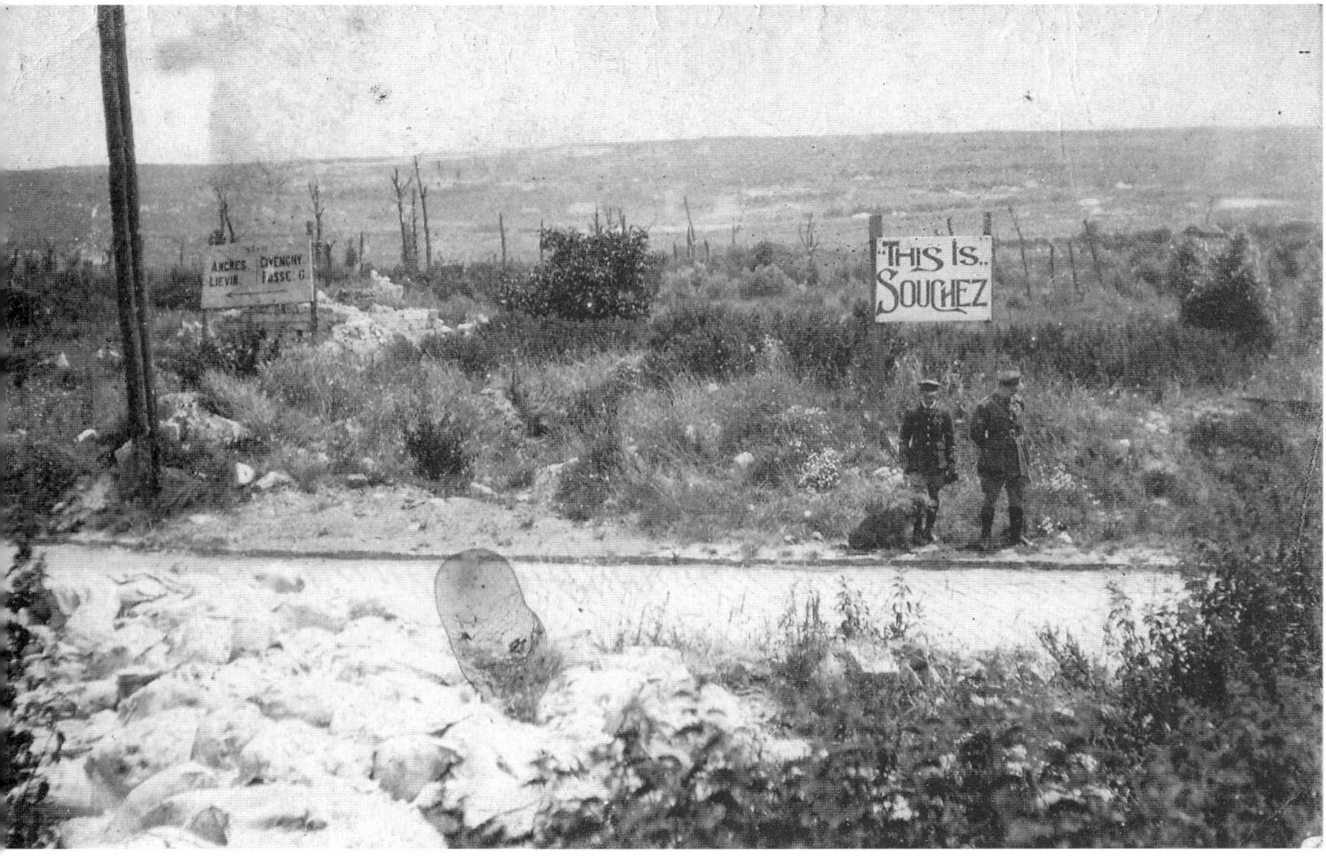

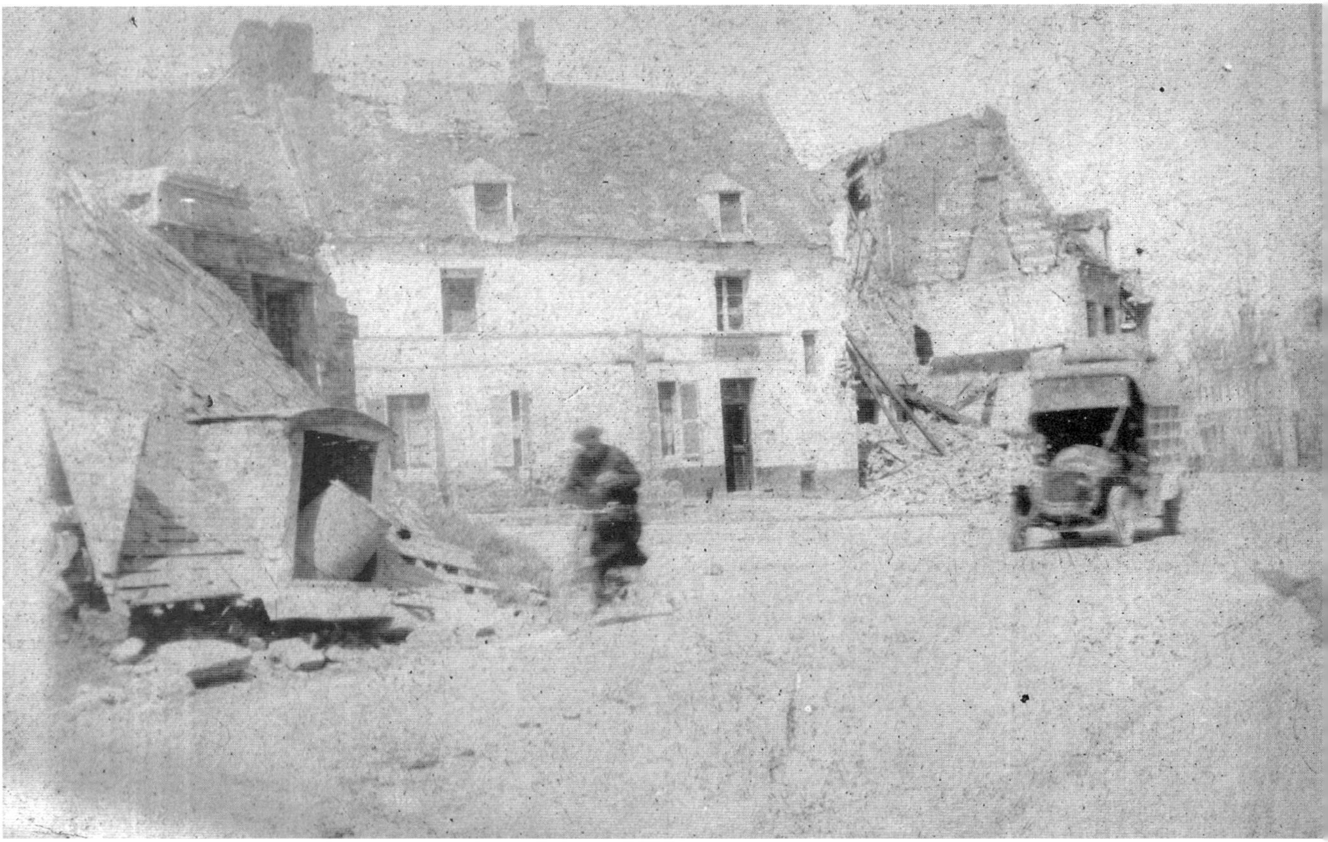

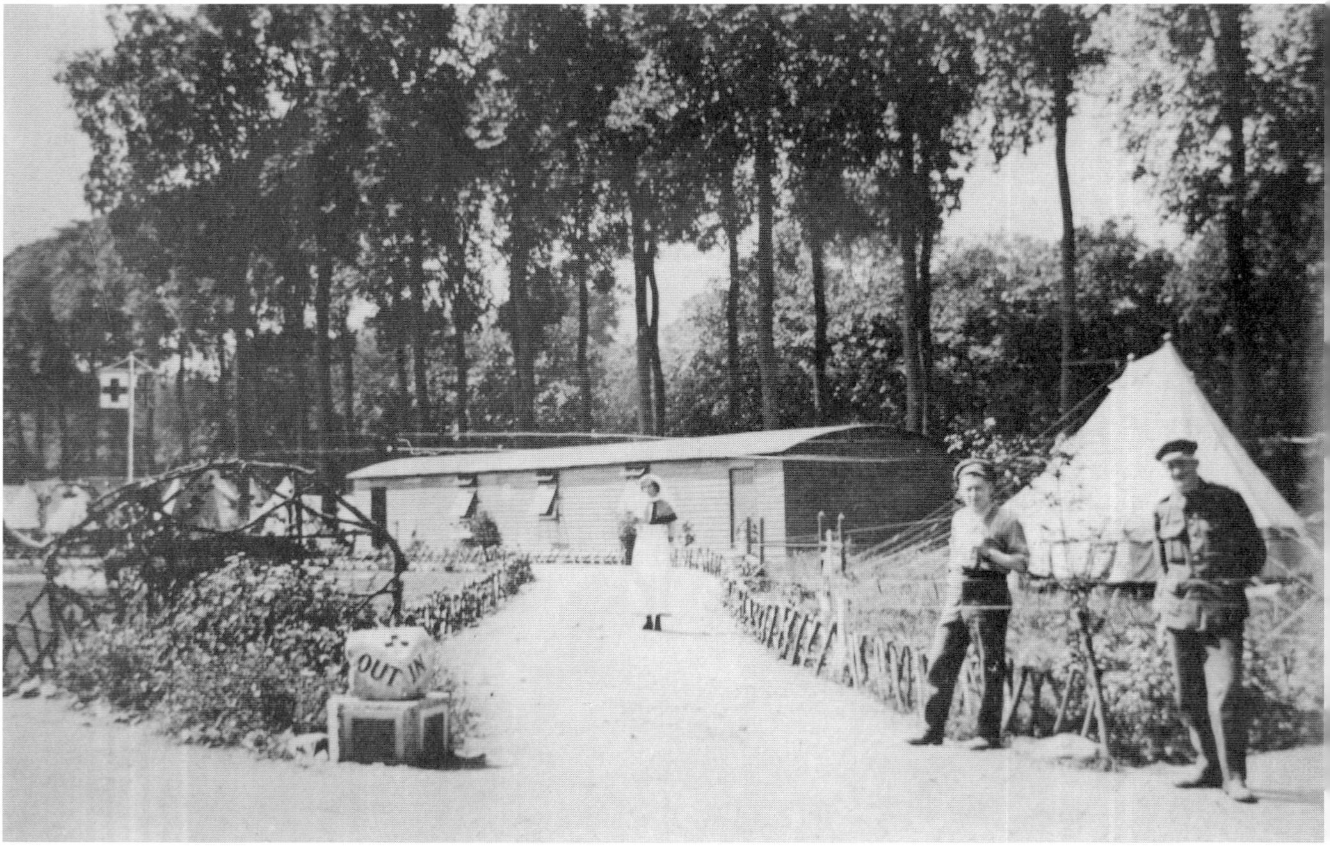

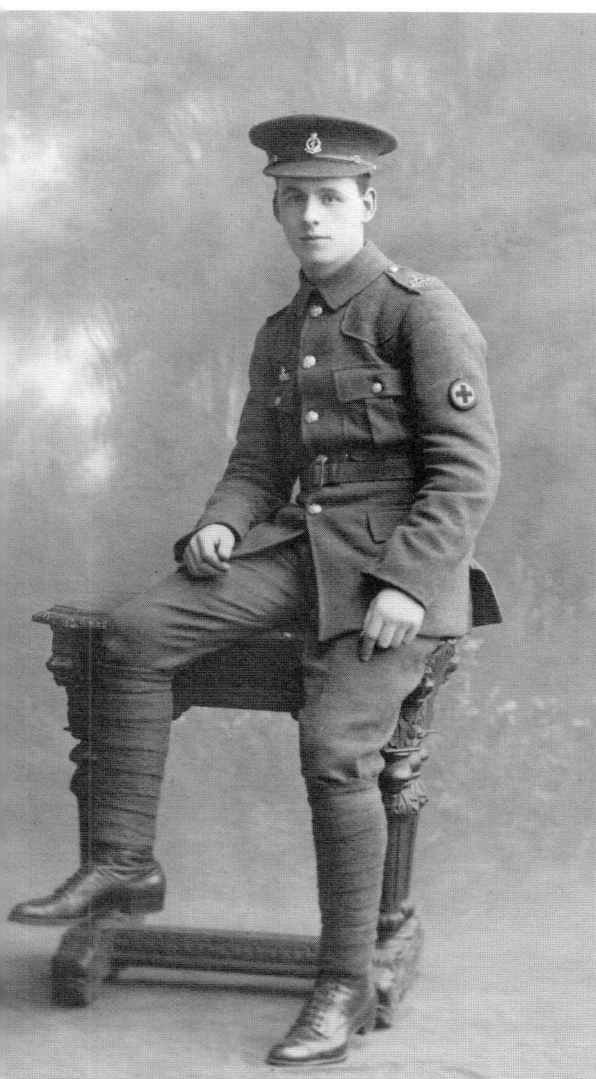 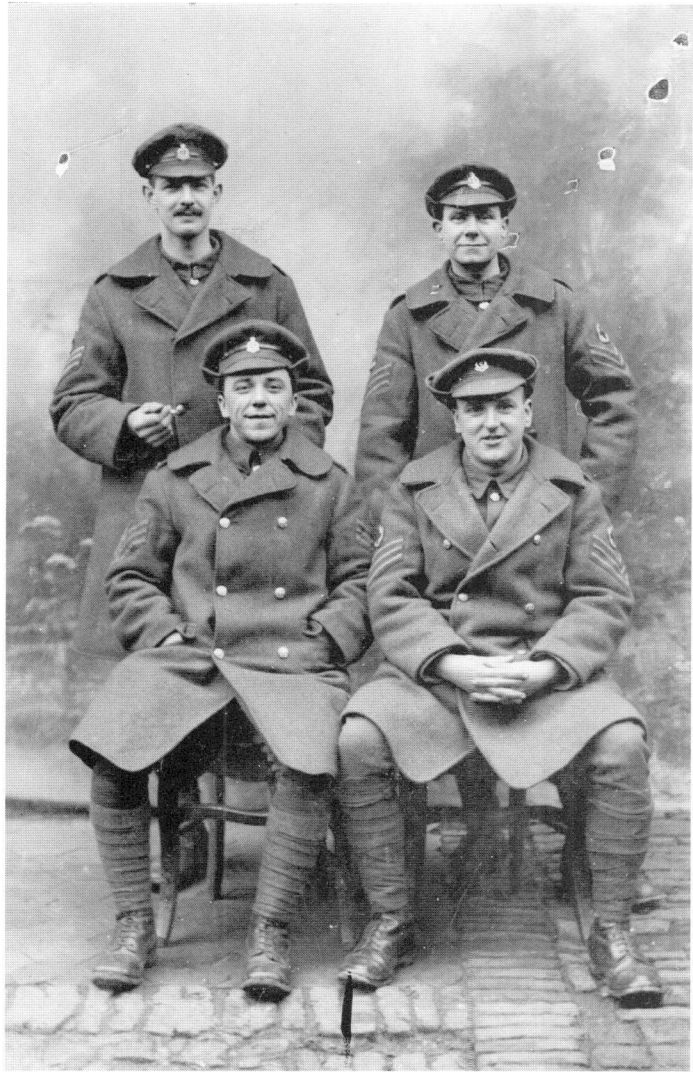

(**Above, left**) A RAMC private serving with a medical unit of the 50th (Northumbrian) Division. The 50th Division served on the Western Front from April 1915; they were one of the first divisions to experience gas warfare at St Julien.

(**Above, right**) A group of RAMC sergeants on the Western Front.

(**Opposite, above**) A war-damaged village on the Western Front, photographed by a member of the 41st Sanitary Section, RAMC.

(**Opposite, below**) The entrance to a medical facility on the Western Front.

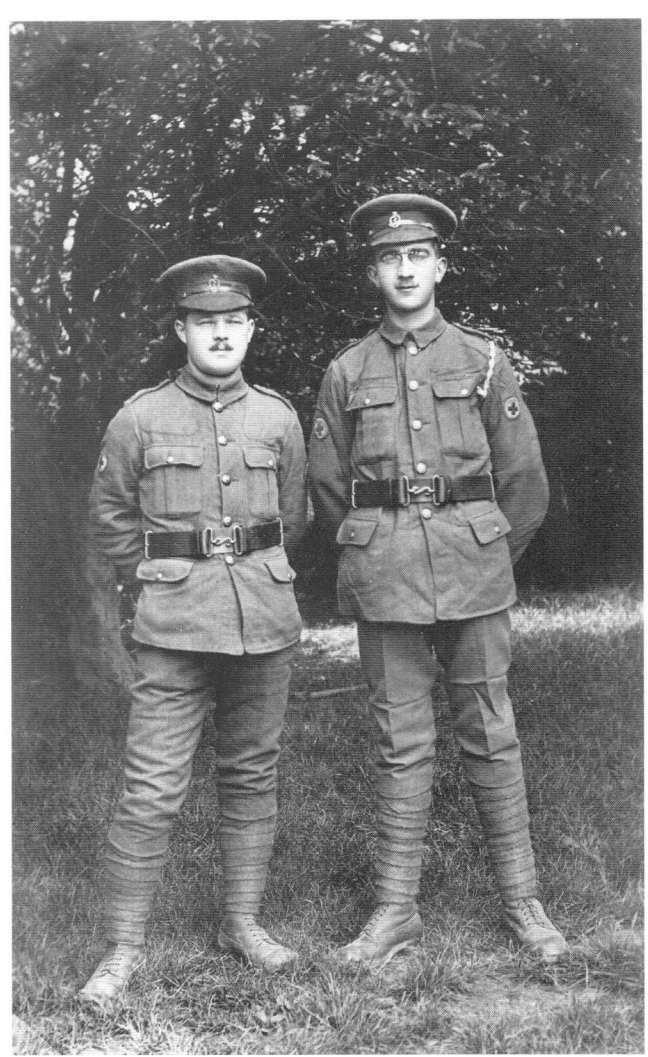 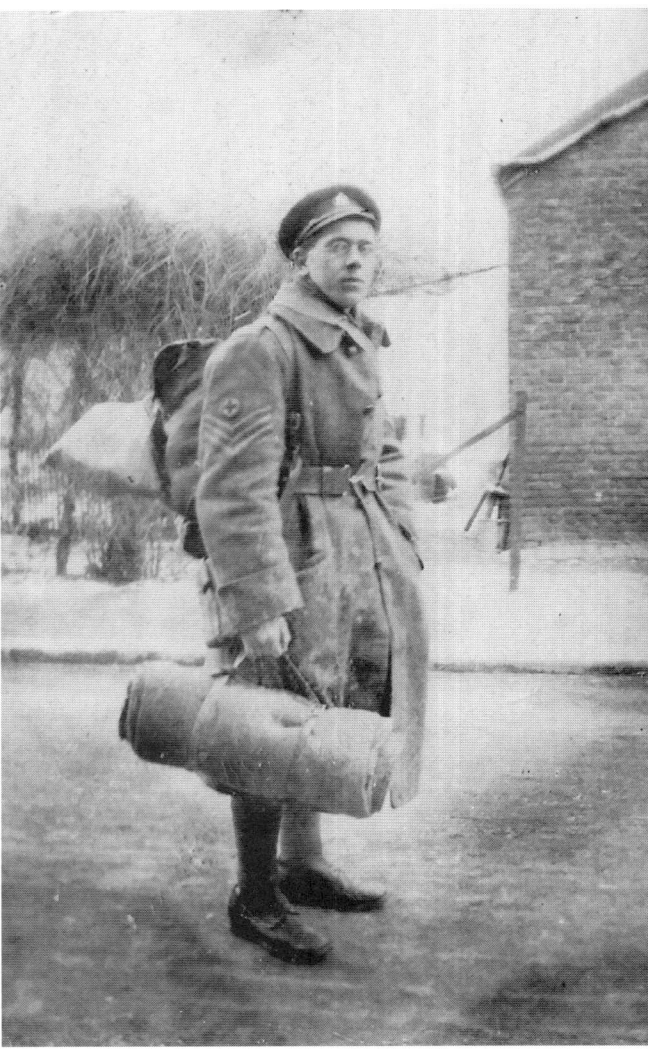

(**Above, left**) Two privates serving with the RAMC in France. The photo is inscribed on the reverse: 'My Pal Snuffy & I taken by a French soldier – it's not up to much though! Abbeville, France 28/7/16'. Several hospitals were based in Abbeville during the First World War.

(**Above, right**) A RAMC sergeant on the Western Front wearing a greatcoat and carrying personal equipment.

(**Opposite, above**) The football team of the West Riding Casualty Clearing Station, RAMC. The unit served on the Western Front from the autumn of 1915.

(**Opposite, below**) The football team of the 2/1st Home Counties Field Ambulance RAMC. The unit served on the Western Front from early 1917 with the 58th (2/1st London) Division.

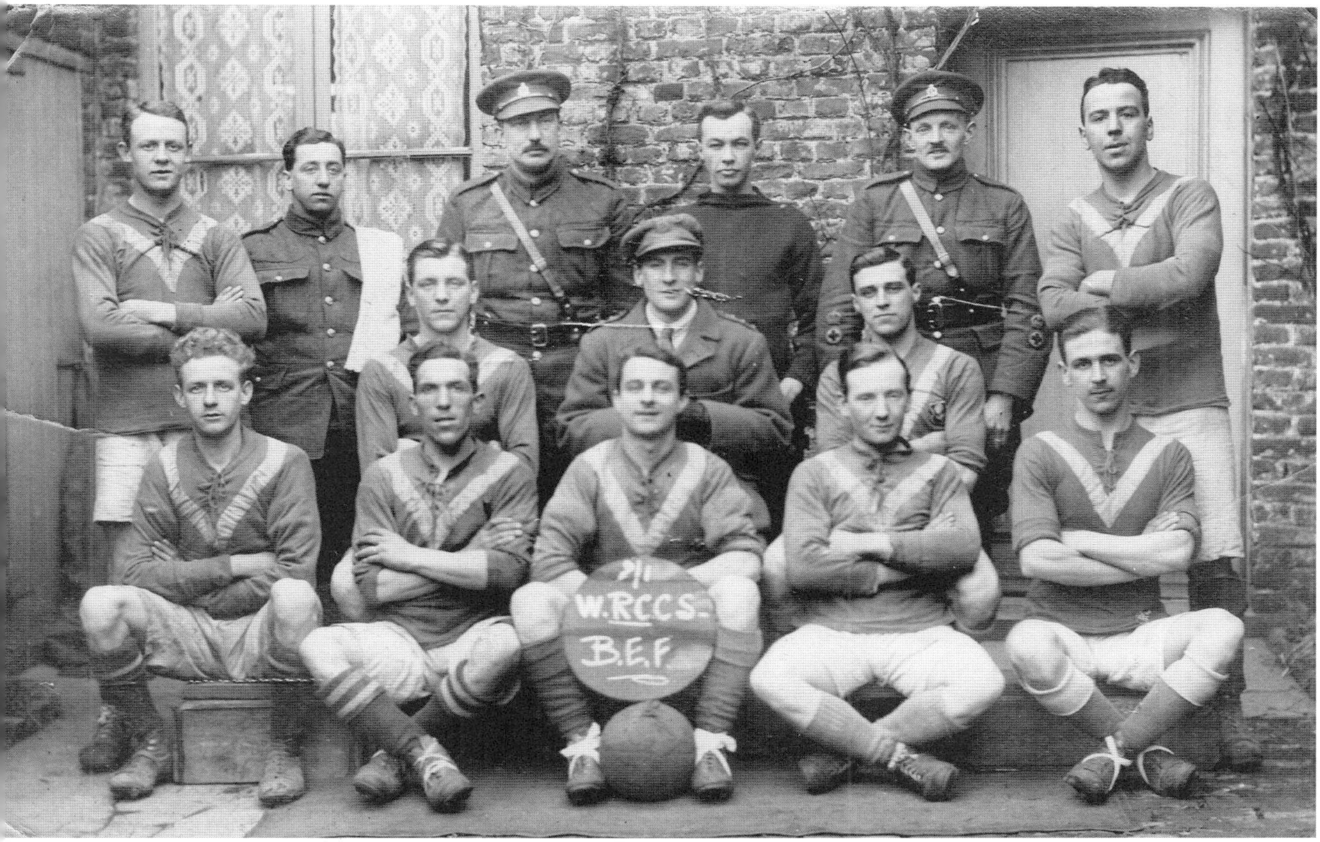

W.R.C.C.S. B.E.F

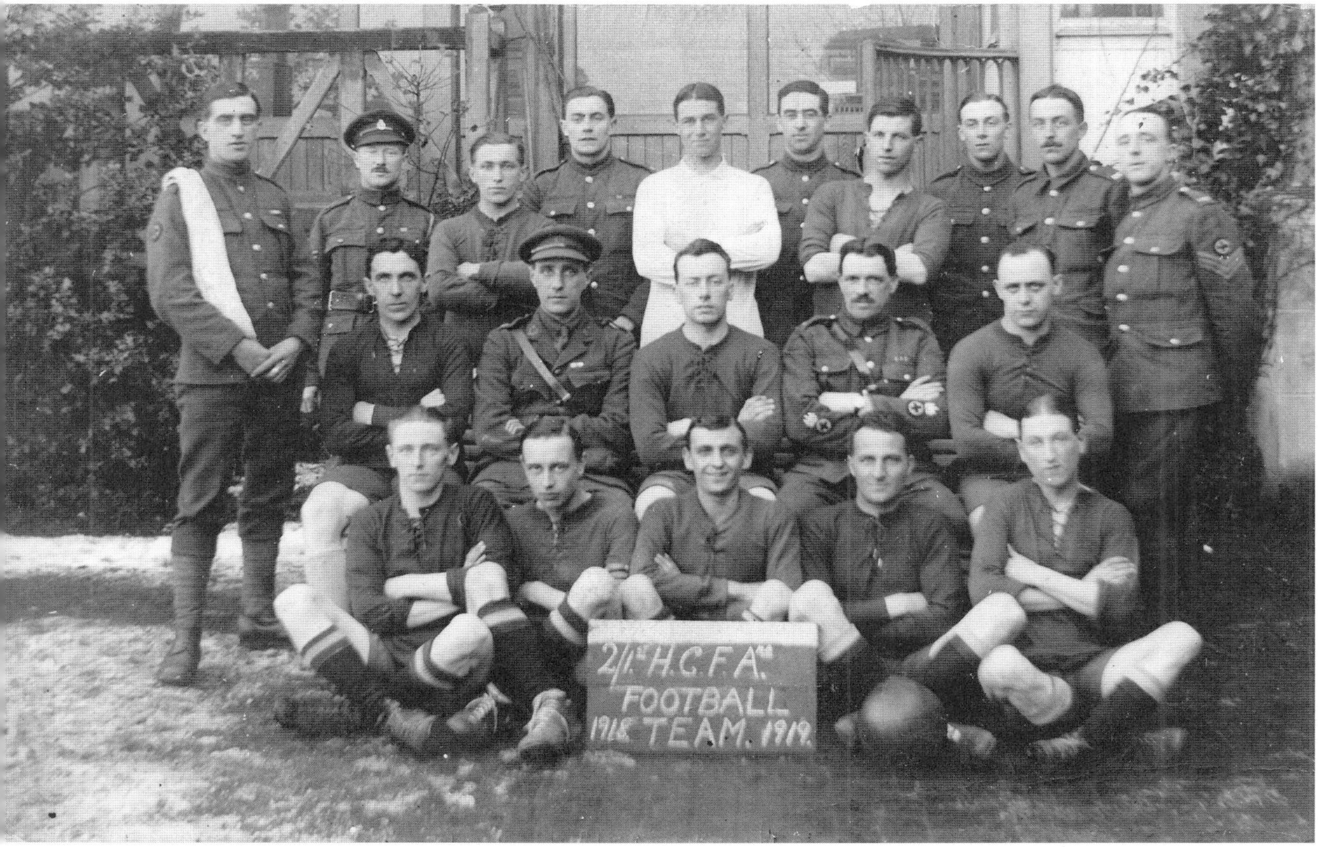

2/1st H.C.F.A. Football Team. 1918. 1919.

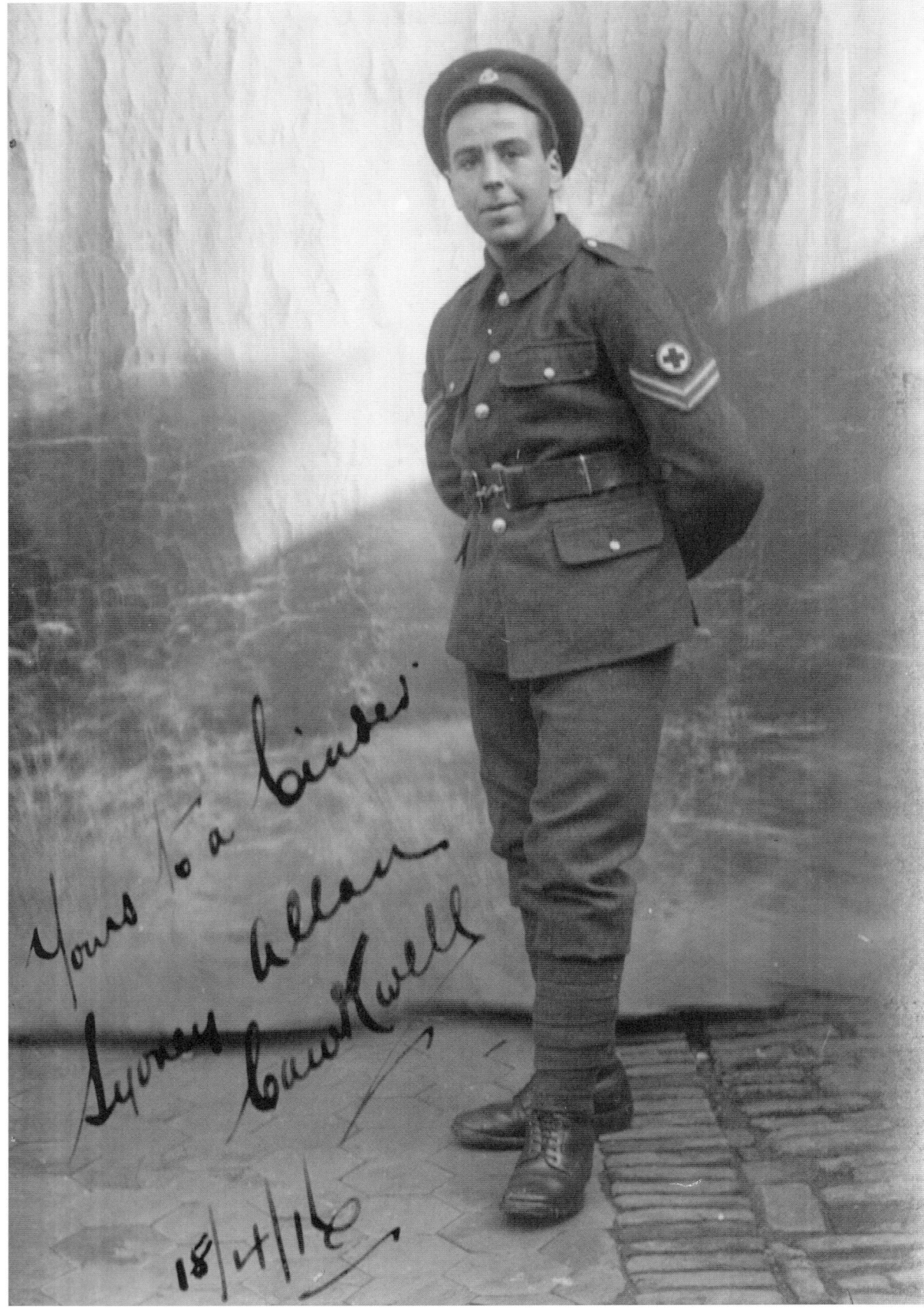

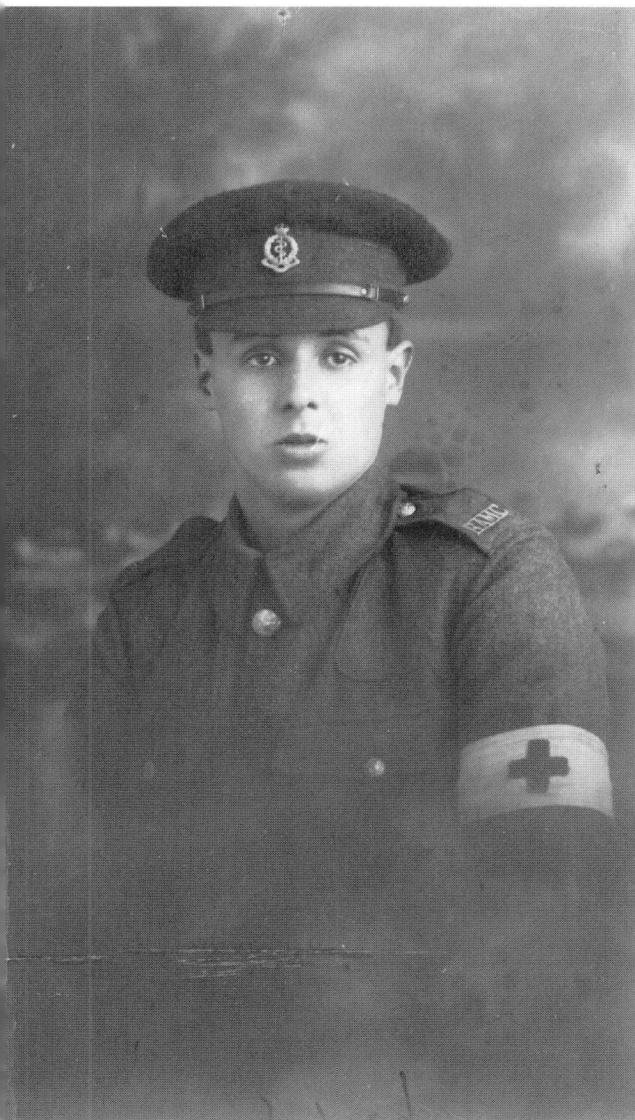 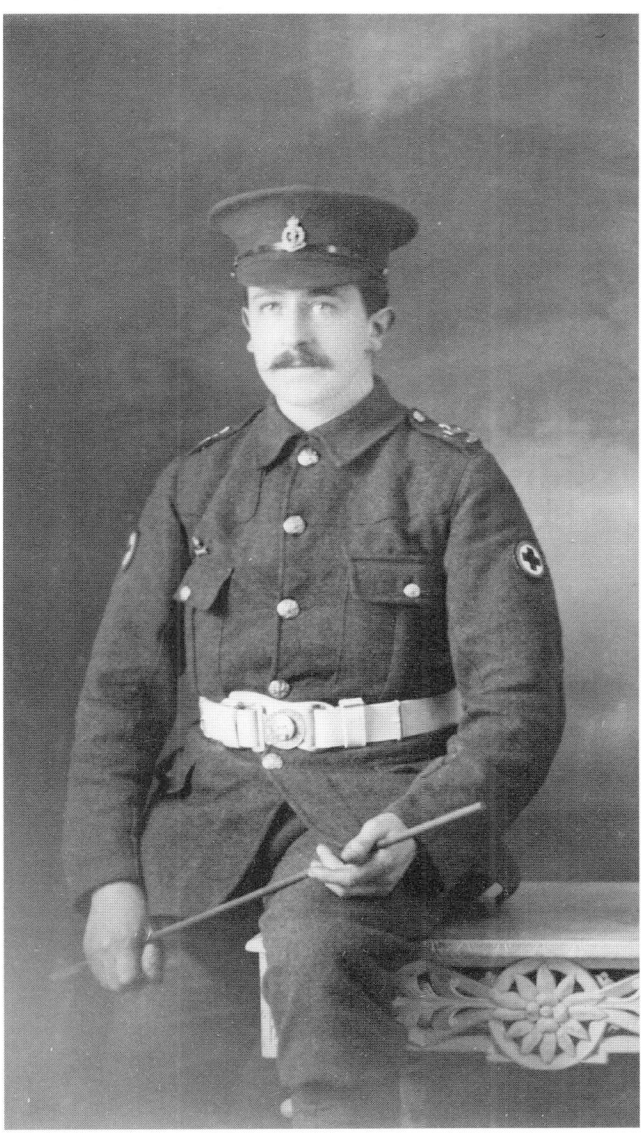

(**Opposite**) 109 Corporal (later Sergeant) Sydney Allan Cawkwell, RAMC. He served in France from 13 April 1915 and was discharged on 31 August 1919. In 1911, aged 18, he was working as a warehouseman and lived with his parents in Bradford. He died in 1979 aged 87.

(**Above, left**) 16434 Private George Robinson Taylor, 16th Field Ambulance, RAMC. The 16th Field Ambulance supported the 6th Division. Private Taylor served on the Western Front from 13 September 1914. During the Battle of the Somme he suffered a gunshot wound to his neck on 27 September 1916.

(**Above, right**) 3069 Private Frederick William Hopkins, 2/2nd Home Counties Field Ambulance, RAMC. This unit served on the Western Front from early 1917 with the 58th (2/1st London) Division.

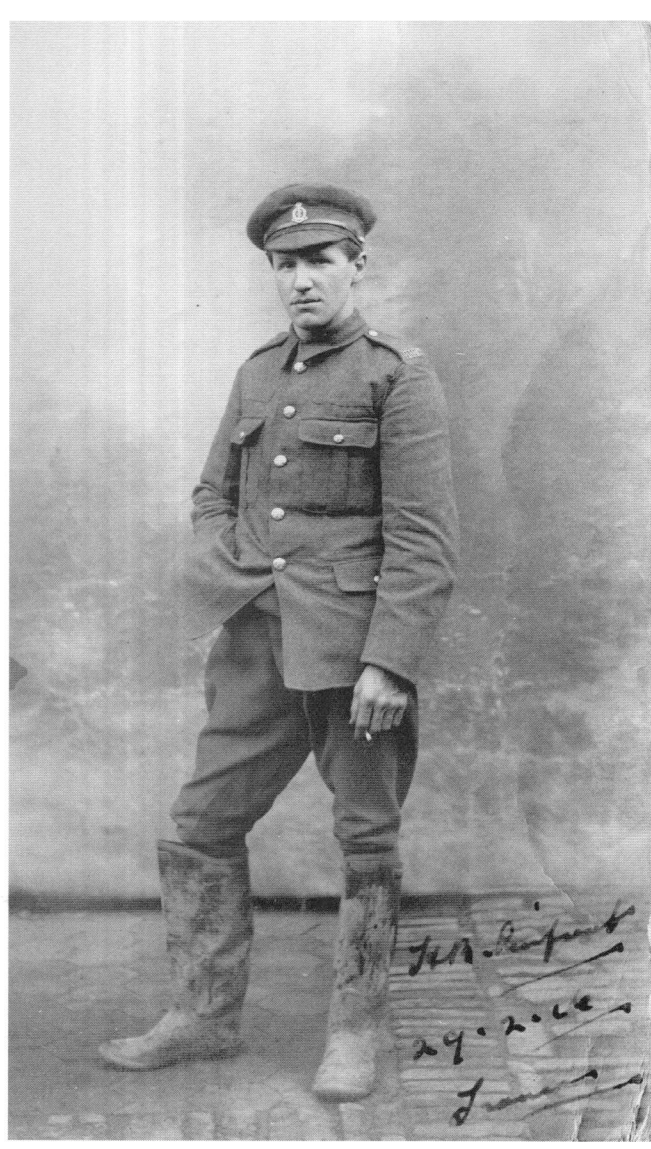 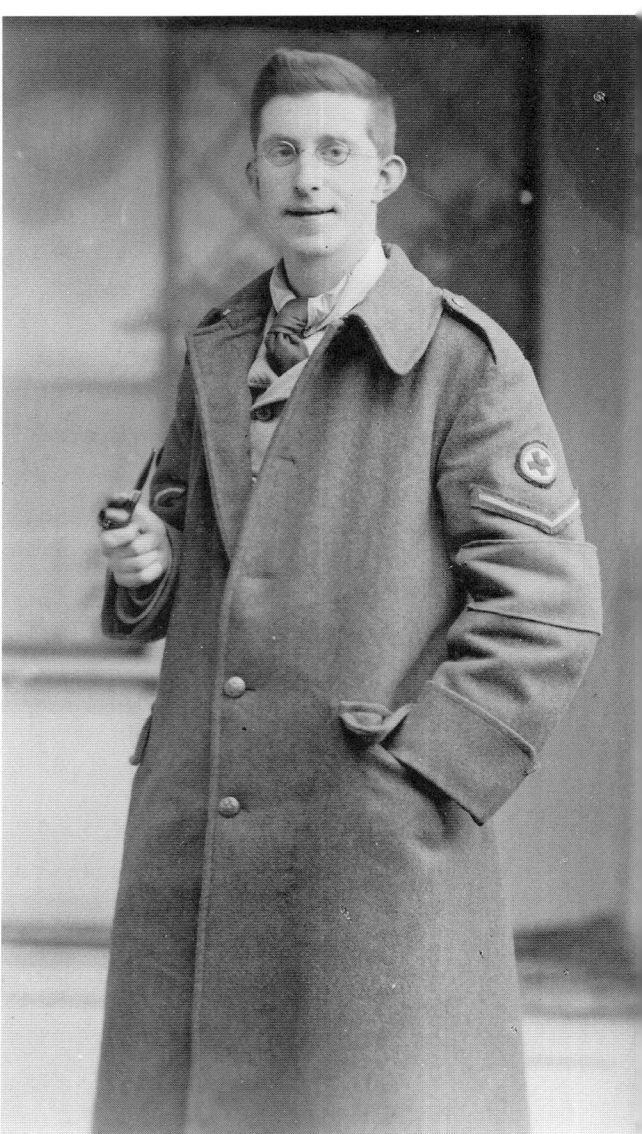

(**Above, left**) An RAMC private wearing waterproof boots, photographed in France on 29 February 1916.

(**Above, right**) A wounded lance corporal serving with the RAMC. He is wearing 'hospital blues' uniform under his greatcoat, showing he was a patient at a military hospital. The photograph was taken in Southwold, Suffolk.

(**Opposite**) A group of senior non-commissioned officers on the Western Front, an RAMC sergeant (left) and warrant officer (right).

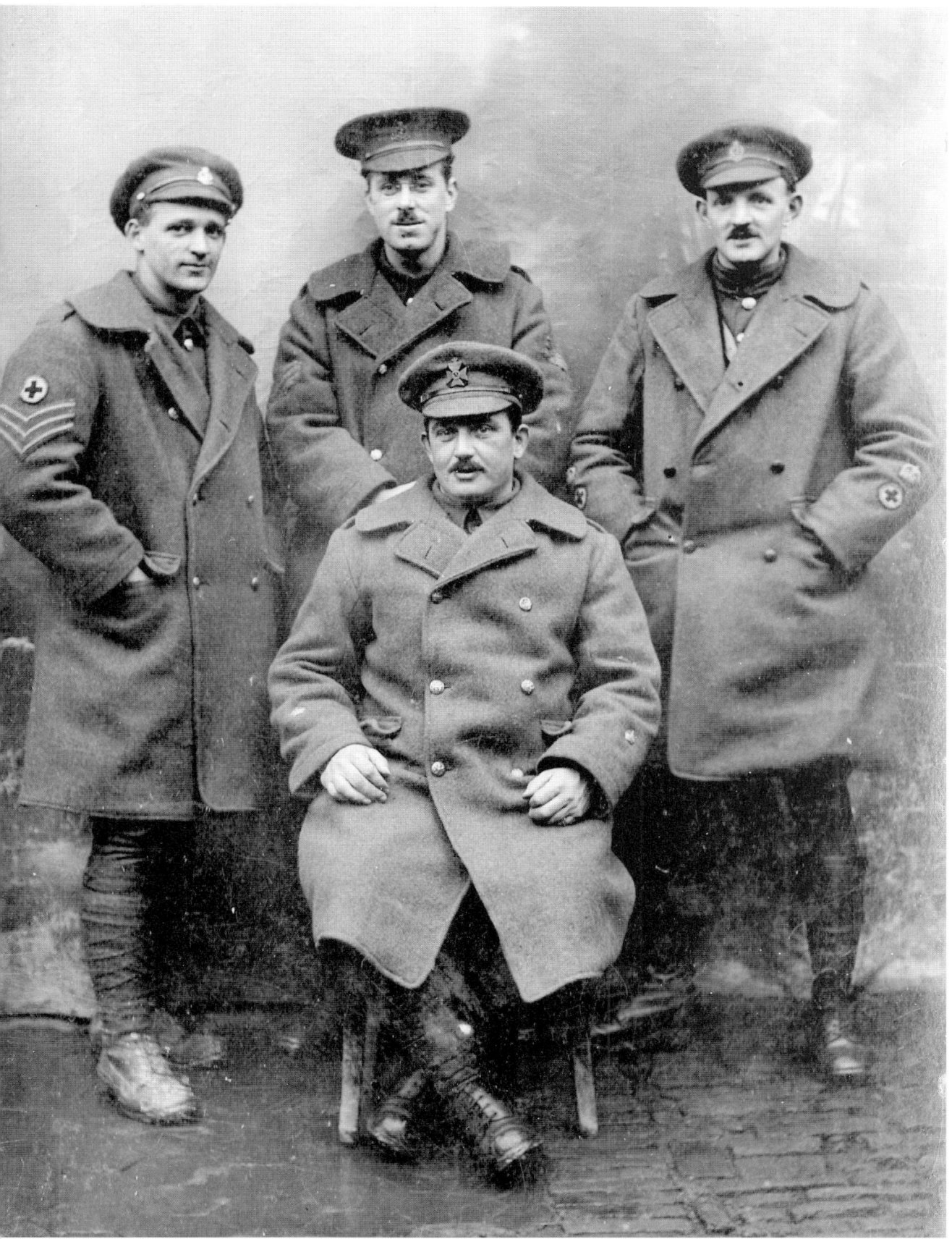

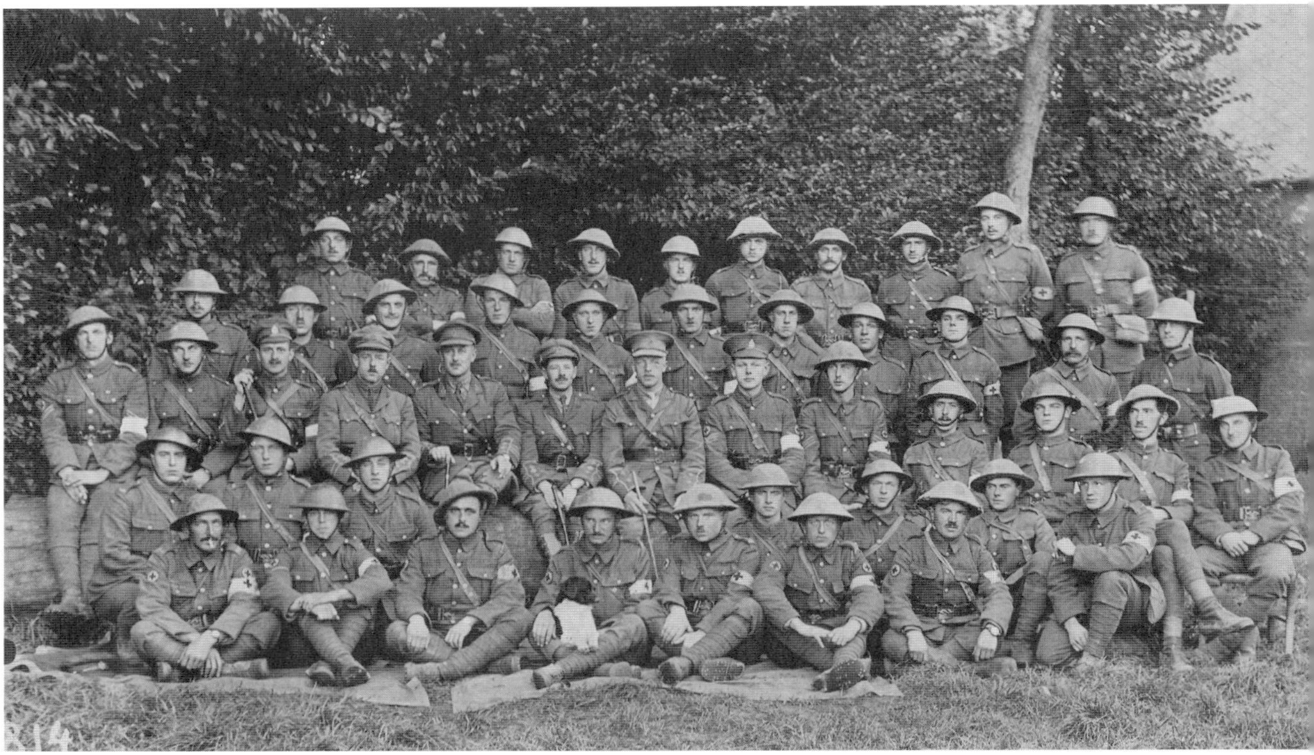

'A' Section, 51st Field Ambulance, RAMC, France, September 1916. The unit served with the 17th (Northern) Division on the Western Front from the summer of 1915.

The band of the 101st Field Ambulance, RAMC which saw service on the Western Front with the 33rd Division from late 1915. Several of the soldiers wear the ribbon of the Military Medal (MM) and 33rd Division patches. The photograph was posted from France on 19 October 1918.

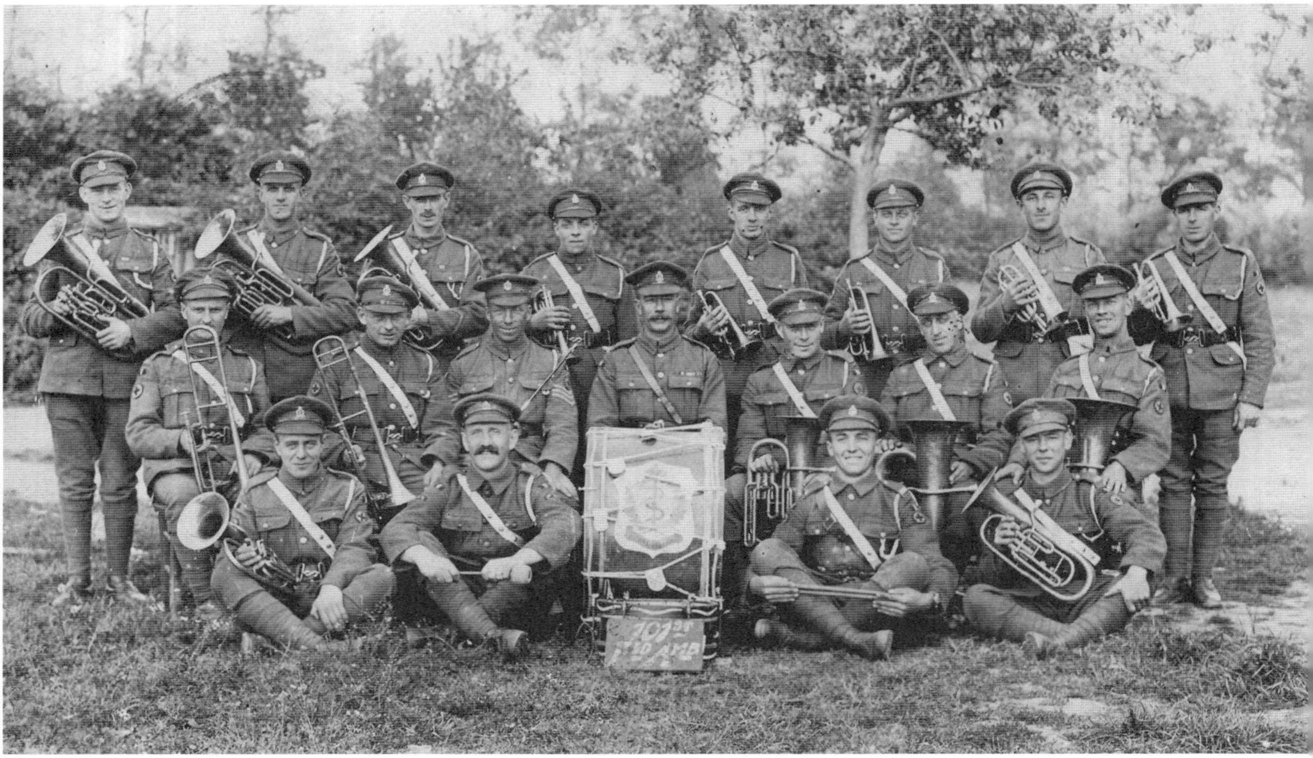

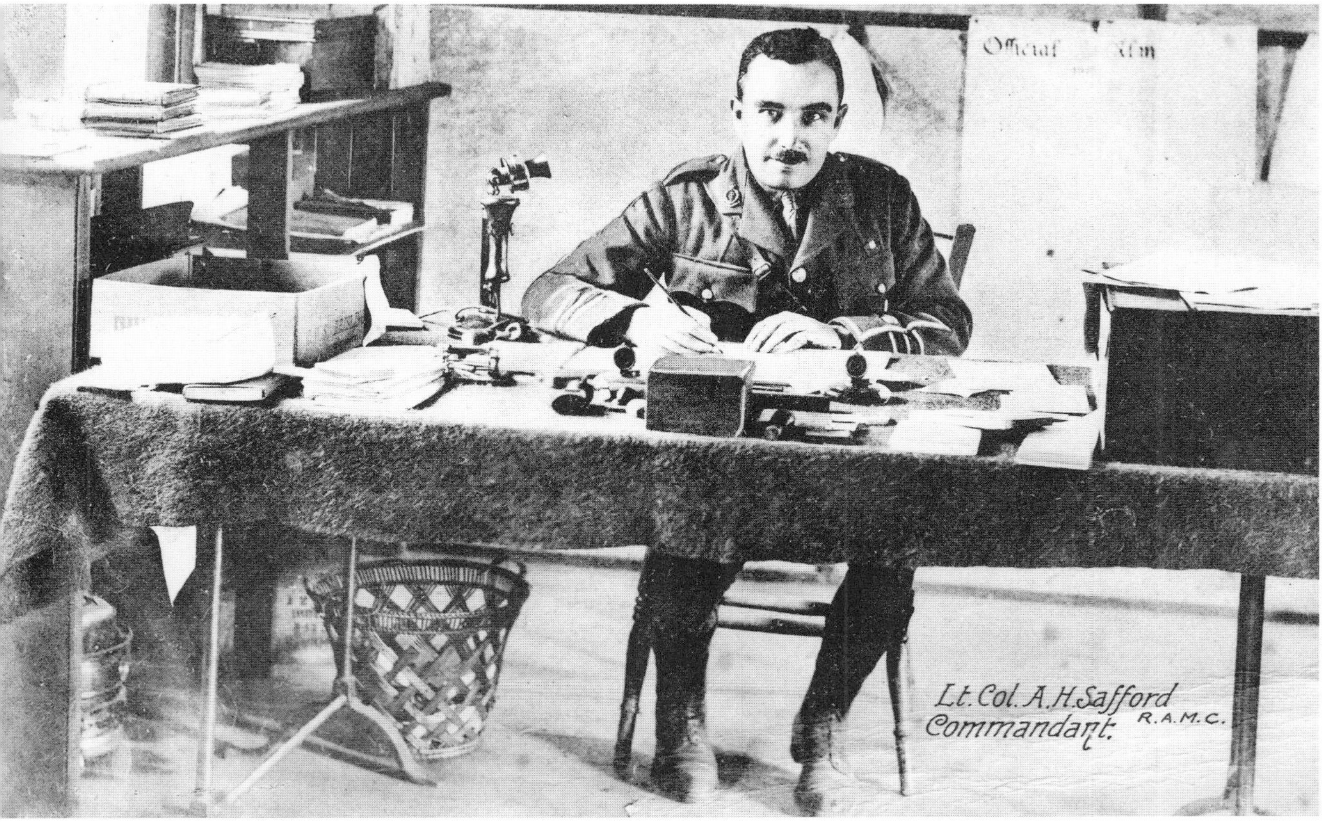

Lieutenant Colonel Arthur Hunt Safford, RAMC, served on the Western Front from 12 March 1917 with the 23rd Casualty Clearing Station and the 2nd Cavalry Division. He later worked in Afghanistan during 1919.

The band of a RAMC unit photographed on the Western Front.

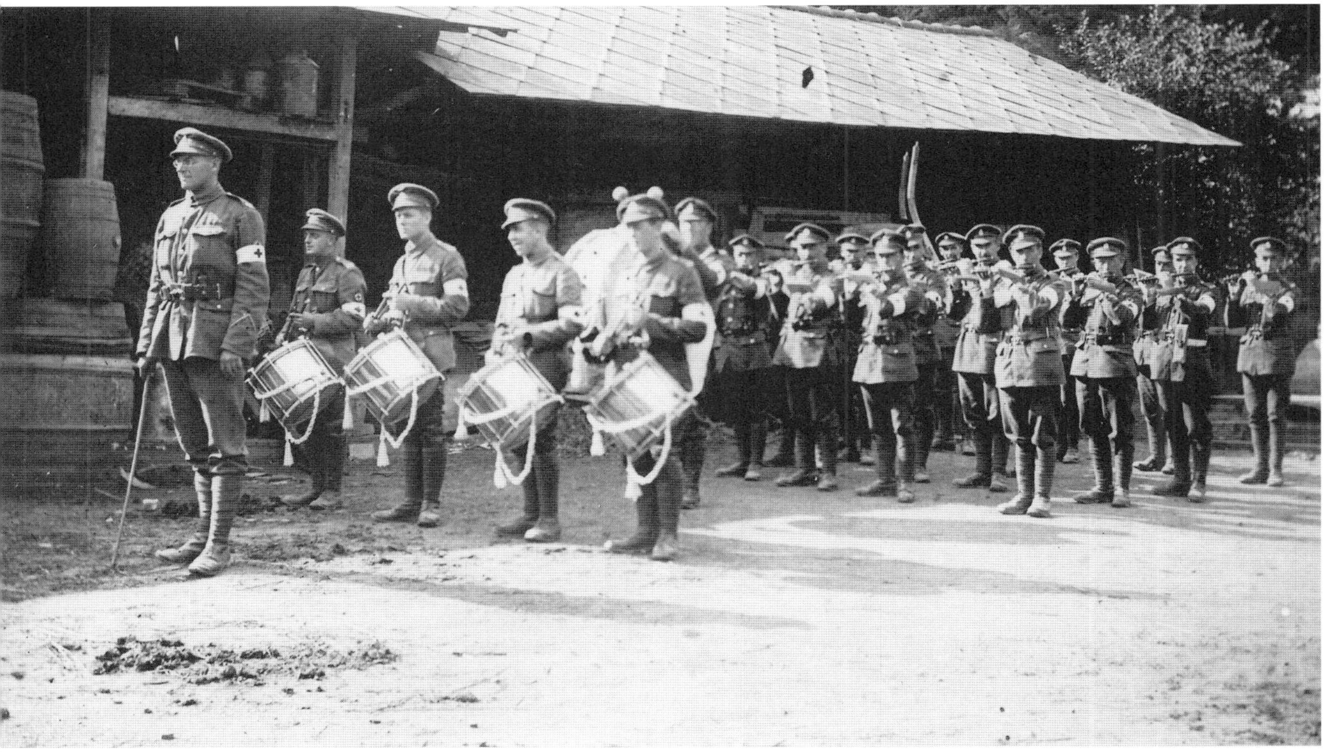

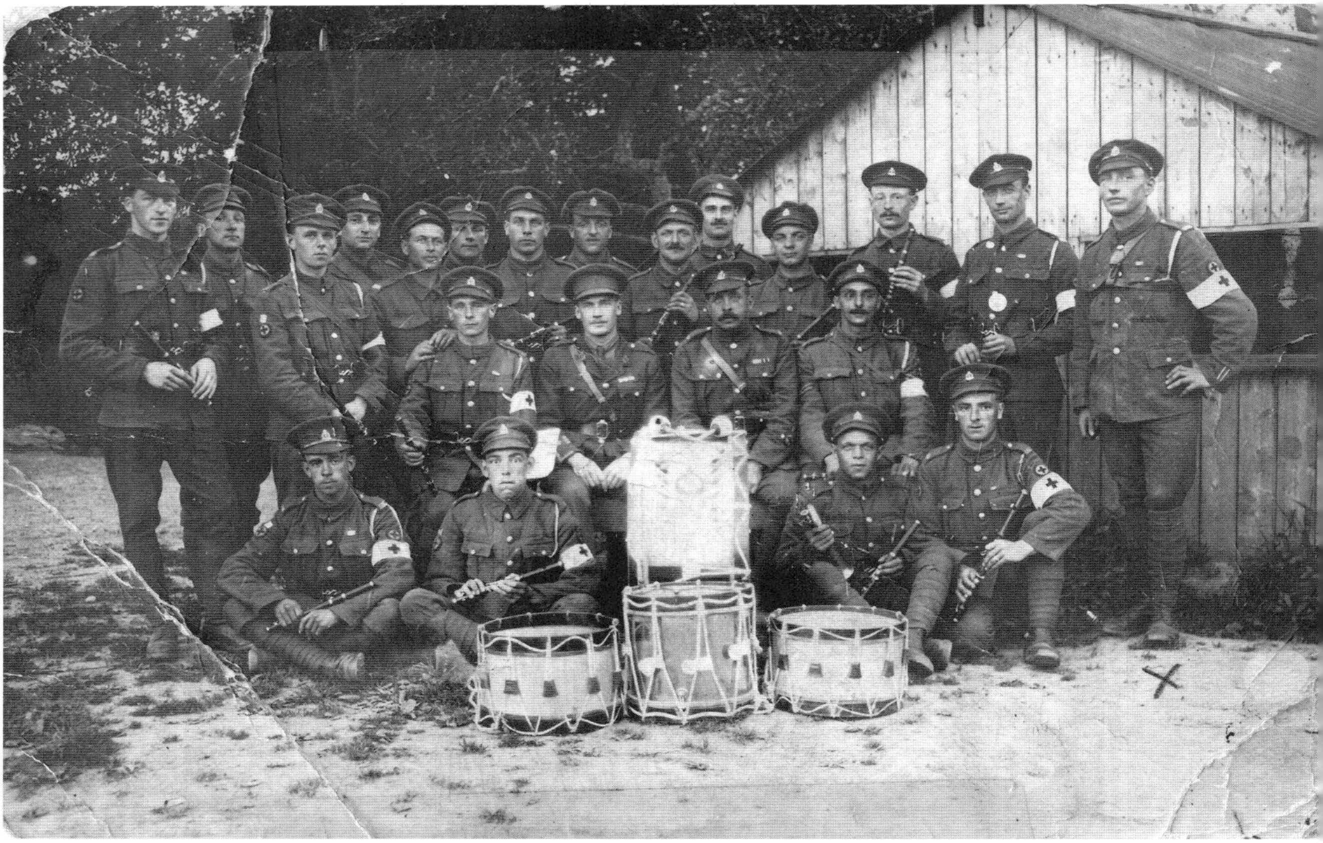

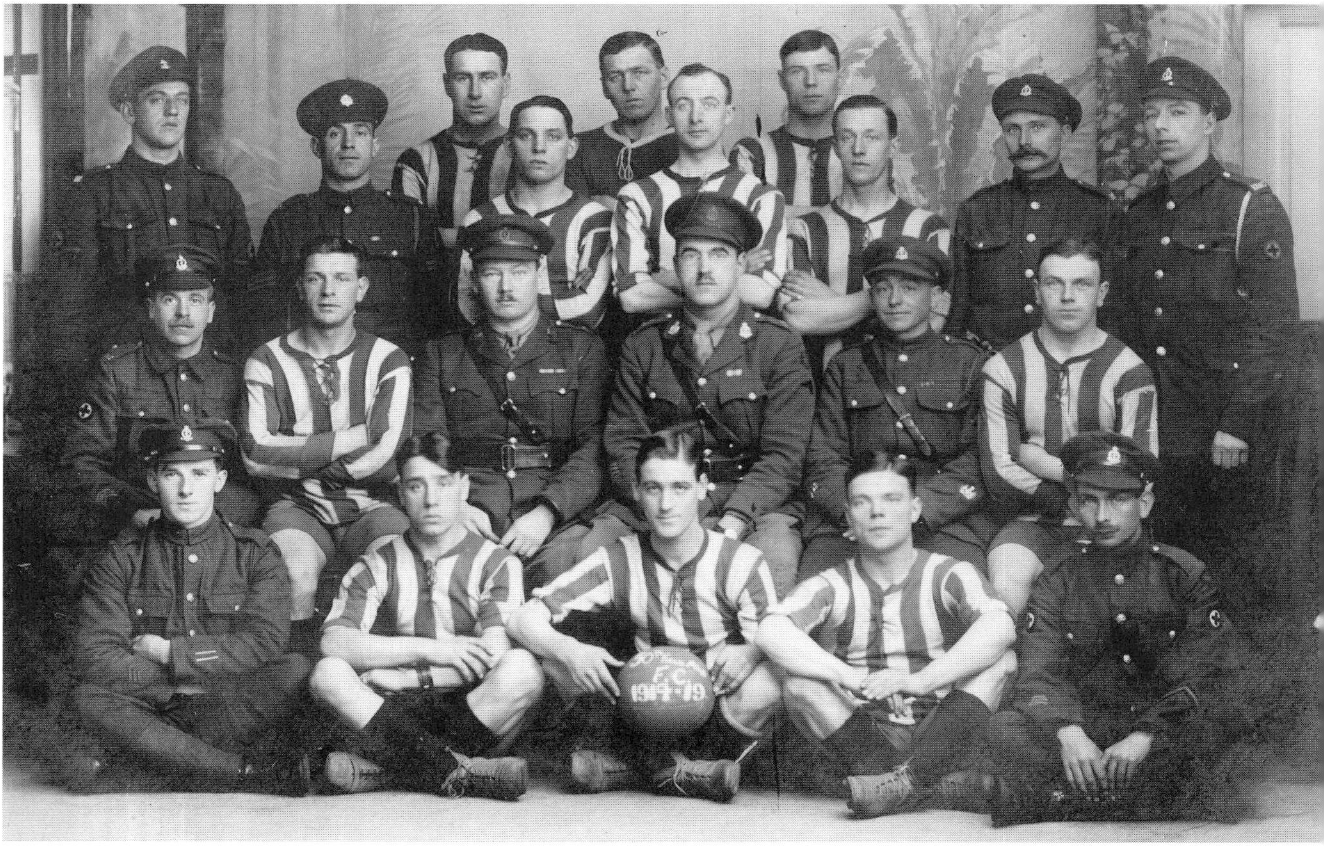

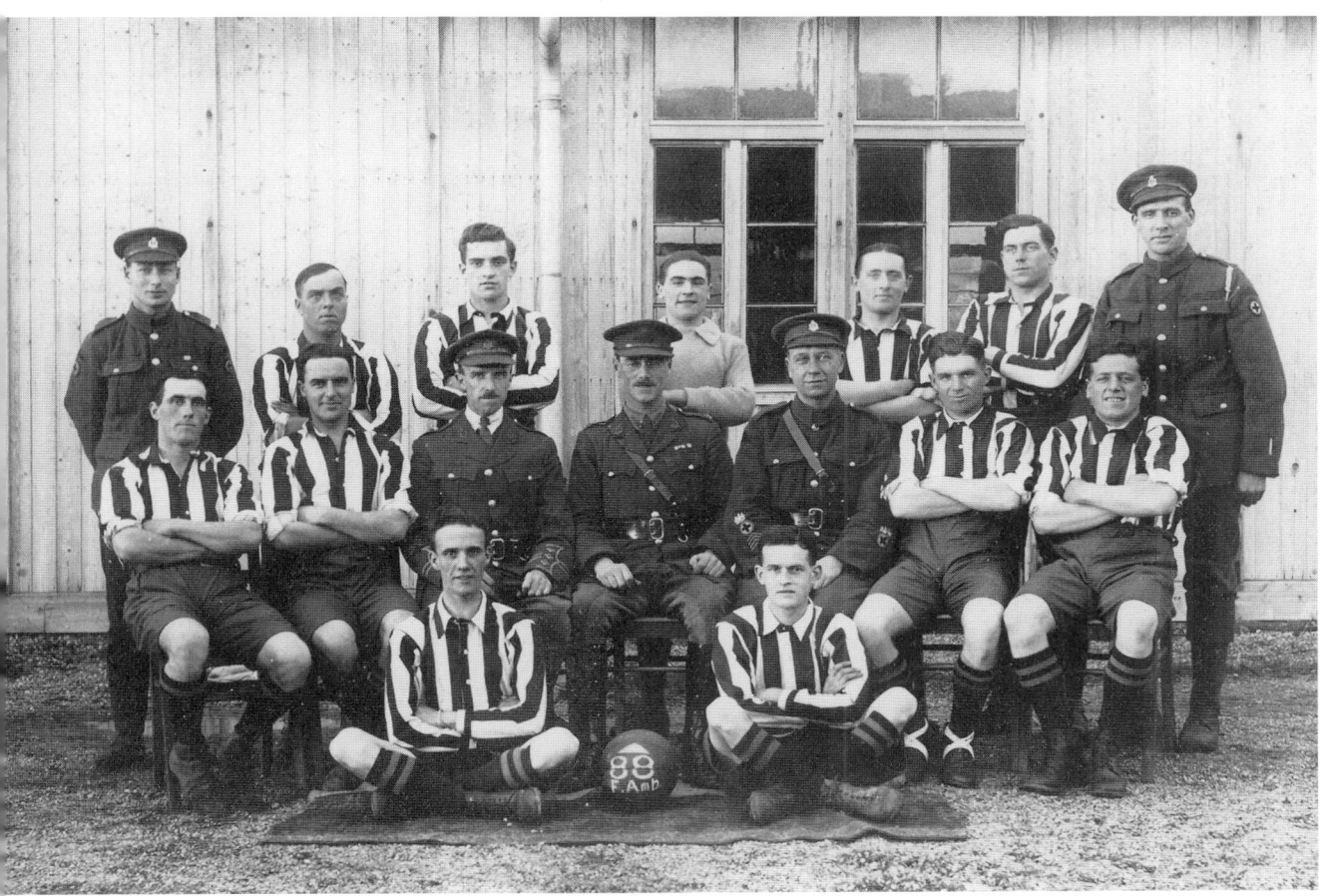

(**Opposite, above**) A RAMC unit band on the Western Front. The private (standing right) wears two wound stripes on his left cuff. The warrant officer (seated middle 2nd right) wears the ribbon of the Meritorious Service Medal (MSM).

(**Opposite, below**) The football team of the 50th Field Ambulance, RAMC. The officers (seated middle centre) both wear Military Cross (MC) ribbons and the warrant officer (seated middle 2nd right) wears the ribbon of the Meritorious Service Medal (MSM). The private (seated front left) has two wound stripes on his left cuff. The 50th Field Ambulance was on the Western Front, with the 37th Division, from the summer of 1915.

(**Above**) The football team of the 88th (1st East Anglian) Field Ambulance, RAMC. The officer (seated centre) wears the ribbon of the Military Cross and Bar (MC). The Field Ambulance served with the 29th Division, a regular army division, at Gallipoli in 1915 and on the Western Front from early 1916. The private (standing right) wears a wound stripe on his left cuff.

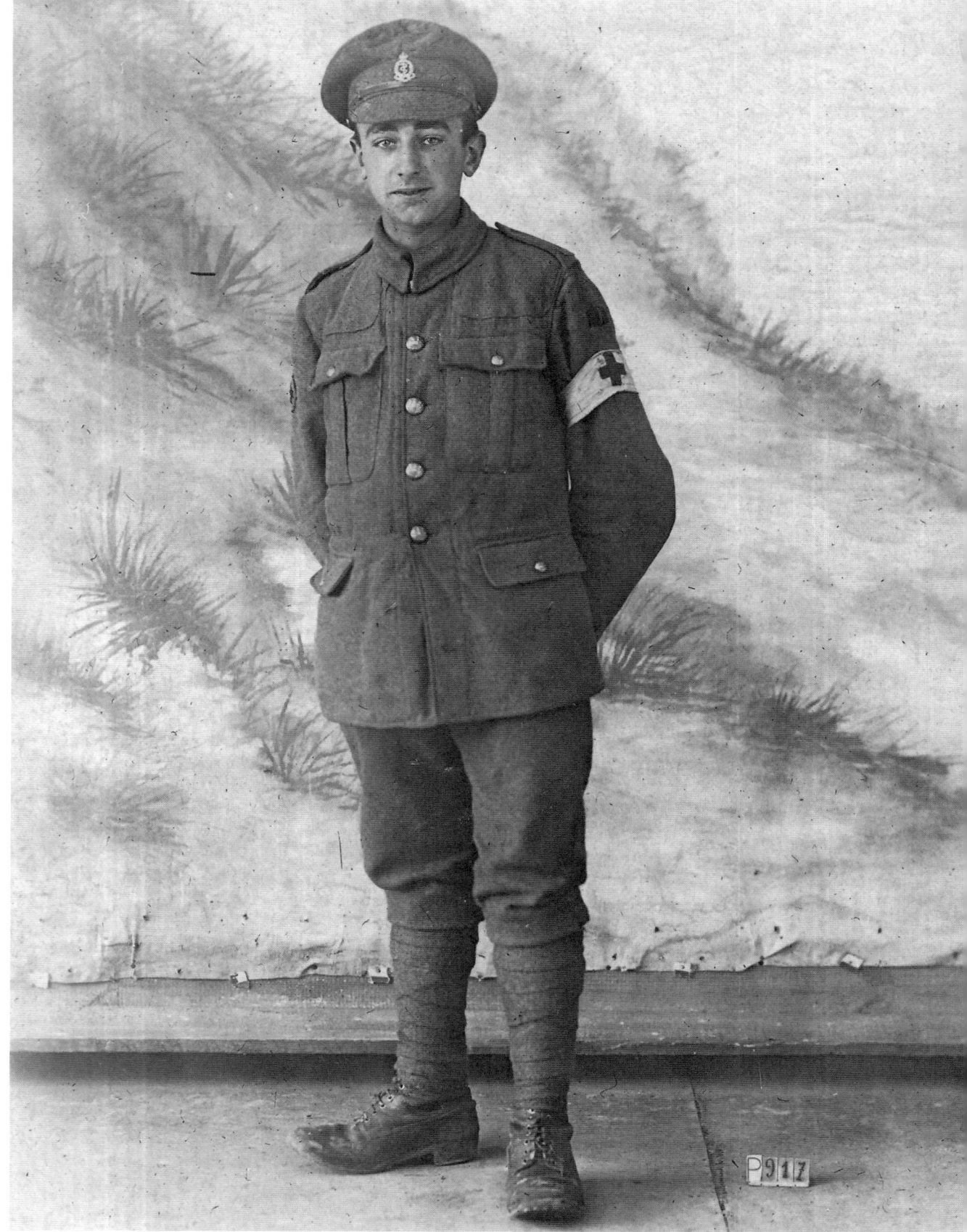

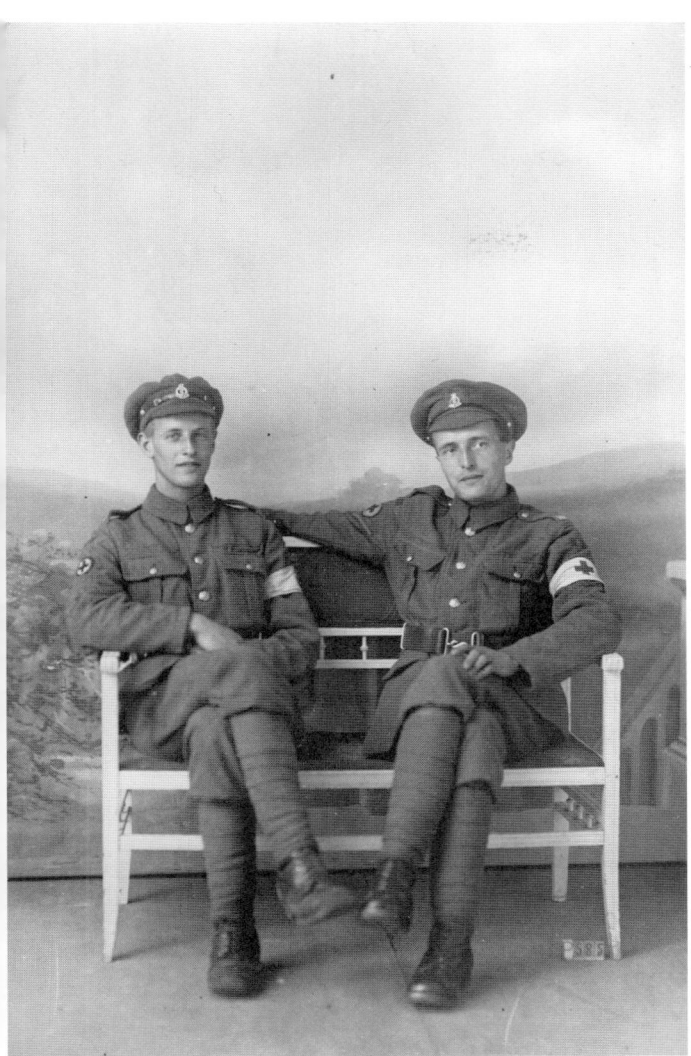 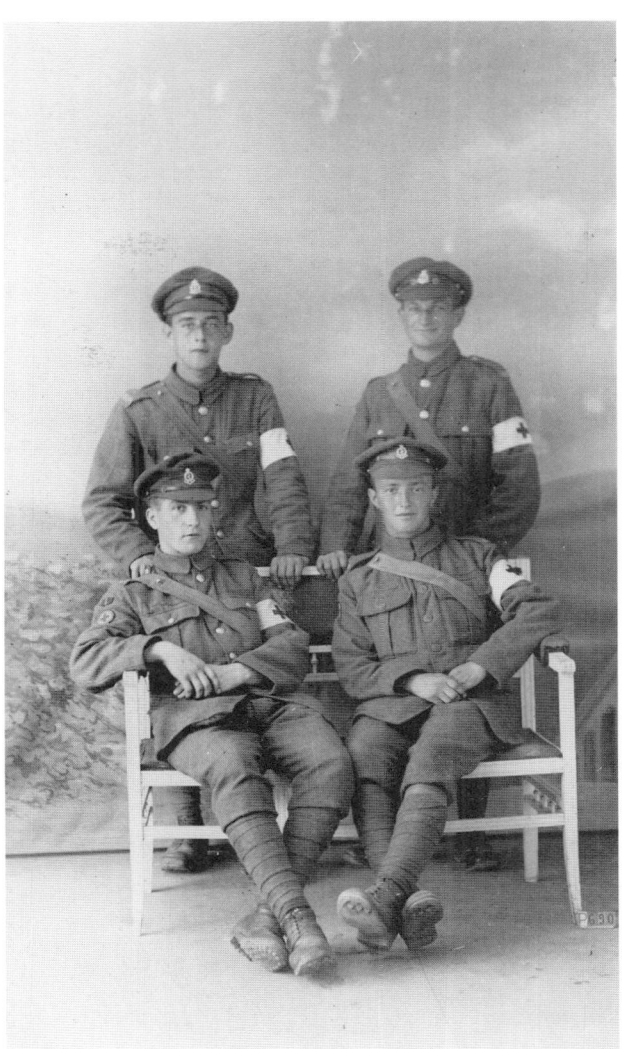

(**Opposite**) A private with the 99th Field Ambulance, RAMC, photographed at Maurepas, France, Christmas Day 1916. This unit was on the Western Front with the 33rd Division from late 1915.

(**Above, left**) A private and lance corporal of the 99th Field Ambulance, RAMC, photographed at Maurepas, France, Christmas Day 1916. Divisional shoulder patches are being worn.

(**Above, right**) No. 1 Squad, 99th Field Ambulance, RAMC, photographed at Maurepas, France, Christmas Day 1916. Standing (back left) is 105667 Private Harry Boothroyd, 99th Field Ambulance, RAMC. He enlisted on 10 December 1915 at Halifax, Yorkshire when his address was 27 Camm Street, Brighouse, and he was a carpet weaver. He served on the Western Front from 2 August 1916 and was posted to the 99th Field Ambulance on 7 August 1916, as a stretcher-bearer. In August 1916 he injured his shoulder whilst jumping into a trench and colliding with an ammunition box. On 22 March 1919 he was posted to the 52nd Stationary Hospital and on 1 August 1919 to the 40th Stationary Hospital.

59192 Private Arthur Lynd Martin, 91st Field Ambulance, RAMC. The 91st Field Ambulance served on the Western Front with the 32nd Division. He was born at Two Mile Hill, Gloucester on 14 March 1877, the son of William Lynd Martin, Commander (retd.) RN, and his wife, Albinia Blanche Vilett. He was educated at the Hill School, Swindon and Edinburgh University. He married Edith Brown at Holy Trinity Church, Fareham on 30 October 1901. In 1902 he was residing at 7 Shakespeare Ave, Portswood, Hampshire. His son, Henry Horace Jack Martin, was born 19 June 1906. His wife died on 30 August 1908. In 1911 he was living with his sister at 1 Milden Hall Road, Lower Clapton where he worked as a clerk at the Rotherhithe Conservative and Unionist Association. Prior to enlistment he was a Special Constable at Rotherhithe. Arthur Lynd Martin volunteered for service in the RAMC in June 1915 and served on the Western Front from 2 October 1915. He died from septicaemia contracted whilst on active service, on 22 August 1917, at No. 53 General Hospital, Wimereux, aged 40. He is buried in Wimereux Communal Cemetery, Pas de Calais, France.

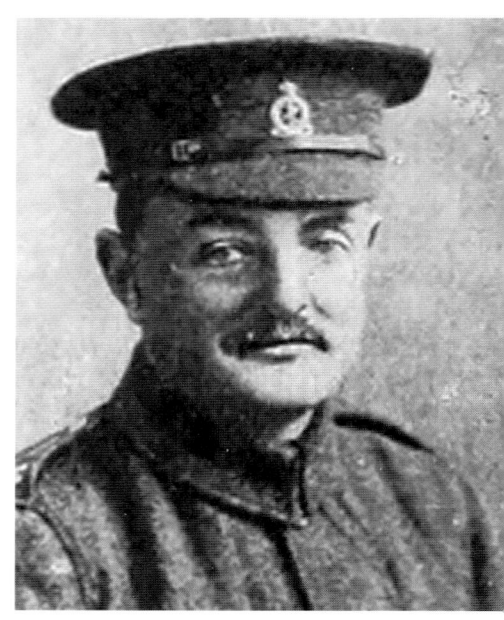

Envelope for a 32nd Division Christmas card sent from the Western Front, December 1916, by Arthur Lynd Martin to his aunt, Mrs A.H. Rolleston in Leamington Spa, Warwickshire.

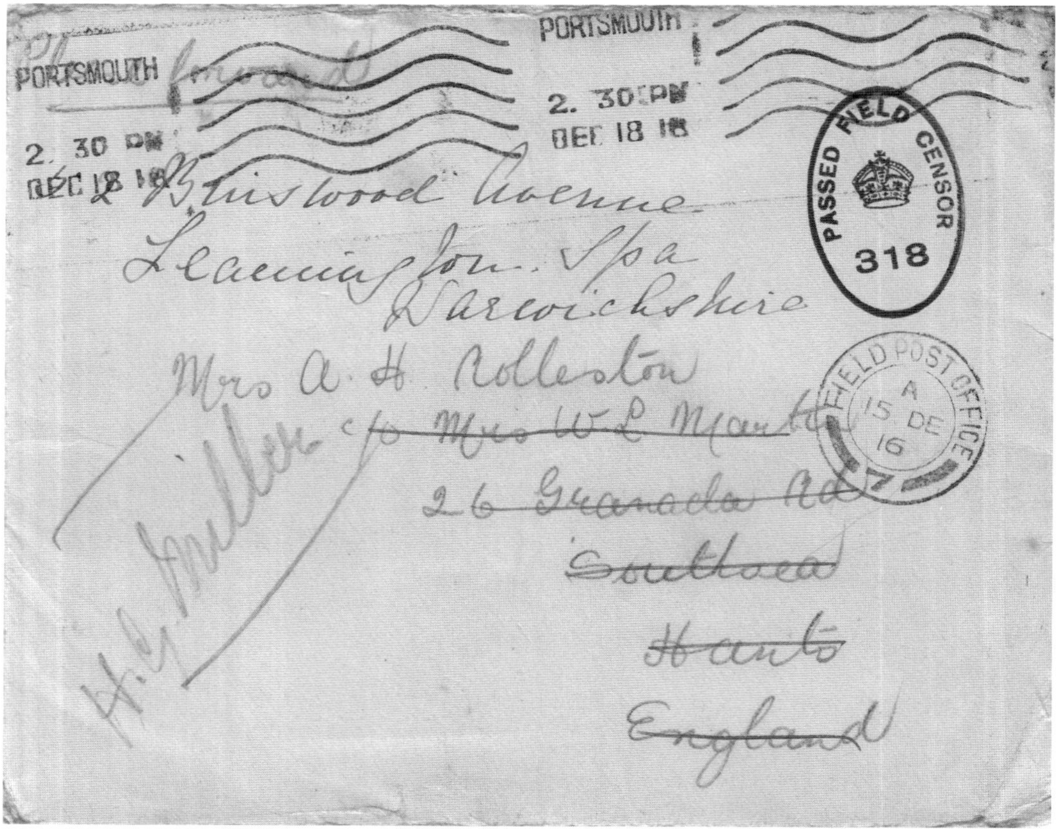

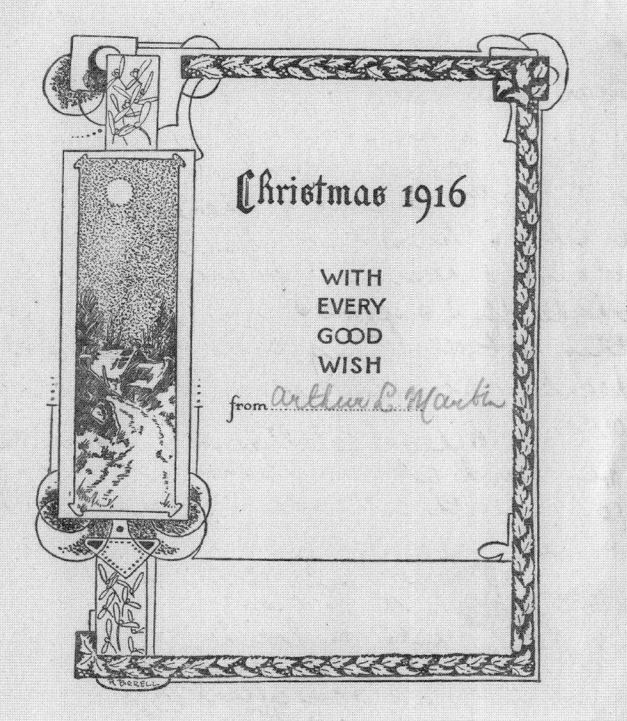

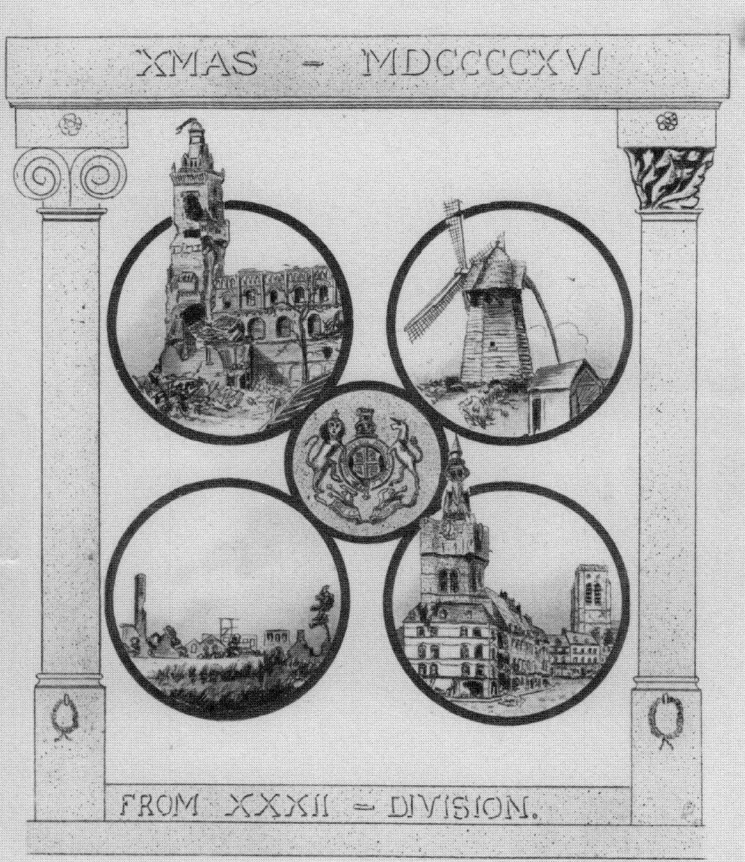

A 32nd Division Christmas card sent from the Western Front, December 1916, by Arthur Lynd Martin to his aunt. He noted in his message: 'I have a cold which I can't shake off; I suppose I am too old for this sort of thing and shall be heartily pleased when it is all over'.

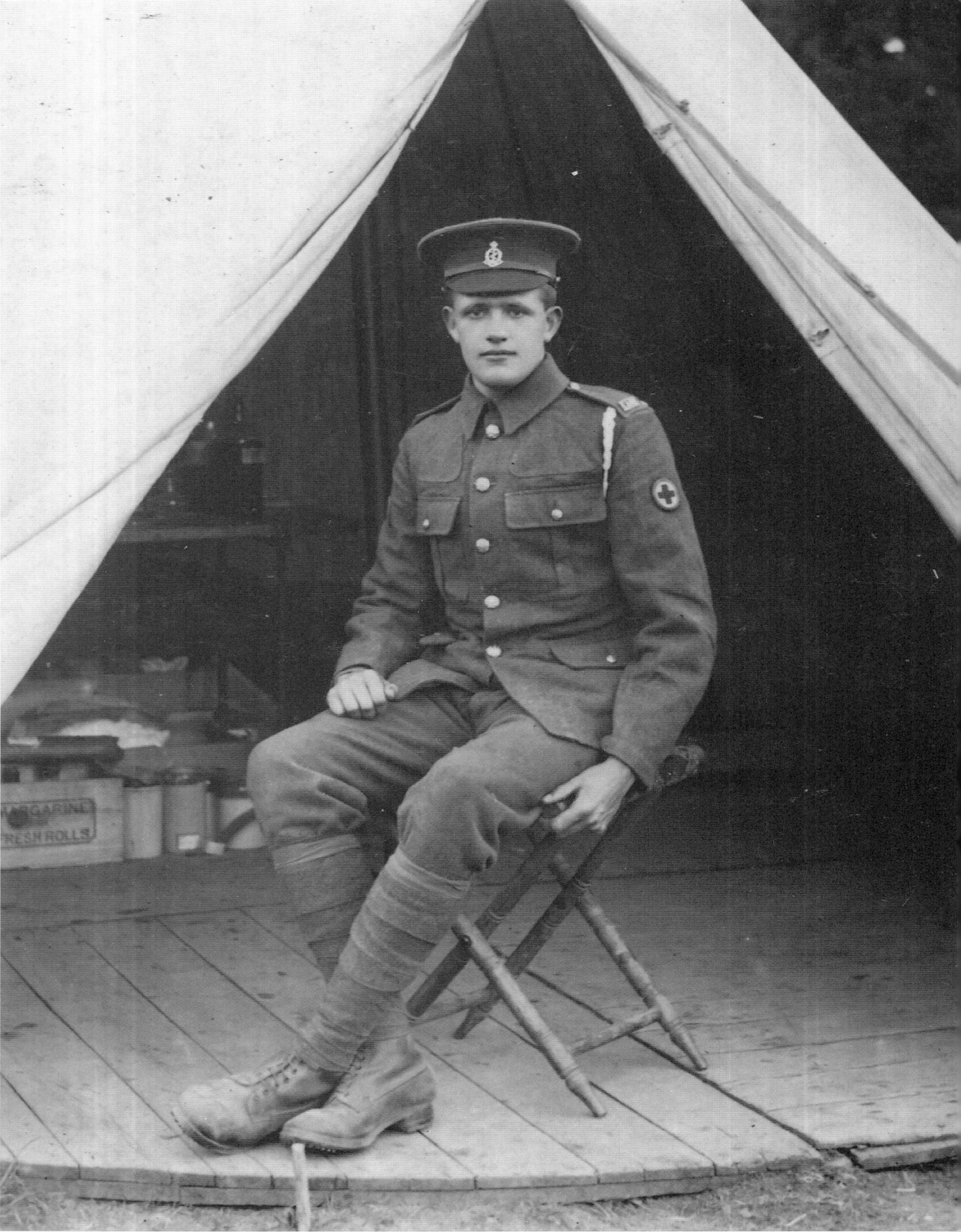

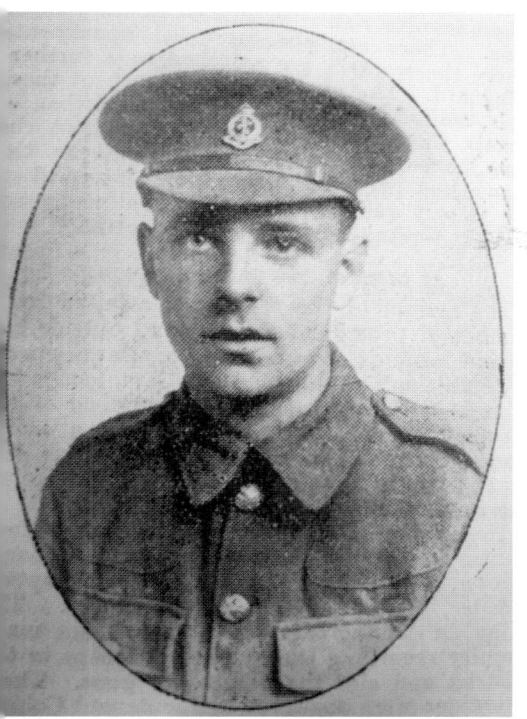 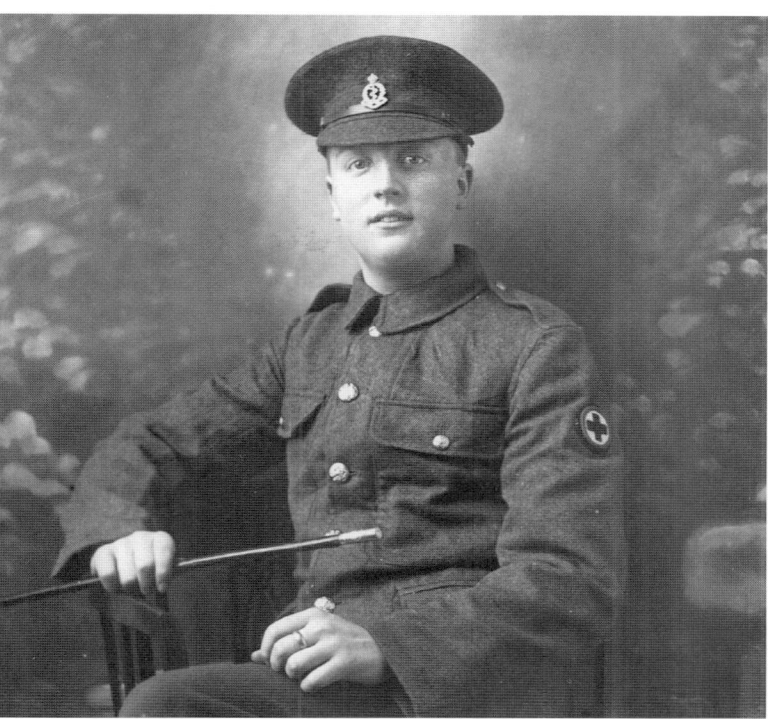

(**Opposite**) 24054 Private Arthur Ernest Gaddass, 74th Field Ambulance, RAMC. This unit served on the Western Front with the 24th Division. He was the son of John Dent Gaddass and Margaret Gaddass, of 24, West Terrace, Billy Row, Crook, Co. Durham. Arthur Ernest Gaddass died of wounds, 28 March 1918, aged 22. He is buried in Namps-au-Val British Cemetery, Somme, France.

(**Above, left**) 30508 Private Archibald Douglas, 8th Field Ambulance, RAMC, was educated at Annan Academy, and served his apprenticeship as a clerk in the office of Messrs. R. Robinson & Sons, Provost Mills, Annan, Dumfriesshire. He afterwards emigrated to Australia. Prior to the outbreak of war he returned to Scotland and was appointed representative for Mr Bell, potato merchant, Annan, in Newcastle and the Midlands. Archibald Douglas enlisted into the RAMC on 13 August 1914, age 22 years and 6 months. After training, on 15 January 1915, he joined the 63rd Field Ambulance. On 19 June 1915 he embarked on the SS *King Edward* at Southampton, disembarking the next day at Rouen. On 5 July 1915, Private Douglas was posted to the command of the 3rd Division's Assistant Director of Medical Services, in the field, and was subsequently attached to the 8th Field Ambulance. He was admitted into the 9th Field Ambulance on 28 January 1917, with an injury to his left foot and was transferred to No. 29 Casualty Clearing Station, where he remained until the 11 February, when he returned to his unit. On 3 May 1917, during the Battle of Arras, Private Douglas was killed in action and is buried in Tilloy British Cemetery, Tilloy-Les-Mofflaines, France. His commanding officer wrote to his family: 'I am more than sorry that his has occurred, for since he has been with this unit, I found him a good, willing and hard-working orderly. There is a great consolation in knowing that he died doing his duty. I hope you will accept my deepest sympathy and that of his comrades'. Archibald Douglas was the second son of Mr and Mrs Douglas of 2 Church Street, Annan, Dumfriesshire. (*Dumfriesshire Newspaper Group*)

(**Above, right**) 72206 Private (later Lance Corporal) Cyril Charles Keech, RAMC. He enlisted on 22 October 1915 and was posted to France in 1916. On 22 April 1916 he fractured his shoulder falling from a troop train at Abbeville, whilst proceeding to the 32nd Division to join 92nd Field Ambulance. He was born on 20 December 1896 and resided at 41 Wellington Street, Kettering. Prior to enlistment he worked as grocer's assistant. He married at Kettering in 1920 and died at Colchester in 1979.

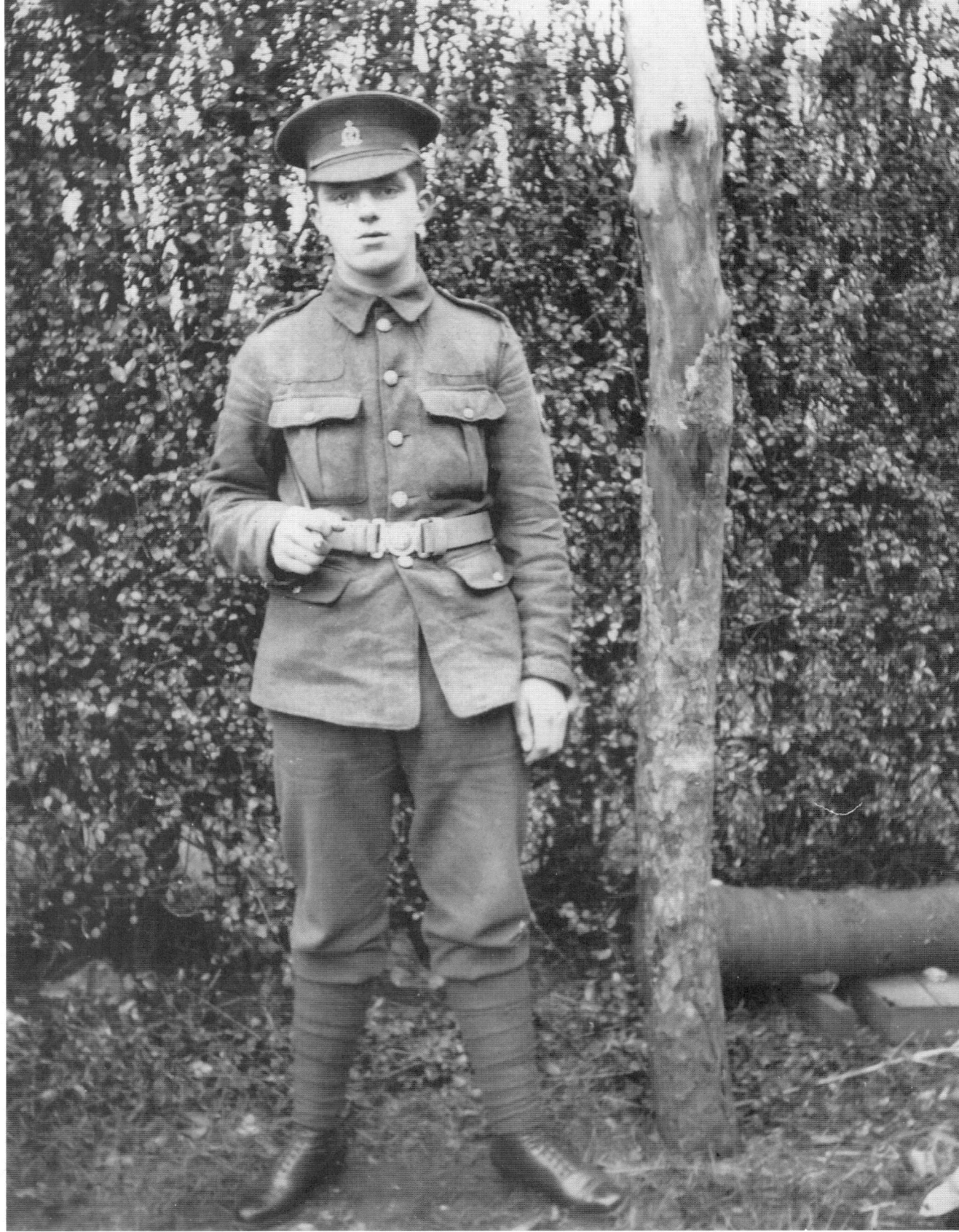

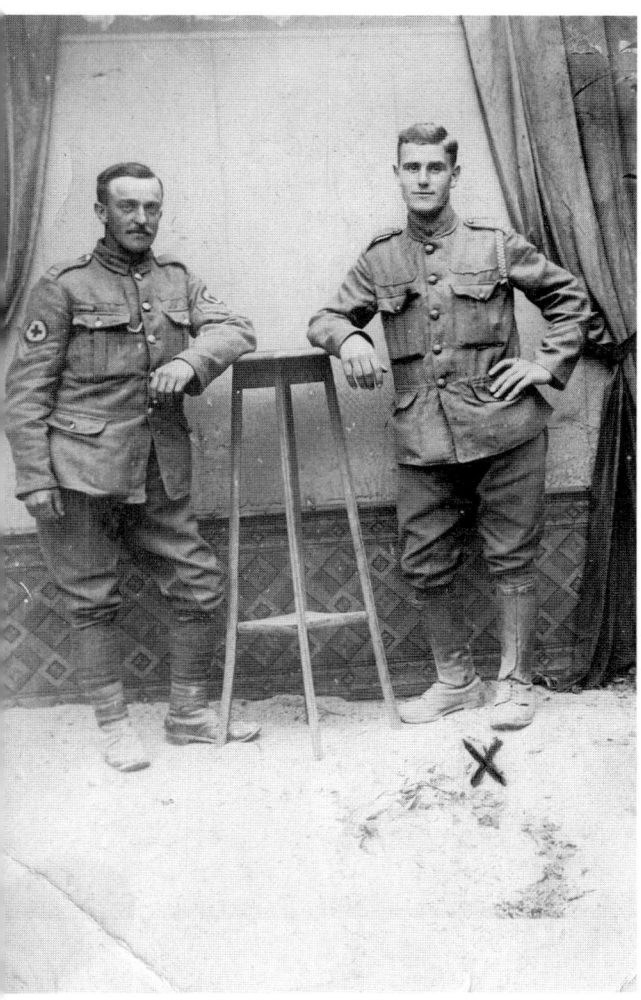 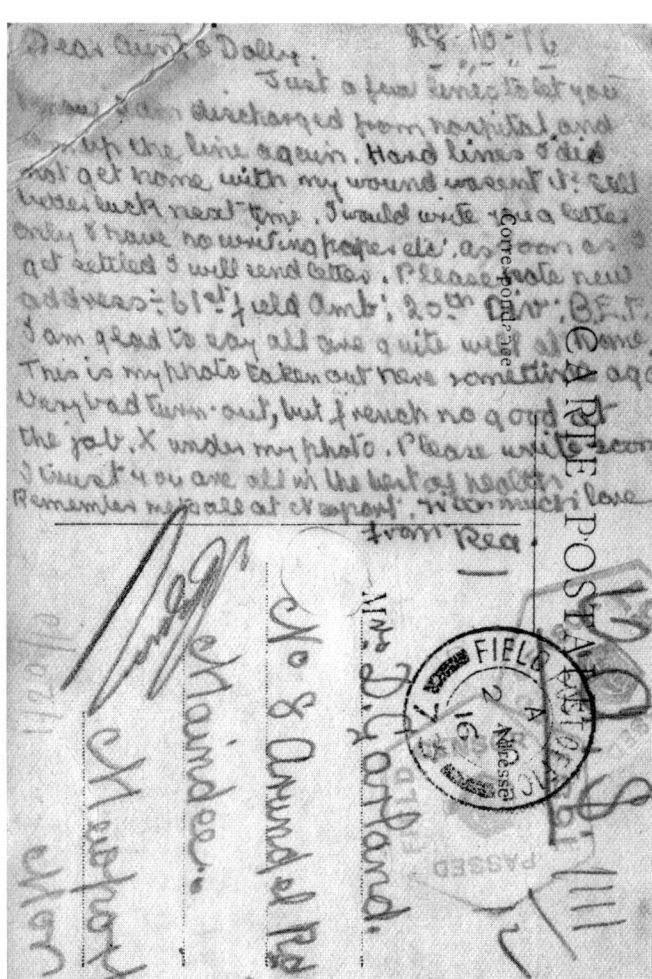

(**Opposite**) 40497 Private George Ernest Cosser, RAMC. He was born in 1896 at Pokesdown, Hampshire and enlisted in the RAMC at Bournemouth on 4 September 1914, his occupation being a surgical boot maker. His last employer prior to enlistment was F. Jenner, 202 Christchurch Road, Boscombe, Bournemouth. Private Cosser was posted to the 12th Field Ambulance, RAMC which served with the 4th Division. He was on the Western Front from 20 May 1915 to 6 July 1916 as a stretcher-bearer. During October 1915 his hand was crushed between a wagon and a wall, and the 3rd finger of his right hand was amputated. Private Cosser was later posted as a nursing orderly to Mesopotamia, from July 1916 to 21 January 1919, with the 3rd Base General Hospital, Basra. From March 1919 he was employed by the Anglo-Persian Oil Company. He married Dora F. Keats in 1932.

(**Above**) 7688 Private Reginald J. Garland, 61st Field Ambulance, RAMC. The unit served with the 20th (Light) Division on the Western Front. The photo was posted by Private Garland to his aunt. His first overseas posting was with the 15th Field Ambulance from 20 August 1914. He was wounded on the Western Front during 1916. On the reverse of the photo he noted in his message: 'Hard lines I did not get home with my wound wasn't it? Well better luck next time.' and 'This is my photo taken out here some time ago. Very bad turn out, but French no good at the job. X under my photo'.

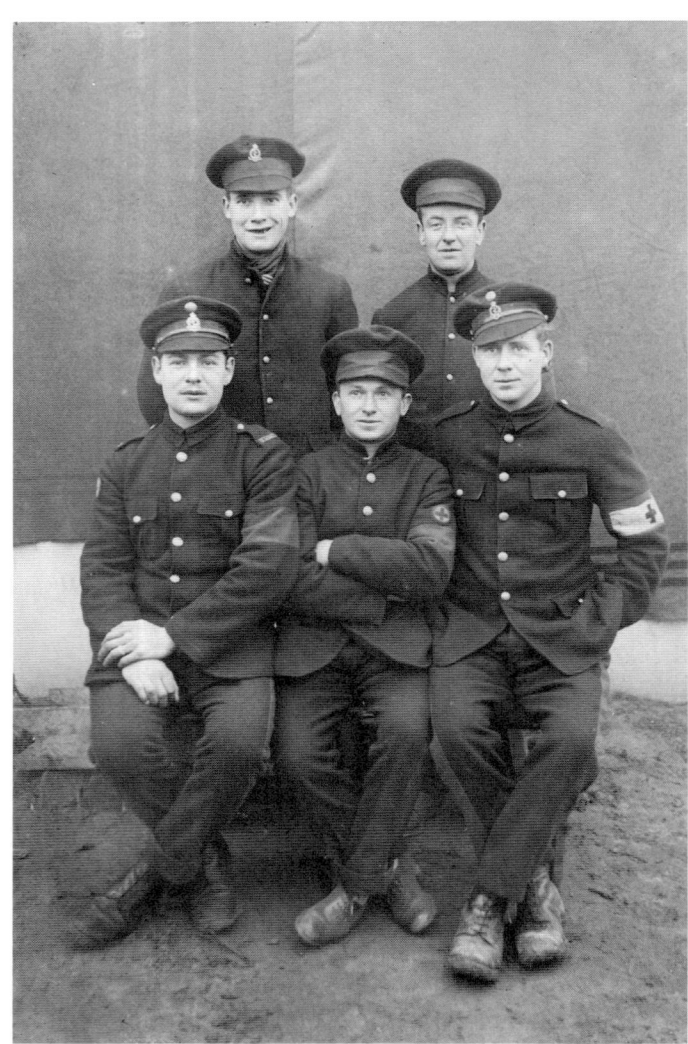 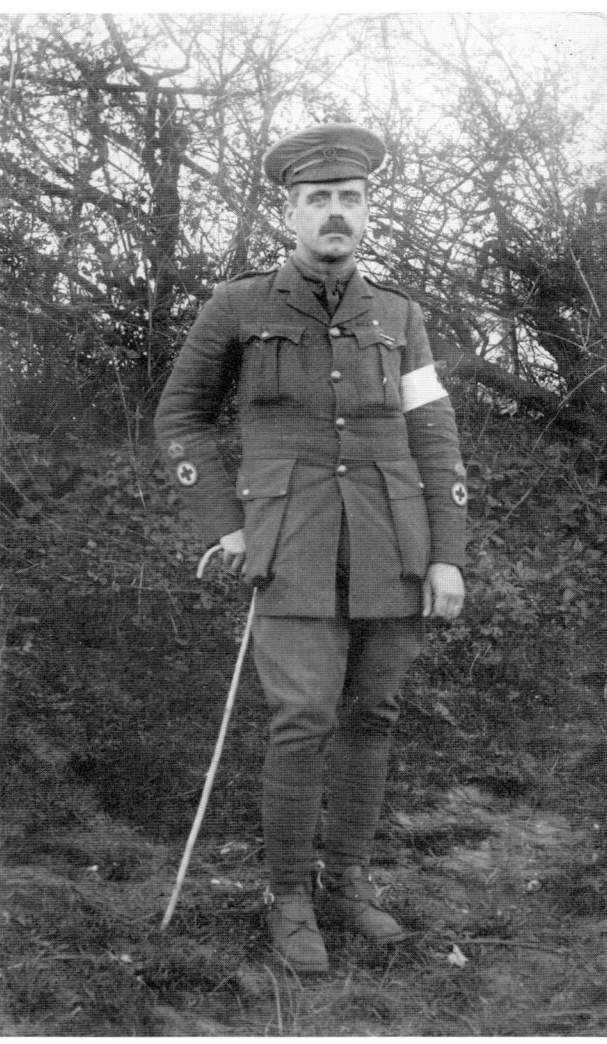

(**Above, left**) A group of RAMC personnel taken prisoner on the Western Front, photographed whilst interned in Germany.

(**Above, right**) A RAMC warrant officer on the Western Front. He wears campaign medal ribbons which signify his service in the 1899-1902 South African War.

(**Opposite, above**) Two RAMC privates taken prisoner on the Western Front and interned at Stendal, Saxony-Anhalt, Germany. The 43rd Field Ambulance served with the 14th (Light) Division.

(**Opposite, below**) RAMC personnel carrying out provost duties, signified by their Military Police armlets.

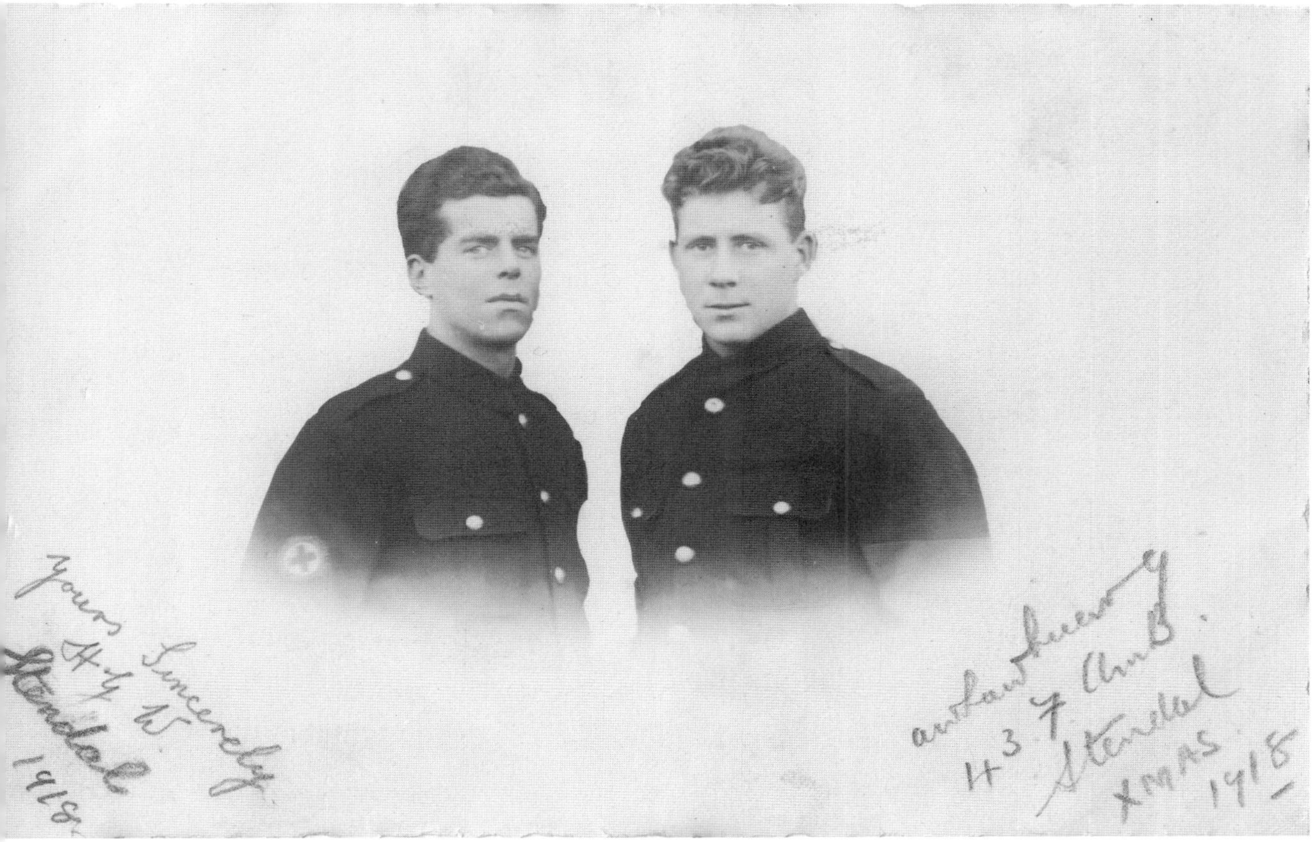
Yours Sincerely
H. J. W.
Stendal
1918
H 3 7
Stendal
XMAS 1918

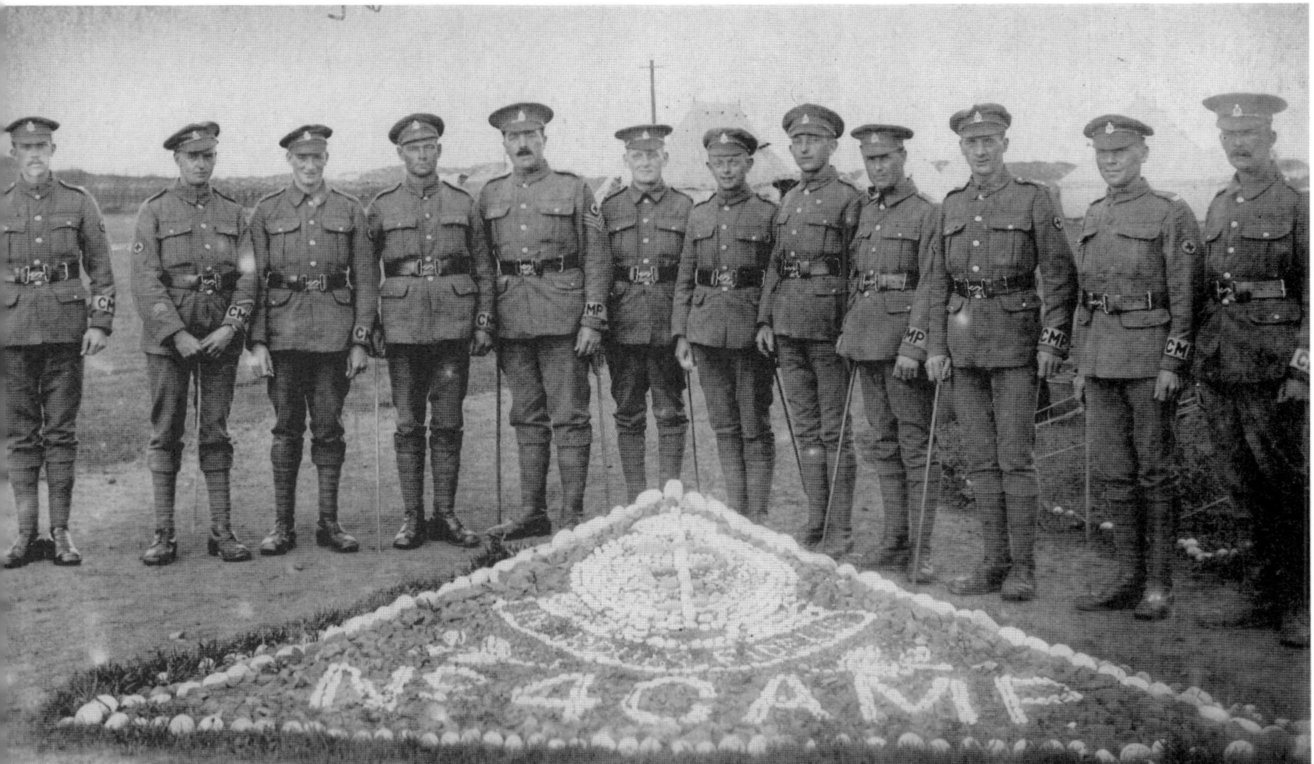
CMP
No 40 AMP

A 1917 Christmas card of the 4th London Field Ambulance, RAMC. This unit was with the 47th (2nd London) Division on the Western Front from spring 1915.

A 1917 Christmas card of the 4th London Field Ambulance, RAMC. The inside of the card shows a building used as an advanced dressing station by the unit.

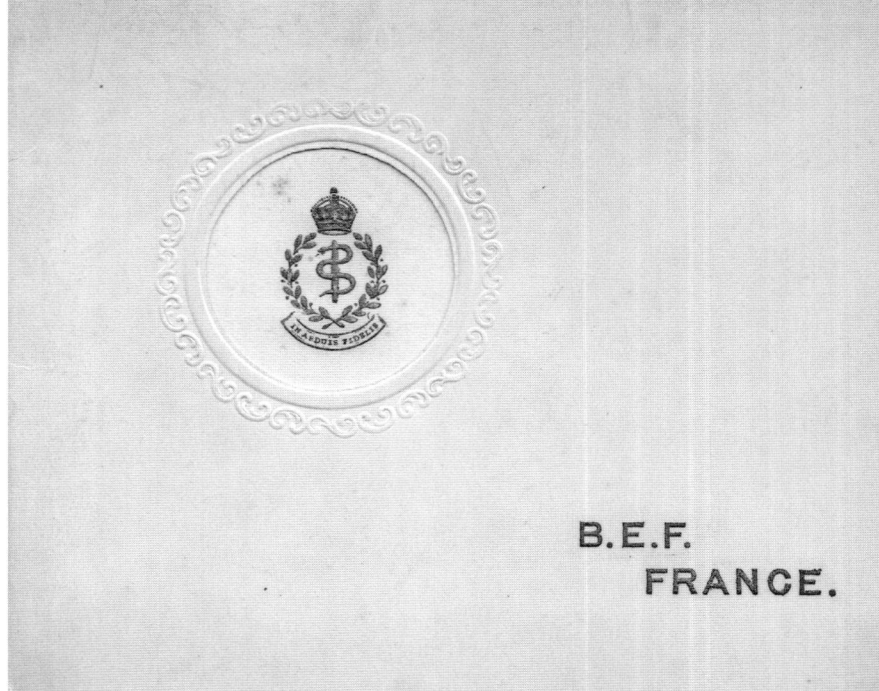

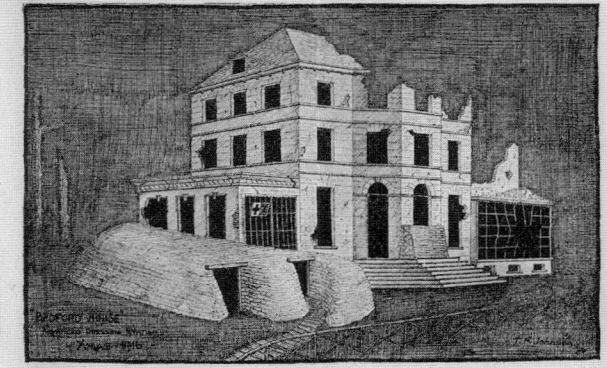

BEDFORD HOUSE, ADVANCED DRESSING STATION, XMAS, 1916.

(**Opposite, above**) A unit greetings card sent by Private E. Long, 92nd Field Ambulance, RAMC. The card was written on 13 May 1918. The 92nd Field Ambulance served on the Western Front from November 1915 with the 32nd Division.

(**Opposite, below**) A group of RAMC soldiers on Western Front. The two privates on the right of the group wear the Red Dragon Divisional Patch of the 38th (Welsh) Division. The division was on the Western Front from December 1915, suffering very heavy casualties at Mametz Wood in July 1916. The division lost over 28,000 killed, wounded and missing on the Western Front.

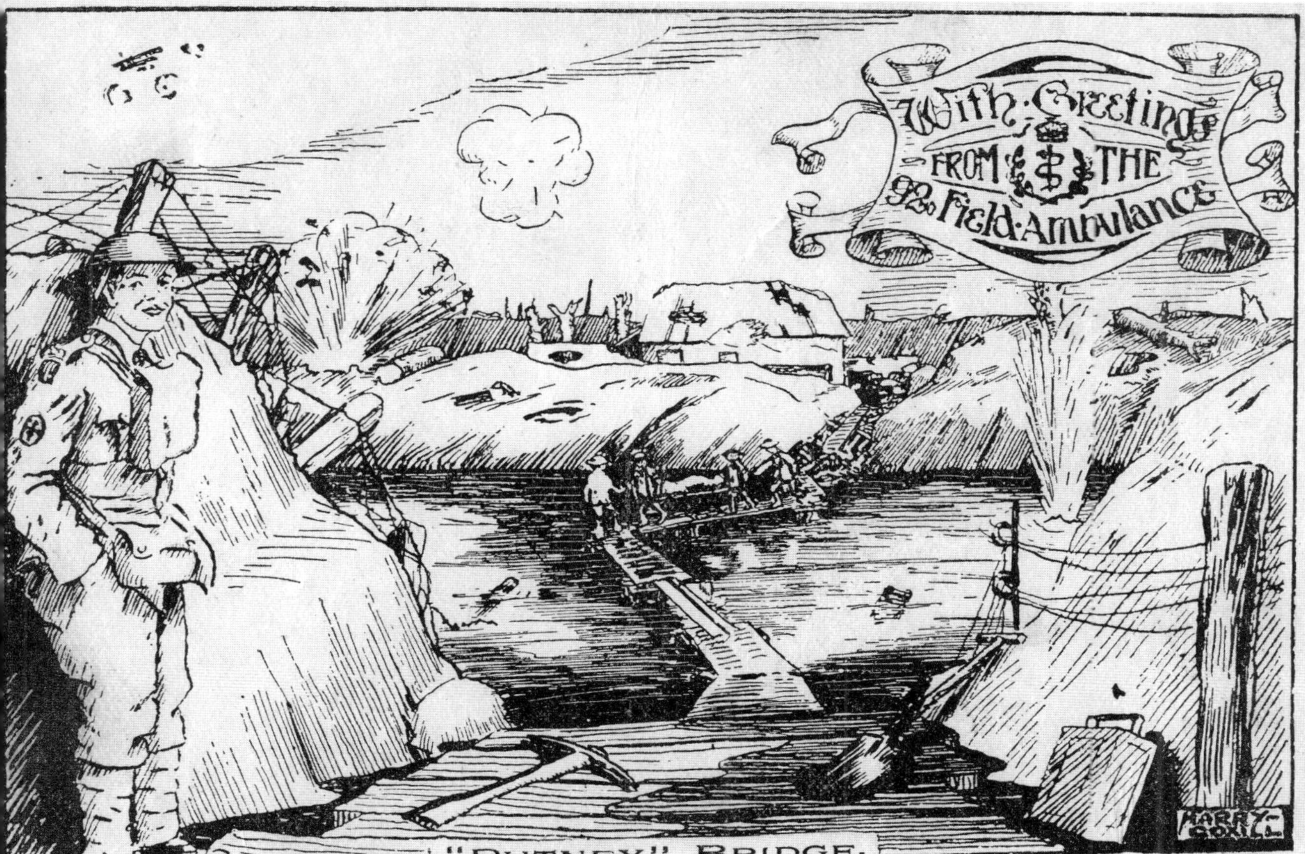

With Greetings
FROM THE
92nd Field Ambulance
HARRY GOXILL

"PUTNEY" BRIDGE.

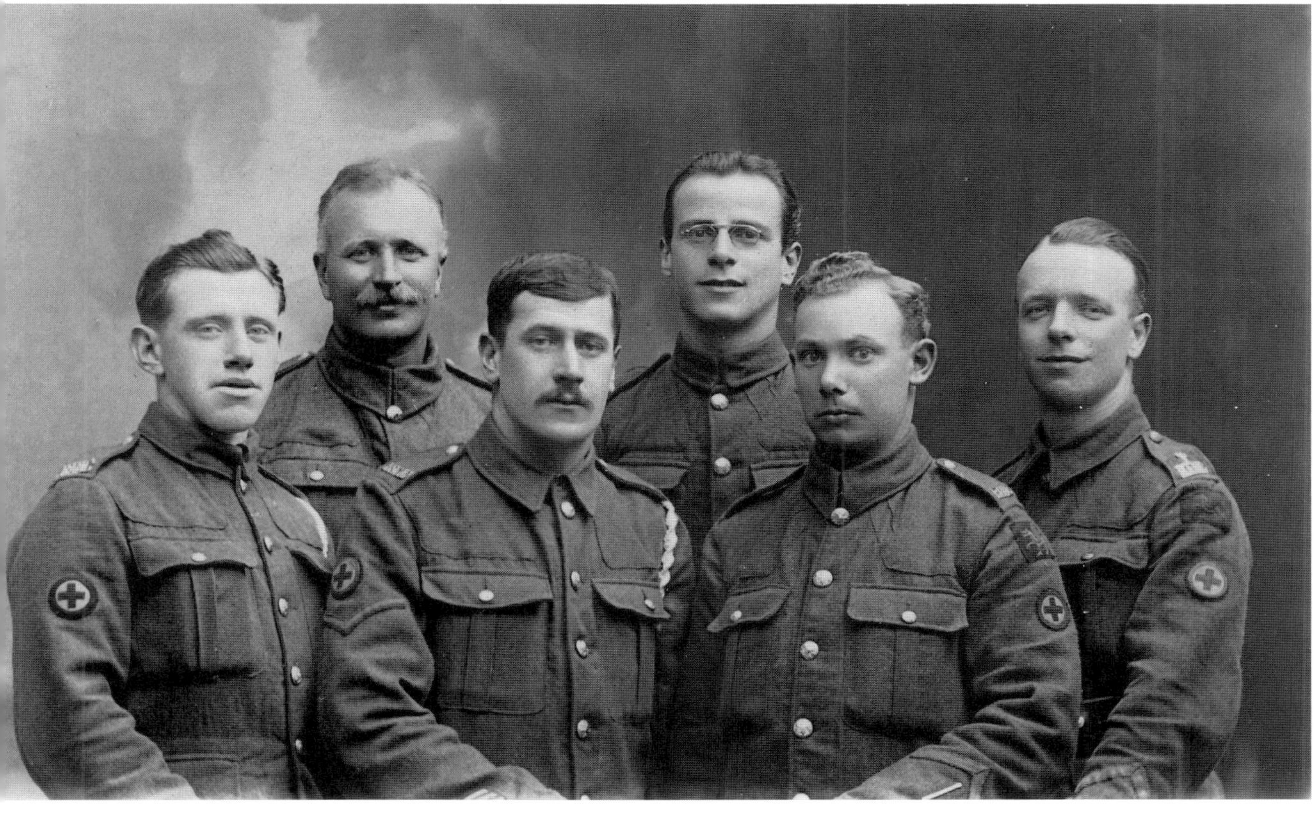

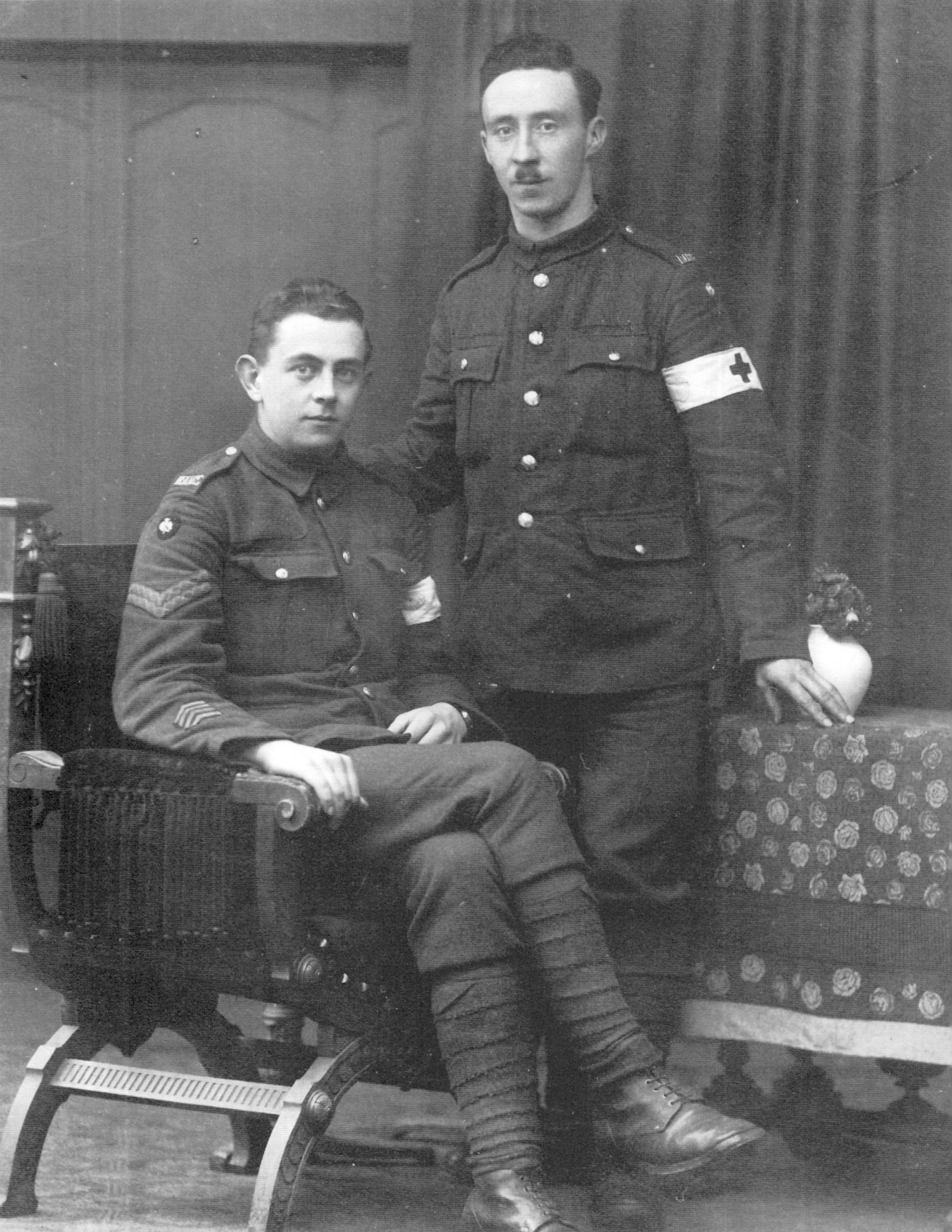

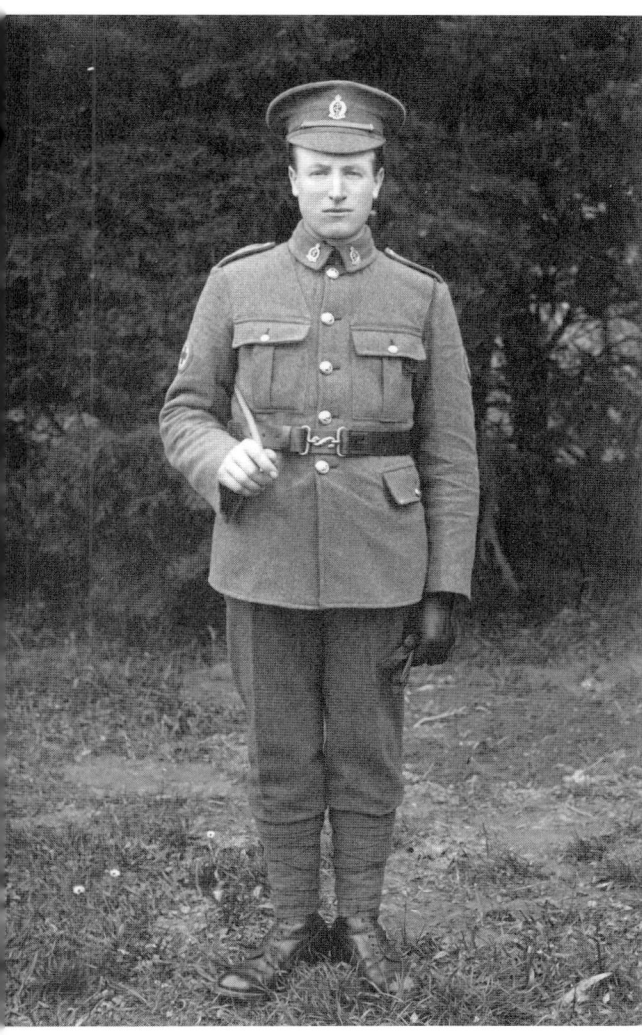
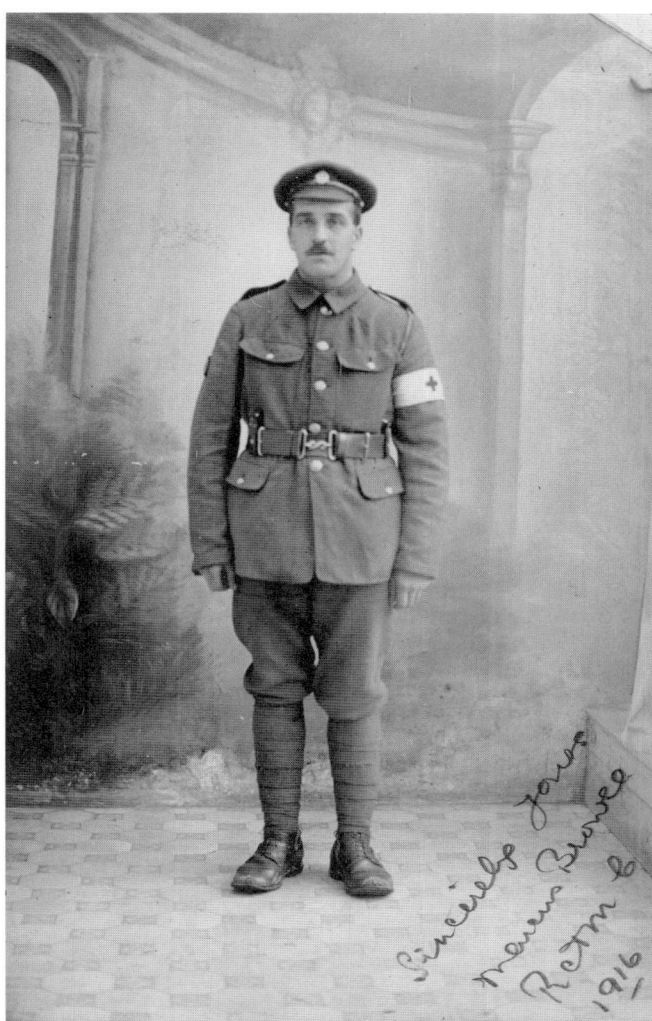

(**Opposite**) 32071 Private Reginald L.D. Crisp, RAMC and 31387 Private George E. Lacey, RAMC. Reginald Crisp was born in Market Harborough, Leicestershire. In 1911 he was a school pupil, aged 14, living with his parents, three sisters and brother in Rugby. Both Reginald Crisp and George Lacey served on the Western Front from 11 May 1915, and wear the Thistle Divisional Patch of the 9th (Scottish) Division. The photo was taken in Solingen, Germany, on 9 February 1919, whilst the division formed part of the Allied occupation forces. The 9th (Scottish) Division was the senior division of the First New Army and was on the Western Front from May 1915. Over 52,000 personnel became casualties (killed, wounded or missing) whilst serving with the division.

(**Above, left**) 538028 Private (later Sergeant) John Stewart, 6th London Field Ambulance, RAMC (TF). John Stewart served on the Western Front with the 6th London Field Ambulance from 15th March 1915. He was awarded the Territorial Efficiency Medal in May 1919. The 6th London Field Ambulance served on the Western Front with the 47th (2nd London) Division.

(**Above, right**) 54465 Private John Marcus Browse, RAMC. He was born in Salcombe on 6 March 1887. In 1891 he was living at 7 Harveys Row, Salcombe. His father Robert Browse was a tailor. In 1911 he was working in Fremington, Devon as a gardener. Private Browse served with the RAMC on the Western Front from 15 May 1915. He married in September 1918 at Paddington, London and died in 1978 at Shillingstone, Dorset.

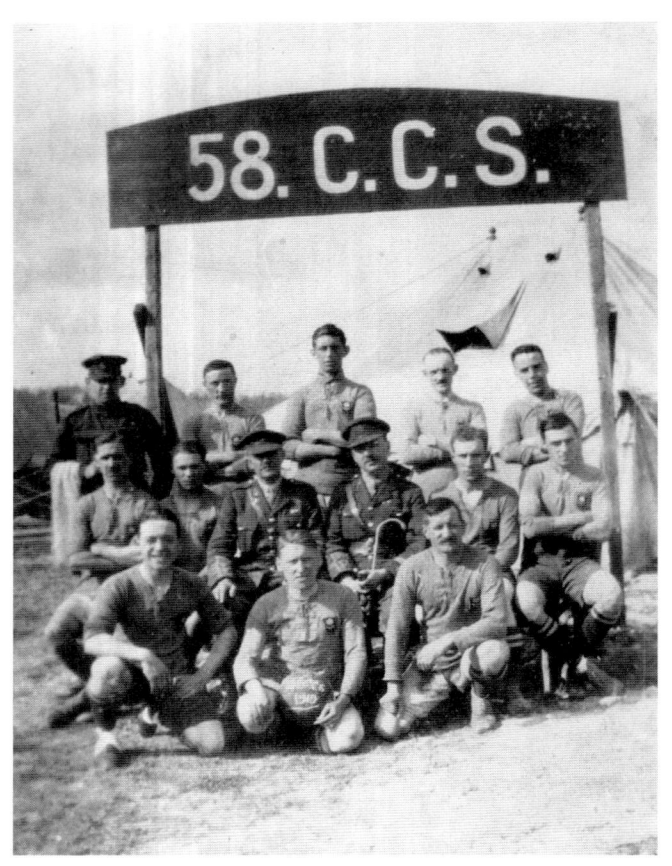

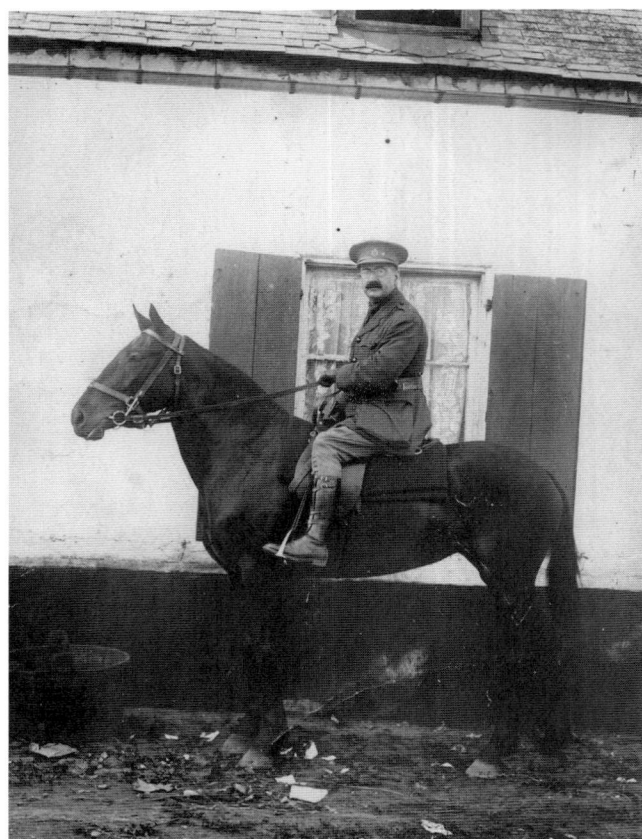

(**Above, left**) Football team of 58th Casualty Clearing Station, RAMC, on the Western Front. Tented medical facilities can be seen in the background.

(**Above, right**) Captain Archibald Farrell Waterhouse, RAMC, photographed on the Western Front. In 1911, aged 27, he was a medical student at Sheffield University and in the same year qualified as a Member of the Royal College of Surgeons and as a Licentiate of the Royal College of Practitioners.

(**Right**) 26913 Warrant Officer James Lamb, 42nd Casualty Clearing Station, RAMC, photographed in France. Warrant Officer Lamb served on the Western Front from 19 December 1915. From March 1916 to 1918 casualties from the 42nd Casualty Clearing Station were buried in Aubigny Communal Cemetery Extension, Pas de Calais, France.

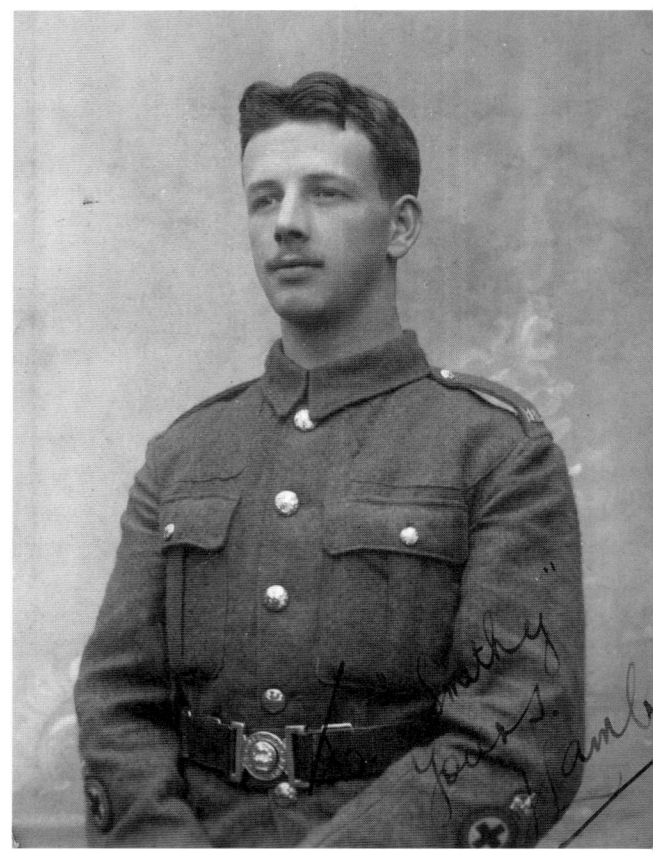

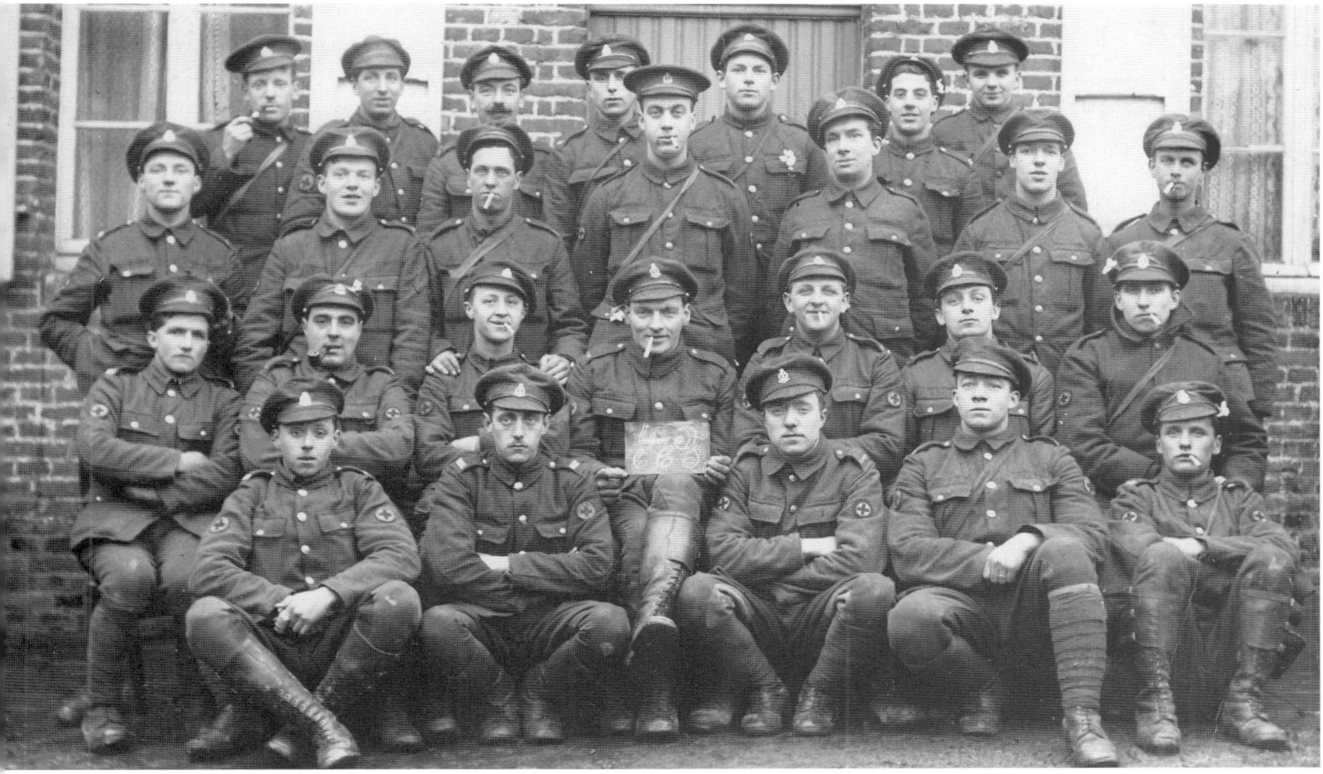

Personnel of 43rd Casualty Clearing Station, RAMC, on the Western Front.

Army Service Corps Motor Transport Drivers attached to the 108th Field Ambulance, RAMC, photographed on the Western Front. The 108th Field Ambulance served with the 36th (Ulster) Division from October 1915, suffering very heavy casualties at Thiepval on 1 July 1916. The division lost over 32,000 killed, wounded and missing.

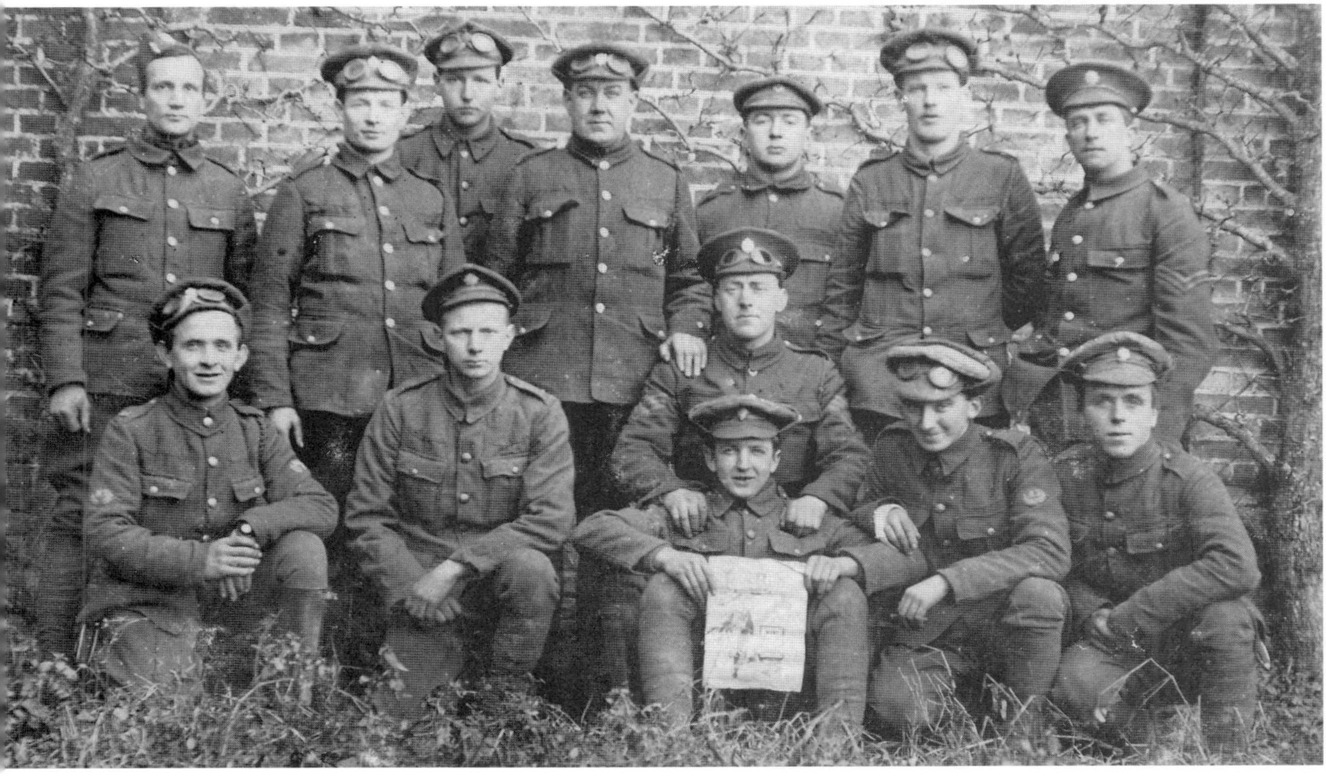

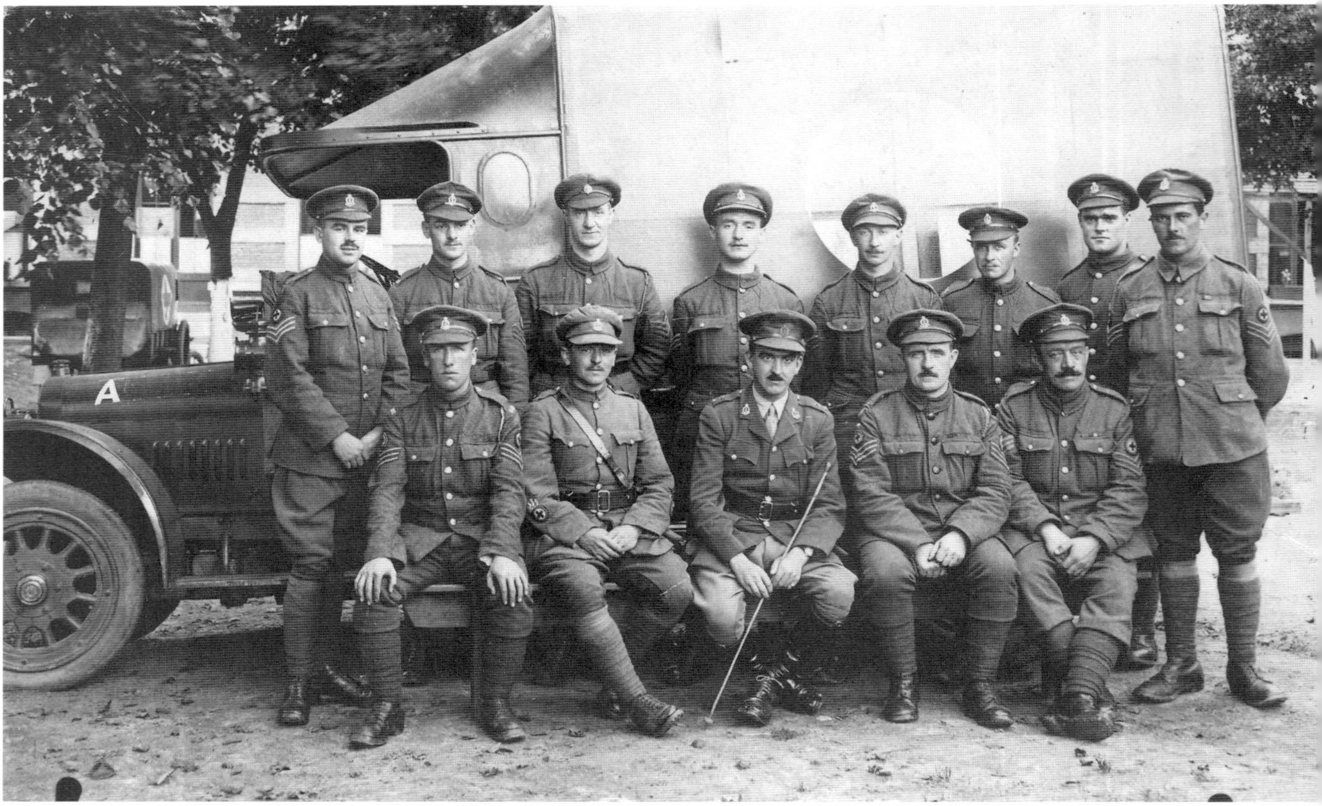

(**Above**) A lieutenant colonel and senior NCOs of a RAMC unit pictured in front of a motor ambulance in France. The sergeant (back right) wears a MM ribbon and the sergeant (front right) wears the ribbons of the Queen's South Africa Medal and King's South Africa Medal.

(**Opposite**) A group of RAMC personnel on the Western Front. Round St John Ambulance badges are worn on the left cuff by several of the soldiers.

(**Right**) 1395 / T4/211754 Private (later Staff Sergeant) Bert Denny, 2/1st East Anglian Field Ambulance, RAMC. He was born in Ipswich in 1894 and enlisted in the East Anglian Field Ambulance RAMC on 10 November 1911. On enlistment he worked as a groom and he lived in Ipswich. He was mobilised in August 1914 with the 2/1st East Anglian Field Ambulance. He later transferred to the Army Service Corps and served with No. 4 Company London Divisional Train ASC and 668 Company ASC. He was in France from 6 September 1916 to May 1920. He was awarded a Territorial Force Efficiency Medal and a Territorial Force War Medal.

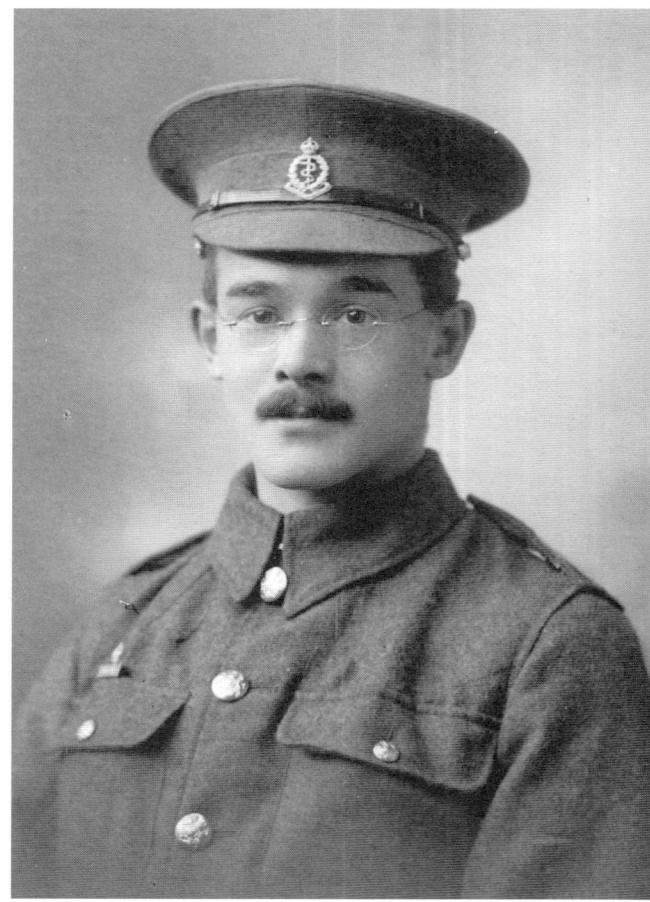

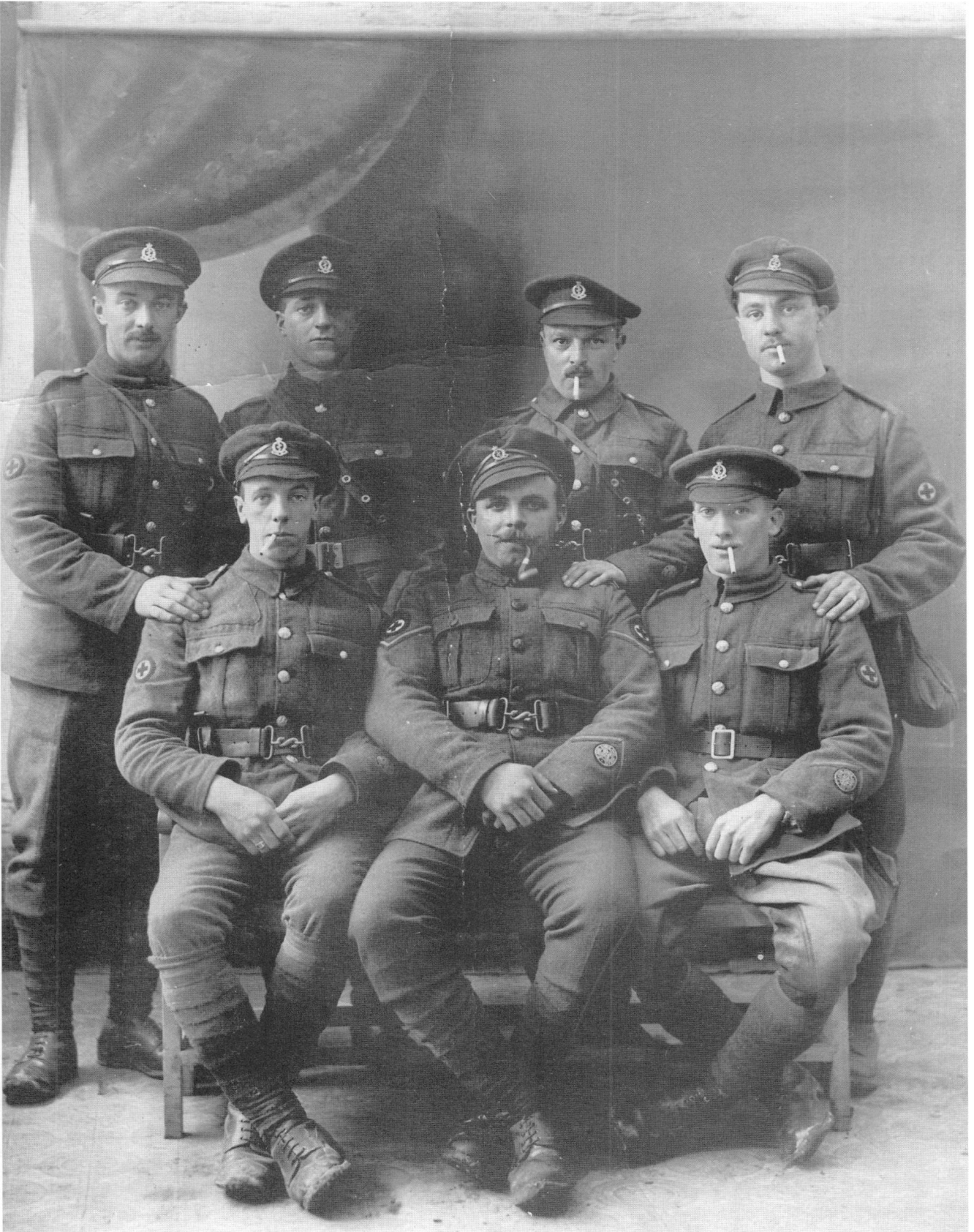

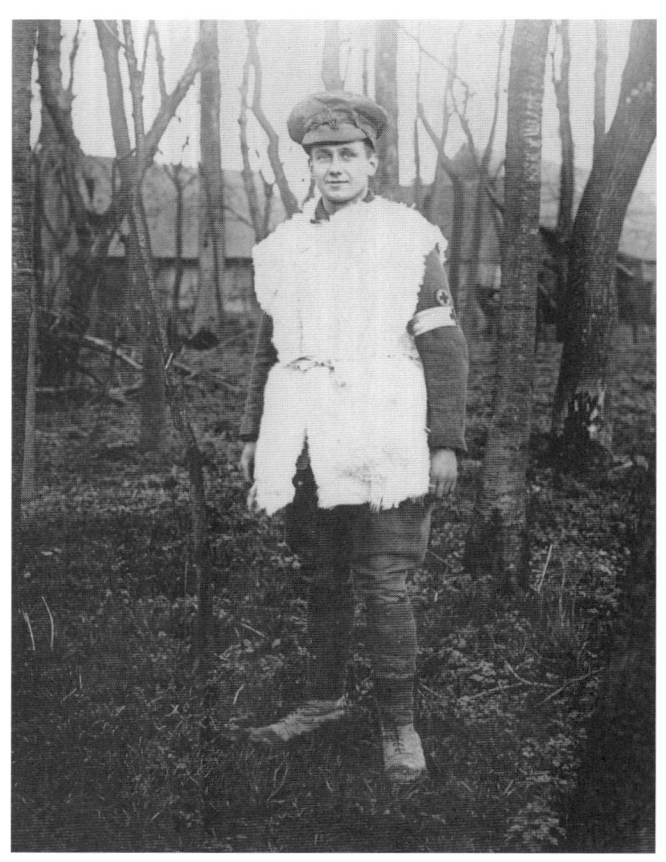

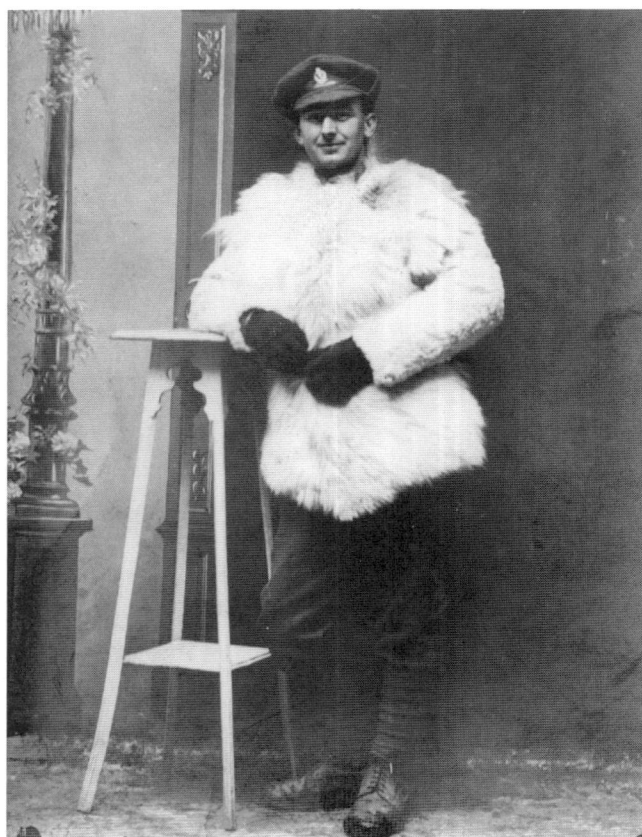

(**Above, left**) A RAMC private wearing winter clothing and waterproof cap cover on the Western Front. In response to the terrible conditions of trench warfare, leather and goatskin tunics were issued.

(**Above, right**) A RAMC soldier in winter clothing on the Western Front. His Red Cross badges and any rank insignia are covered by the goatskin coat he is wearing.

(**Right**) A RAMC private wearing a goatskin tunic on the Western Front. The reverse of the photo is dated 20 January 1917.

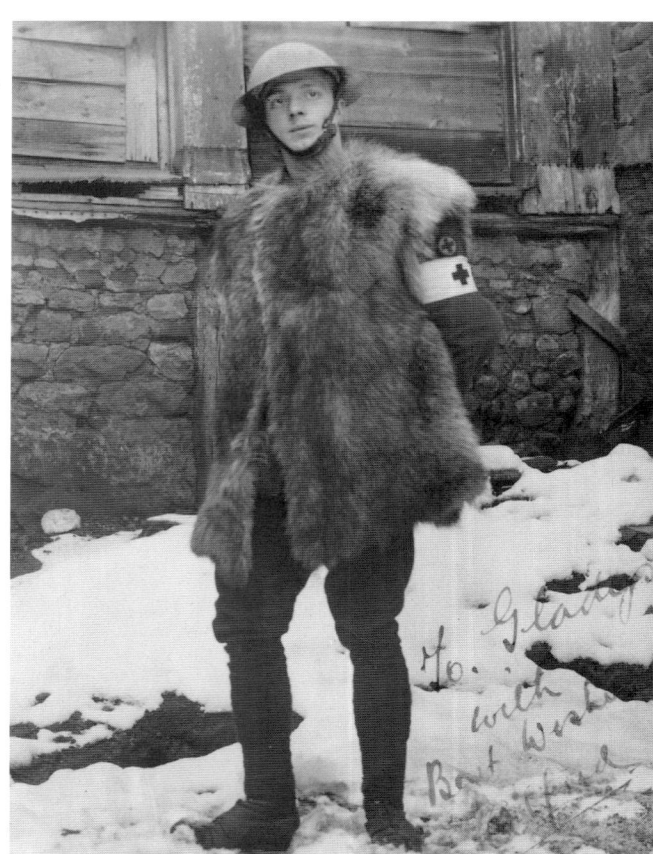

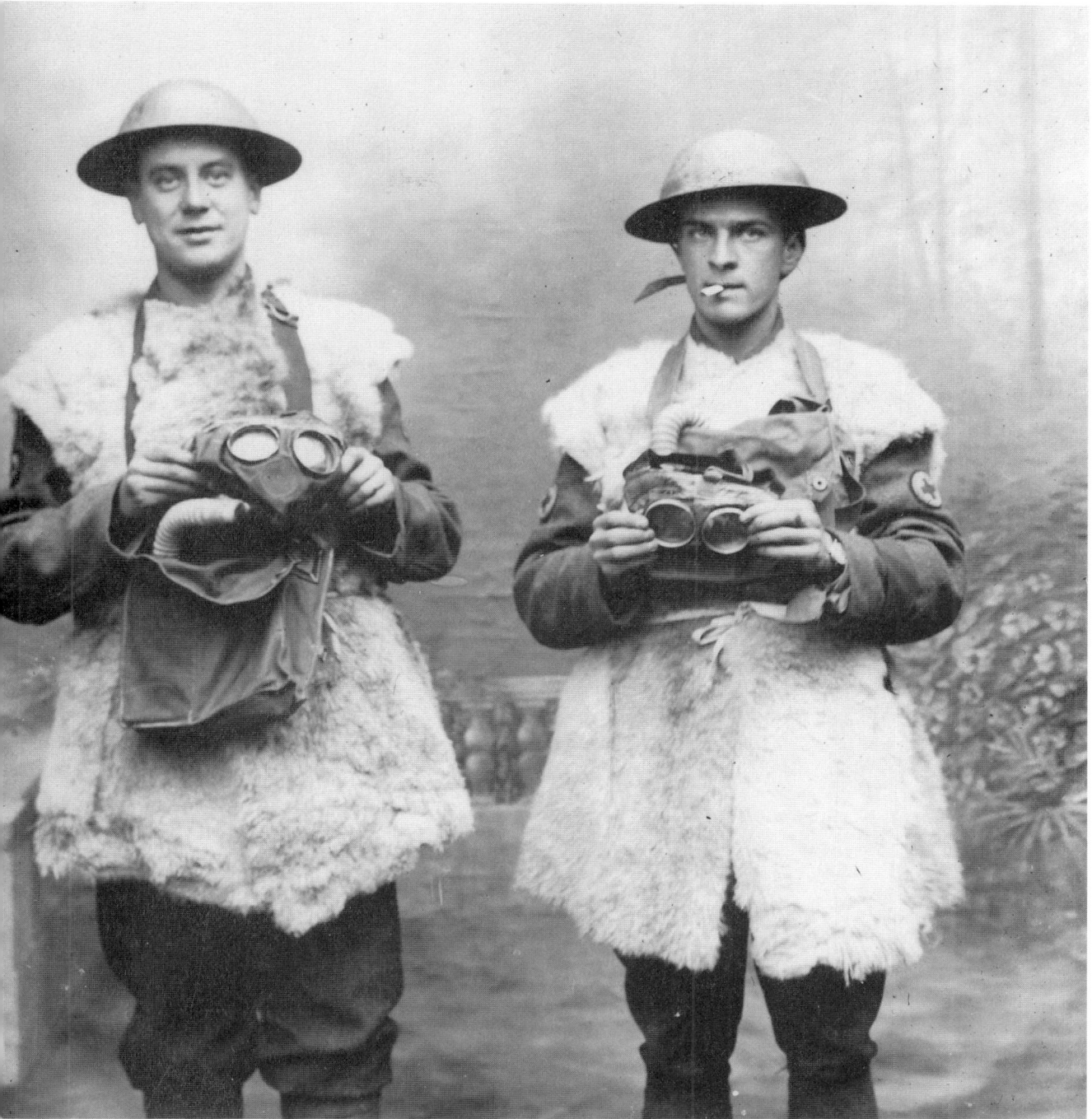

RAMC personnel on the Western Front, wearing goatskin tunics and with Small Box Respirators. The Small Box Respirator was first introduced in August 1916 and was standard issue by the spring of 1917. It consisted of a face mask with glass eye-pieces, which was connected to a metal 'small box' filter (containing active charcoal and granules) with a flexible hose. The contents of the filter provided protection against the concentrations of different gases likely to be encountered in combat. Worn on the chest in the 'alert' position, the pack could be opened and the mask worn quickly, saving vital time during a gas attack.

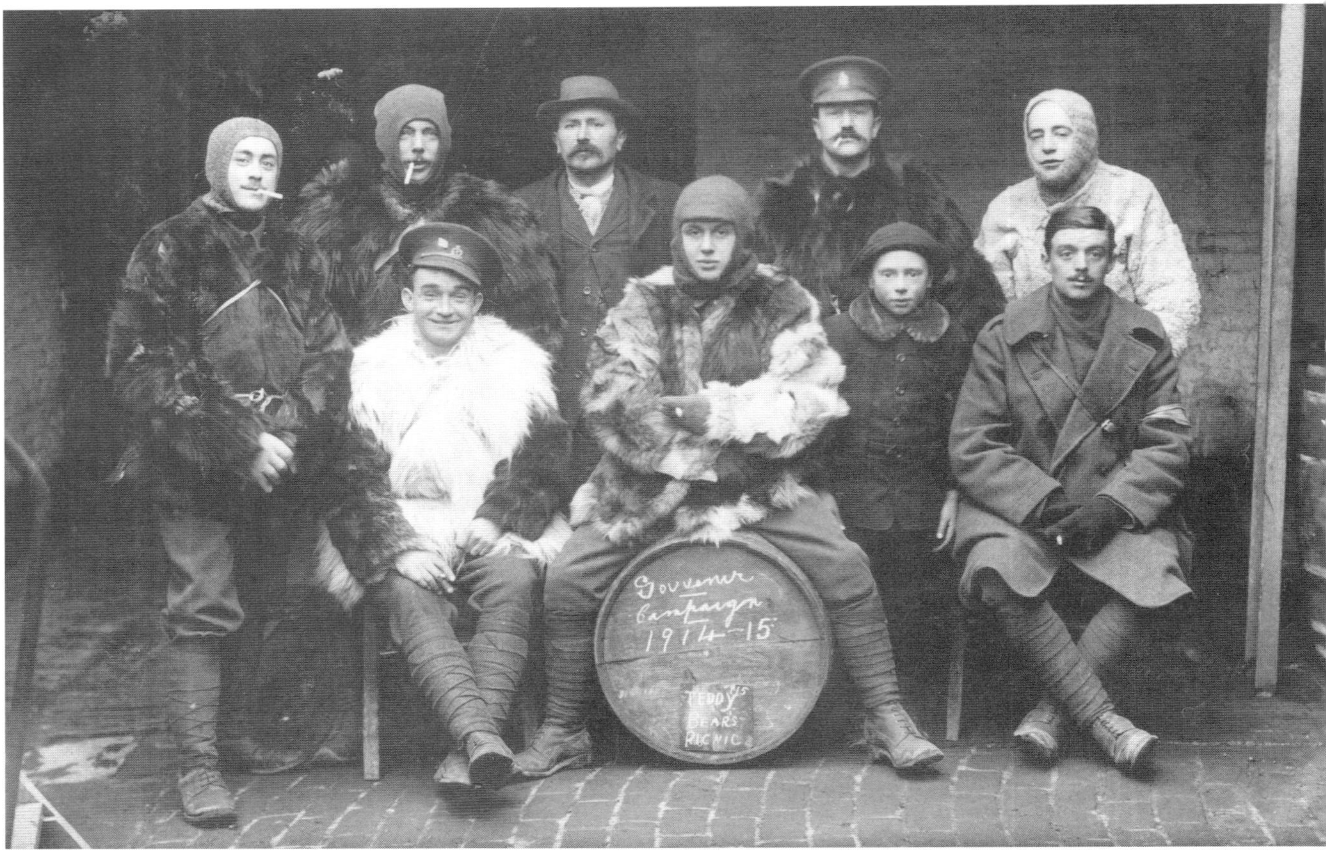

RAMC personnel in France wearing winter goatskins and caps. On the barrel is inscribed 'Souvenir Campaign 1914–15' and 'Teddy Bears Picnic'. Also photographed with the group are local French civilians. *(Mr Andrew Read)*

RAMC personnel at Vignacourt, France, 1916. A chaplain is seated in the centre of the group.

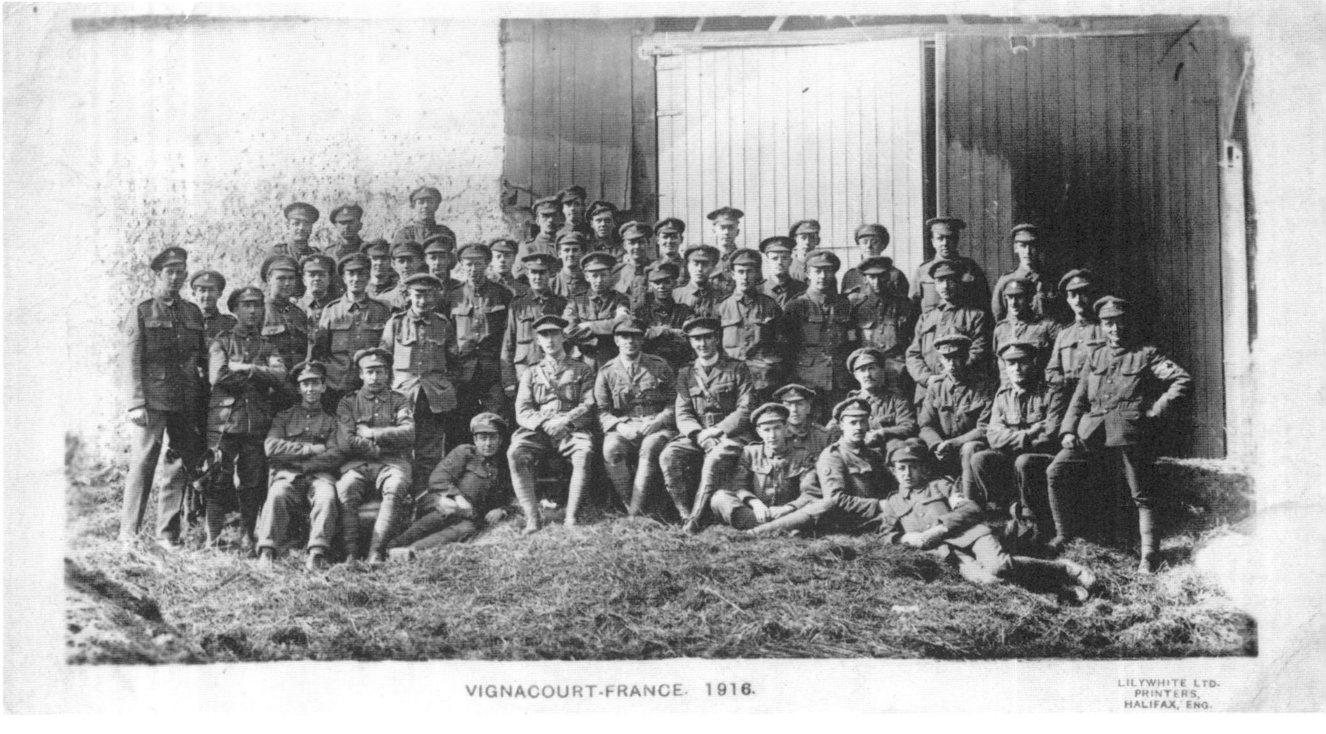

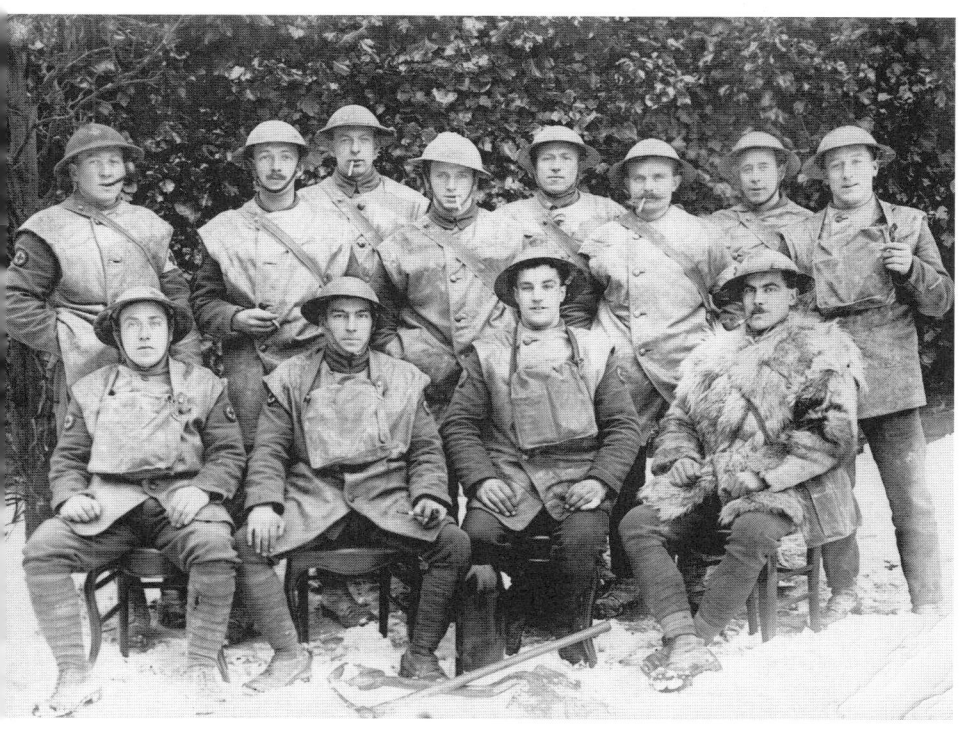

RAMC personnel, of the 36th Field Ambulance, wearing jerkins and with Small Box Respirators. Inscribed on the reverse: '36 FA, 'A' Sec Working Party attached to New Zealand Tunnelling Company at work in Caves at Arras'.
(Mr Andrew Read)

The 103rd Field Ambulance, RAMC, November 1918. The soldiers wear the square chequered divisional patches of 34th Division below their shoulders. This division served on the Western Front from January 1916, suffering very heavy casualties at La Boiselle on 1 July 1916. The division included the Tyneside Scottish Brigade and the Tyneside Irish Brigade. The 34th Division lost over 41,000 killed, wounded and missing on the Western Front.

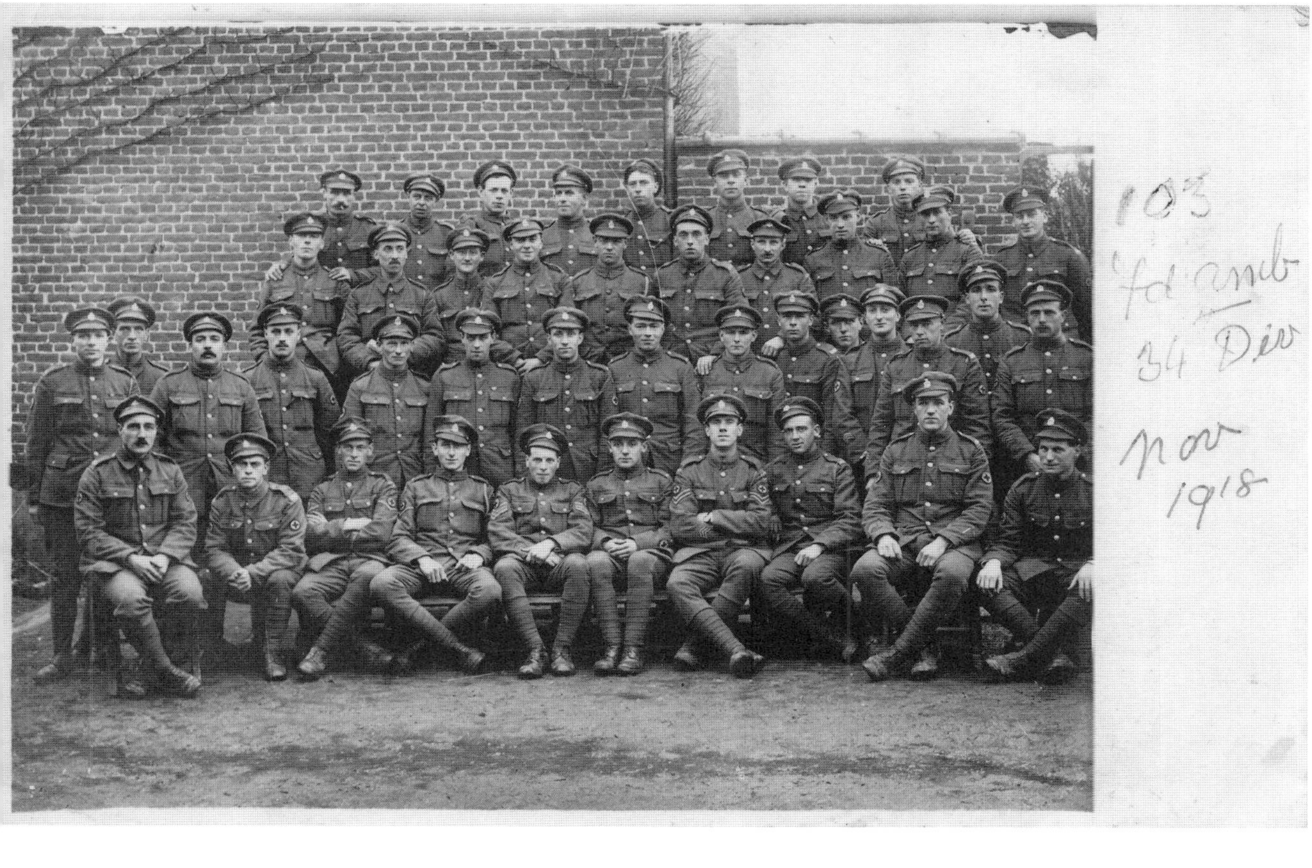

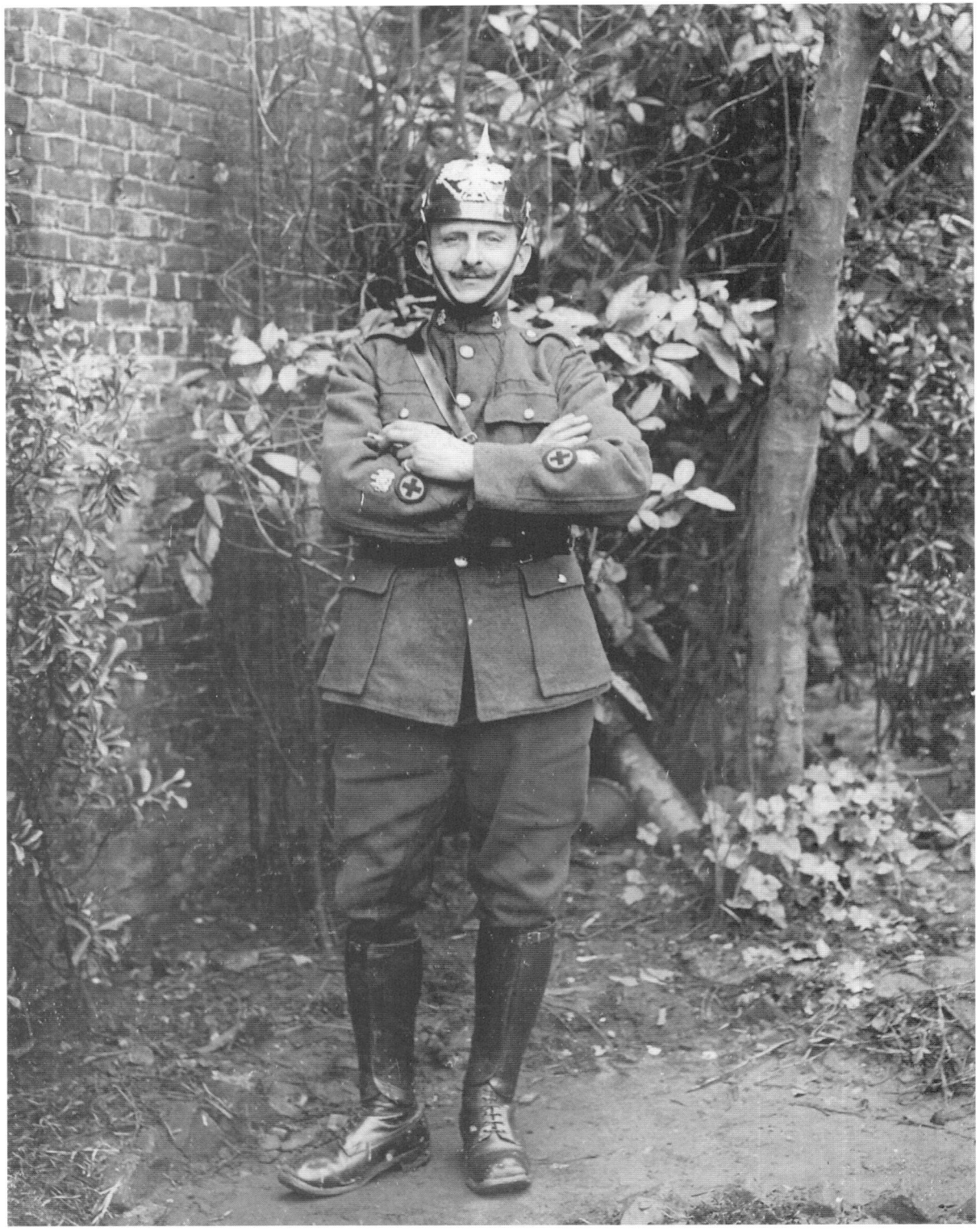
A RAMC warrant officer on the Western Front, wearing a German pickelhaube.

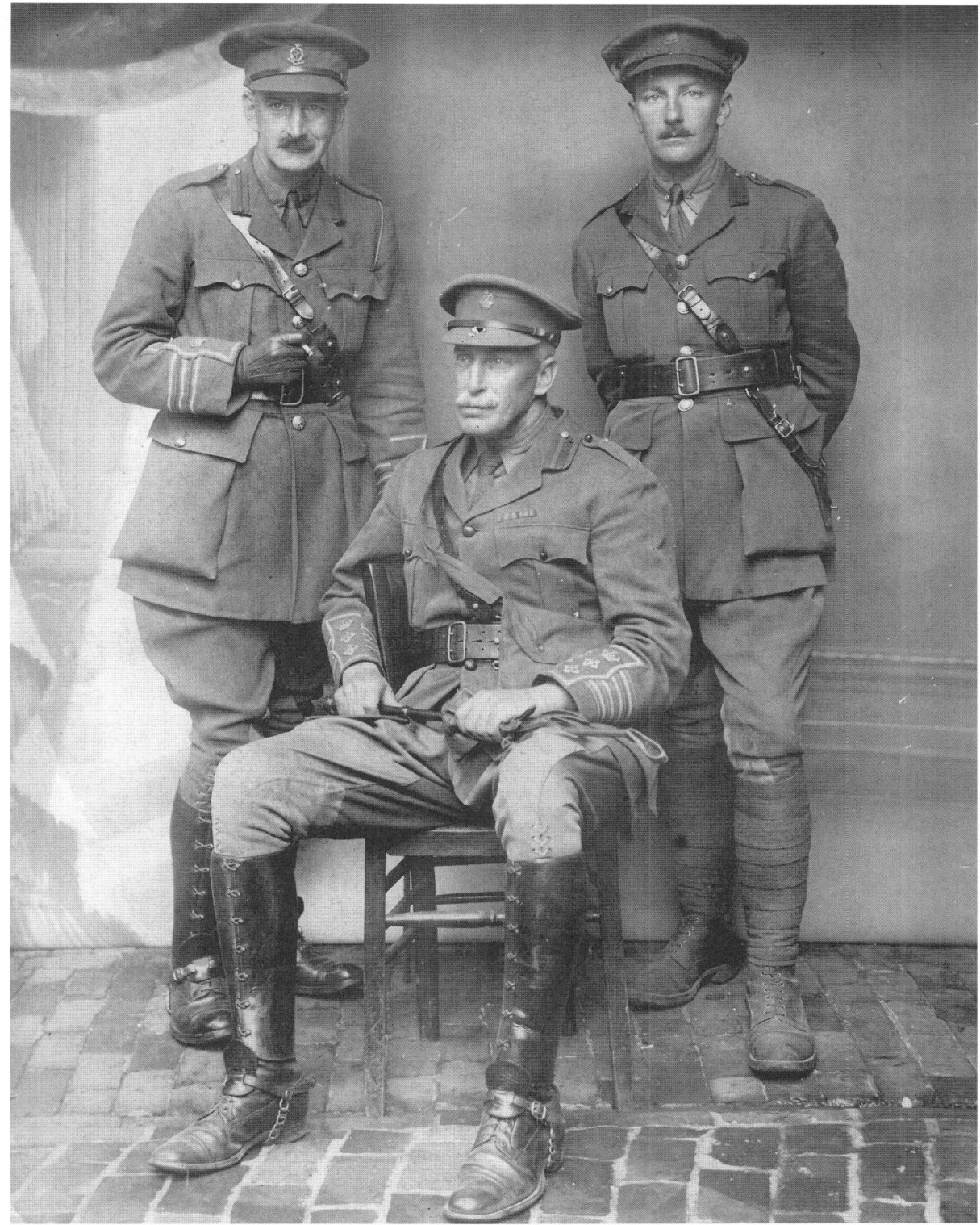
Three staff officers on the Western Front. To the left is a RAMC major and a staff officer, with the rank of colonel, is seated.

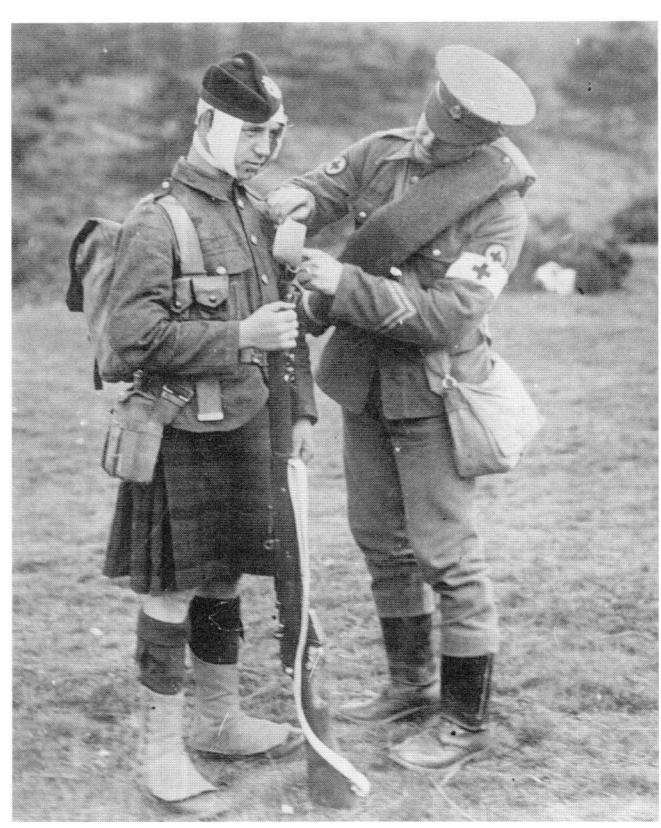

A soldier serving with the Cameron Highlanders having a Field Medical Card attached by a RAMC orderly, photographed in Belgium. (*Mr Andrew Read*)

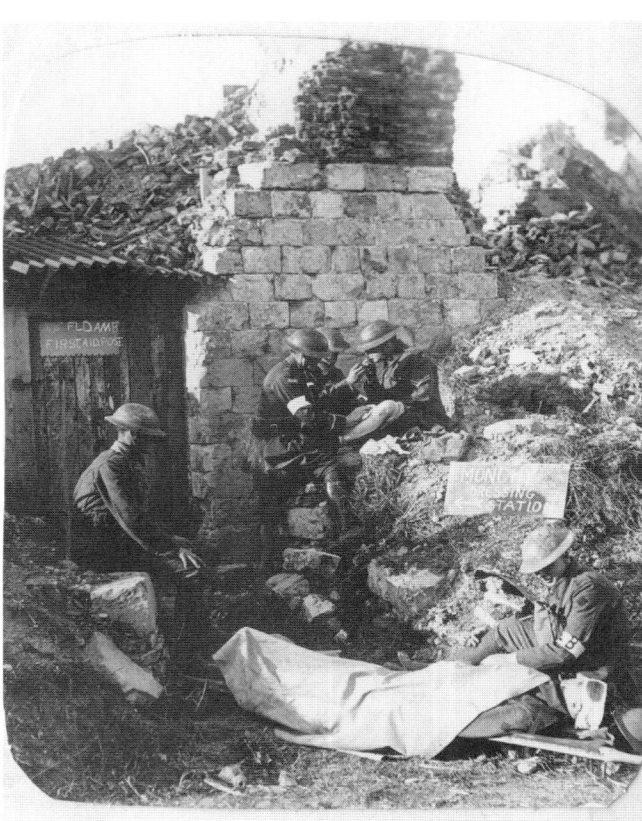

A dressing Station of 46th Field Ambulance RAMC, Monchy, France. (*Mr Andrew Read*)

RAMC stretcher bearers with a casualty, photographed in Belgium. (*Mr Andrew Read*)

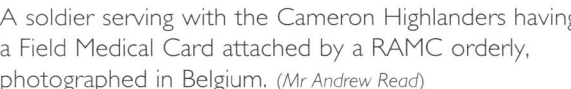

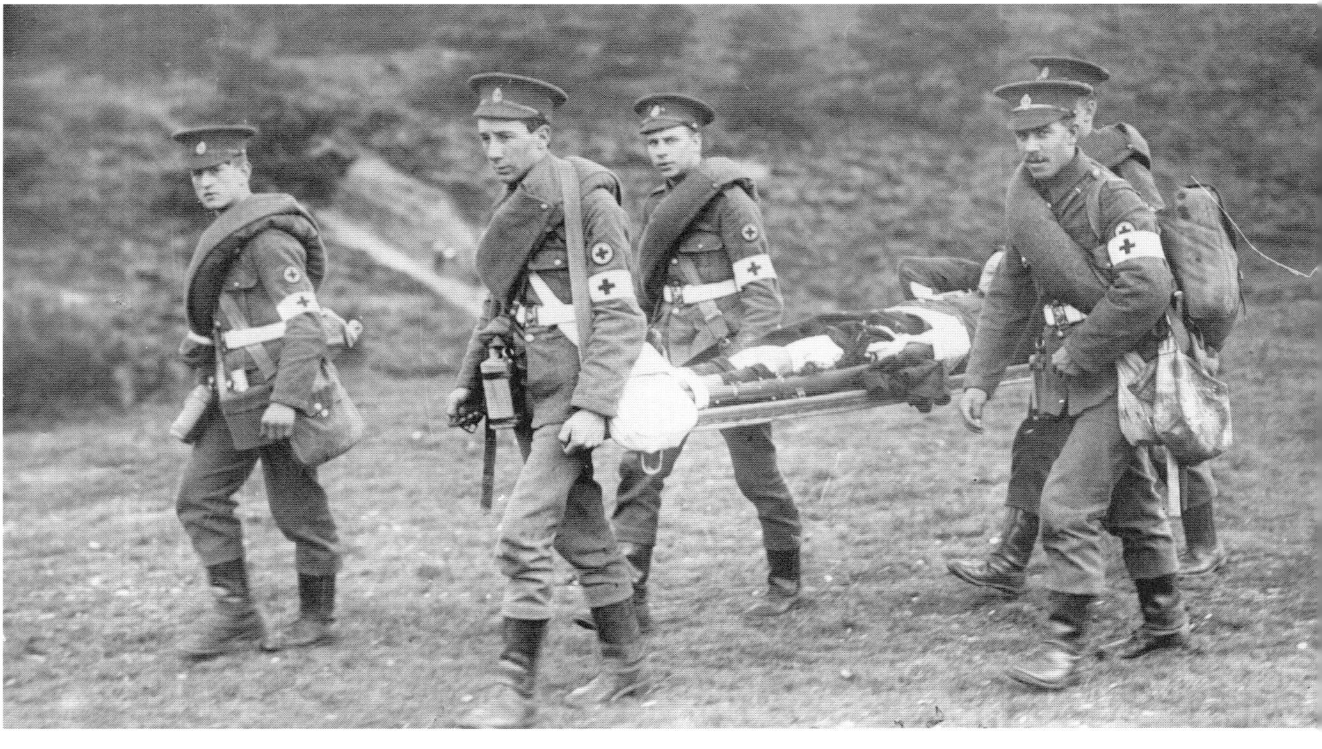

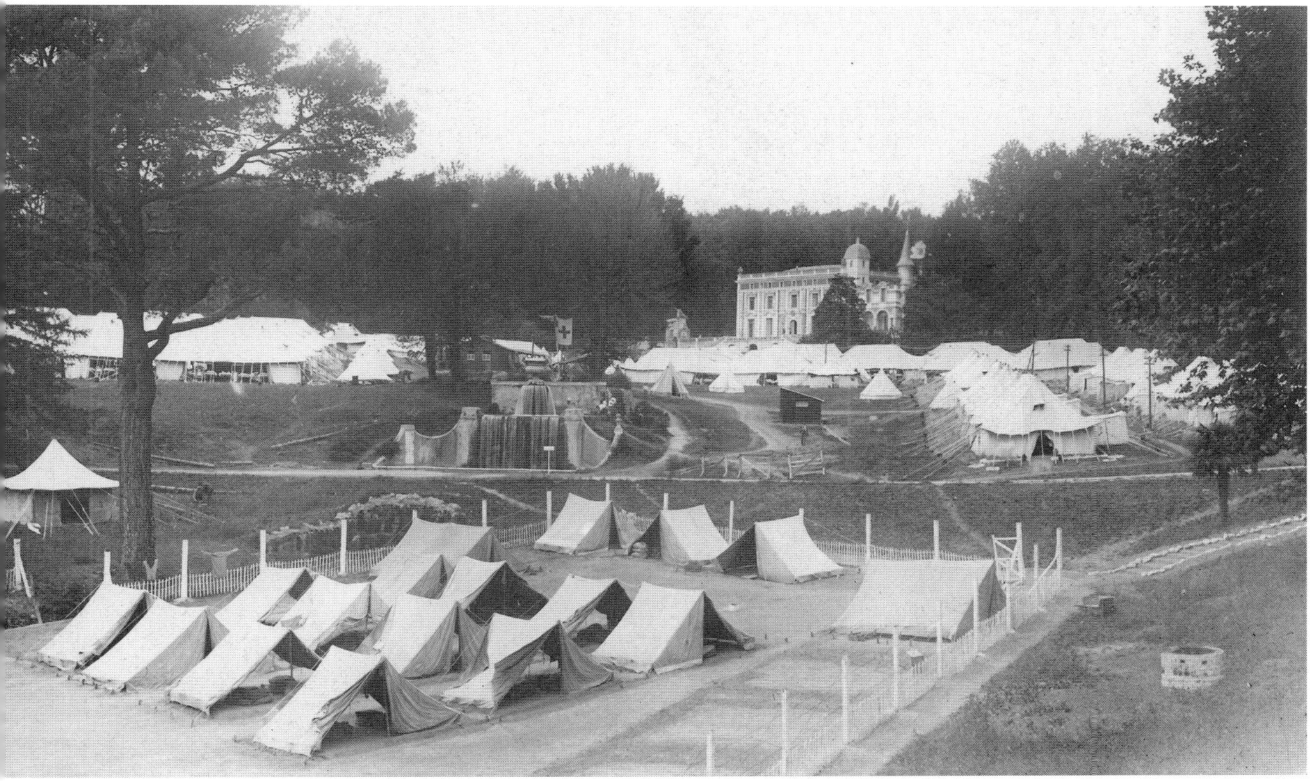

A British field medical facility on the Western Front.

Nurses serving with Queens Alexandra's Imperial Military Nursing Service (QAIMNS), at a Western Front field medical facility.

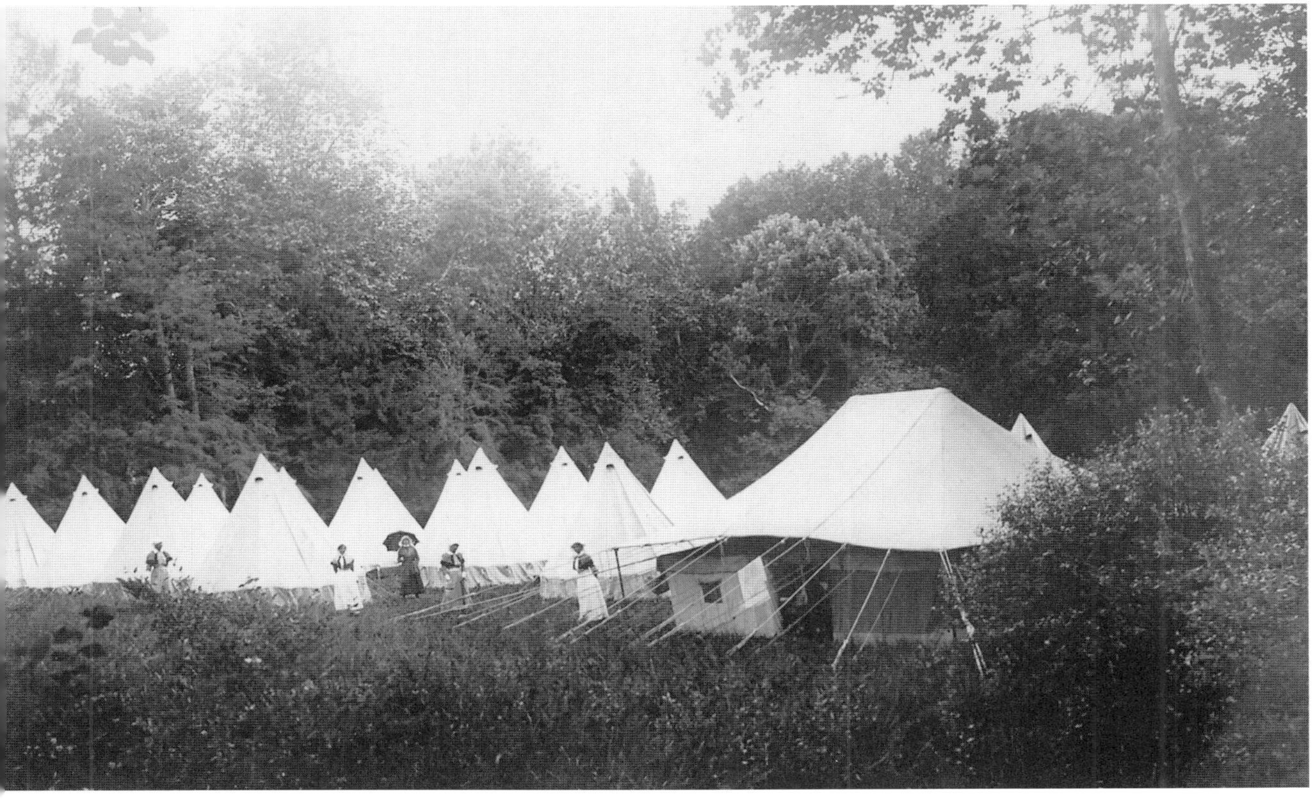

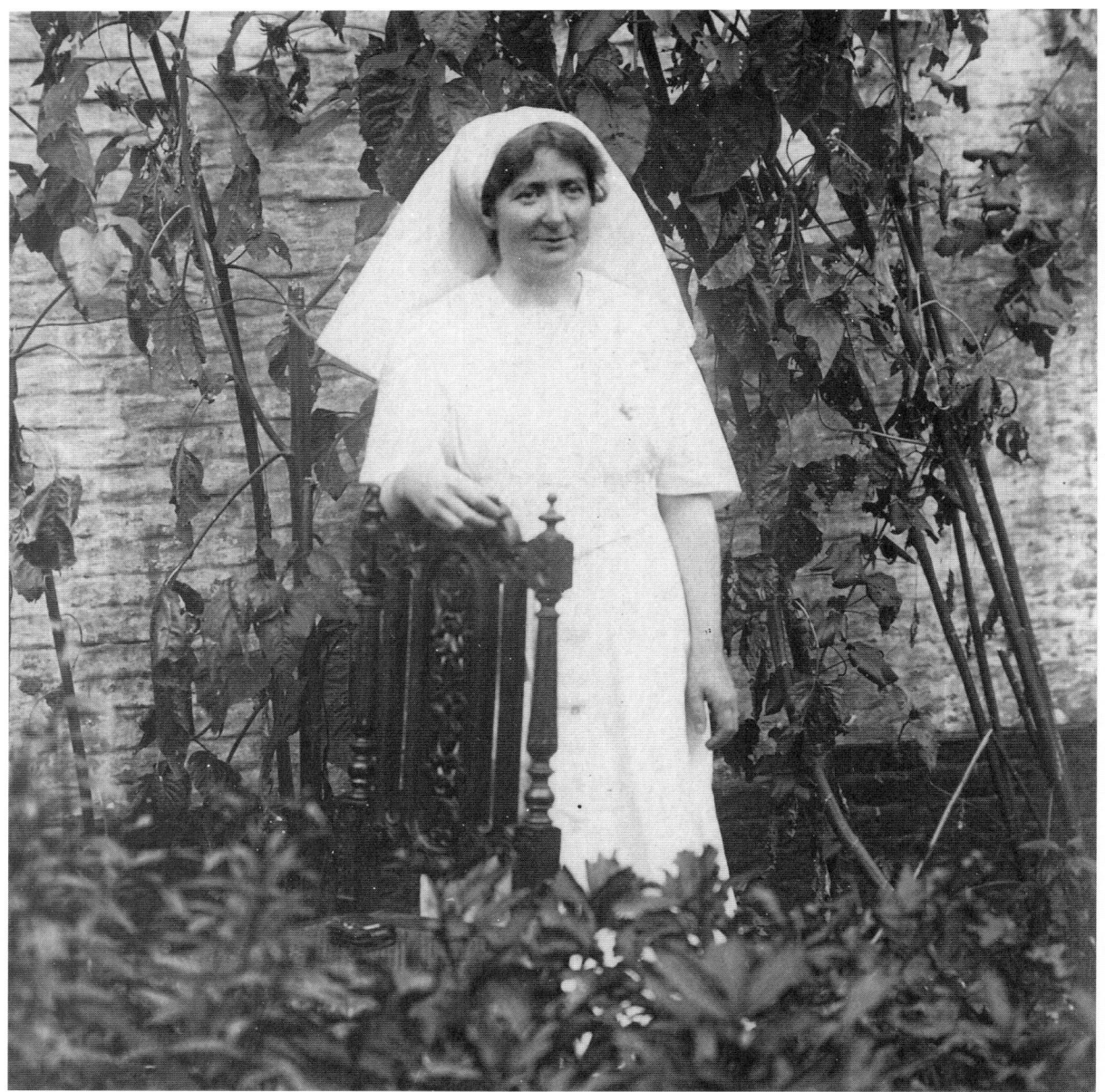

Sister Enid Rose Pilson, Royal Red Cross (RRC), Territorial Force Nursing Service (TFNS), photographed on the Western Front where she was an operating theatre sister. Living in London, Sister Pilson served at the 4th London General Hospital, RAMC (TF) located at Denmark Hill, London. She joined the TFNS in 1909 and was mobilised for war service on 17 August 1914. Sister Pilson served on the Western Front from 20 January 1915 and was attached to the 2nd Casualty Clearing Station RAMC and, later, the 1st Portuguese General Hospital. On 29 November 1917 she was admitted to the 10th Stationary Hospital, St Omer, from the 54th Casualty Clearing Station, suffering from tonsillitis. Sister Pilson was demobilised on 25 April 1919. She was awarded the Royal Red Cross (First Class) in June 1919 for her good work and valuable nursing services during the First World War. She was also awarded the *Médaille de la Reconnaissance Française en Bronze*, by the French Government, for devoted services to French civilians during the First World War. In 1920 she moved to South Africa to live with her sister. In 1921 Sister Pilson was working at the Nightingale Nursing Home, East London, Cape Province, South Africa.

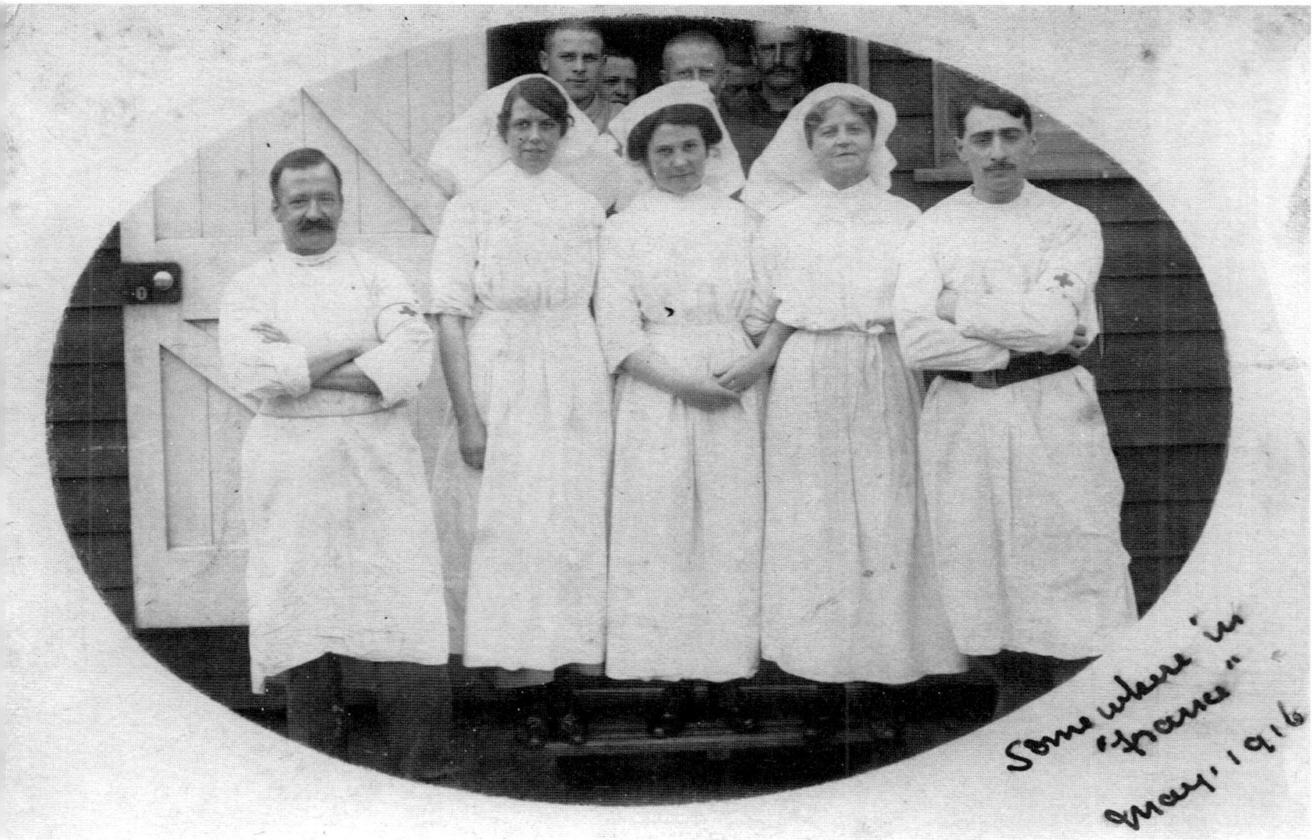

Nurses and RAMC personnel wearing surgical gowns photographed in France, May 1916.

Ambulances damaged by shellfire on the Western Front, 22 March 1918, during the Spring Offensive. (*Mr Andrew Read*)

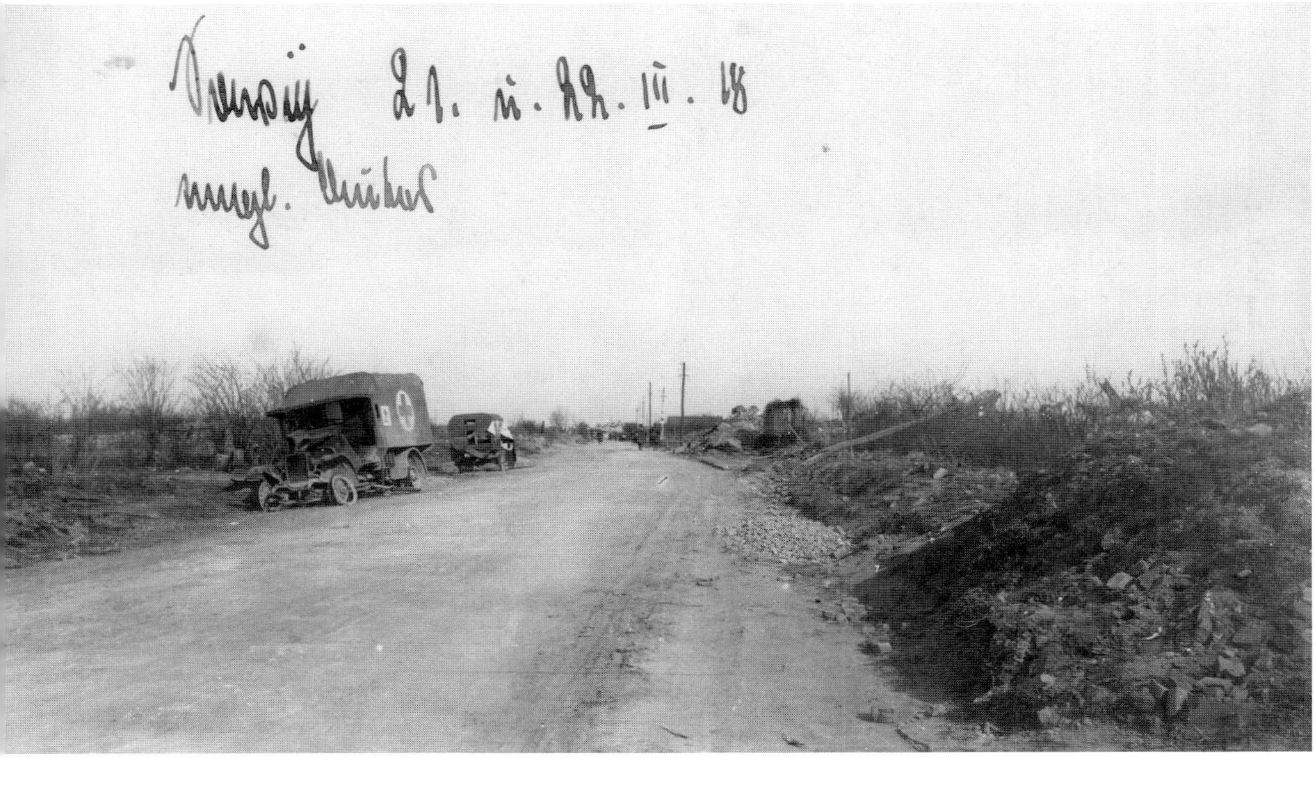

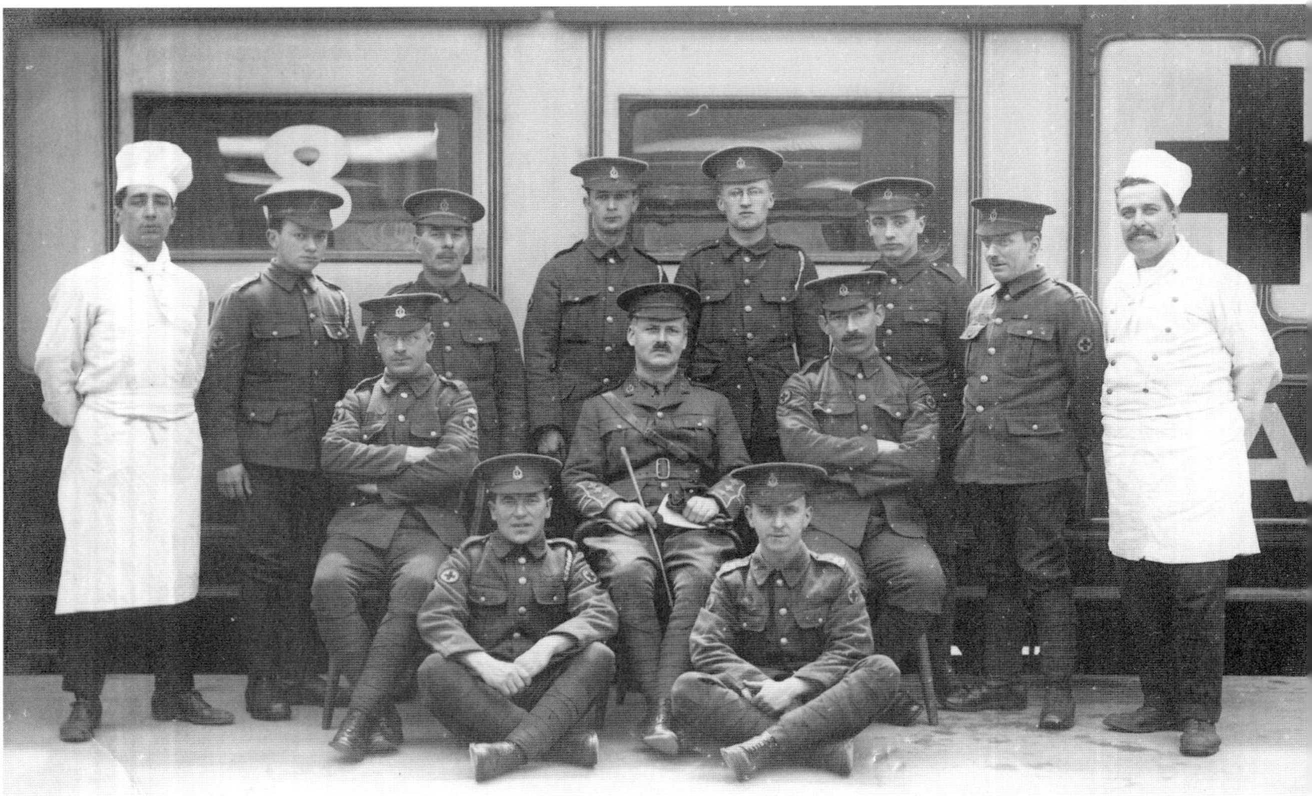

RAMC personnel in front of an ambulance train carriage.

The interior of an ambulance train carriage.

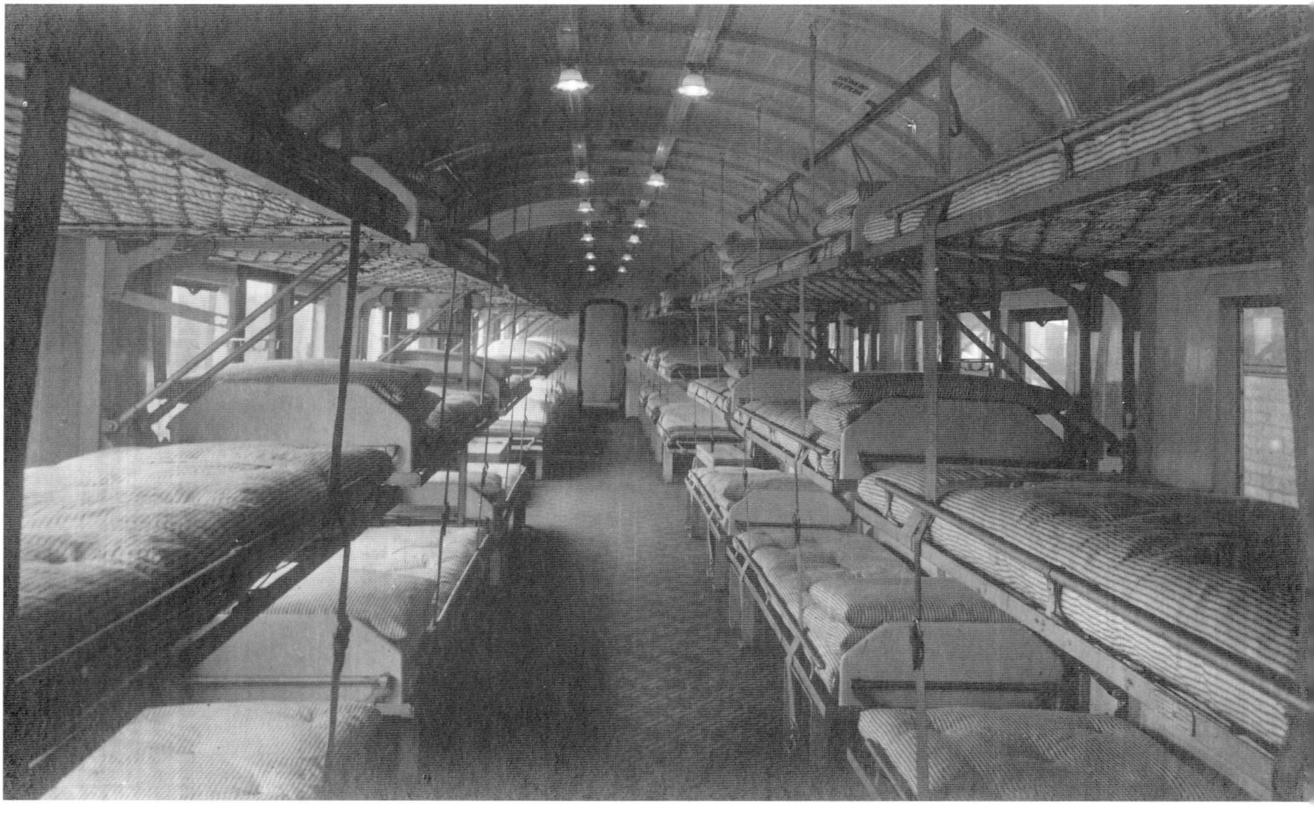

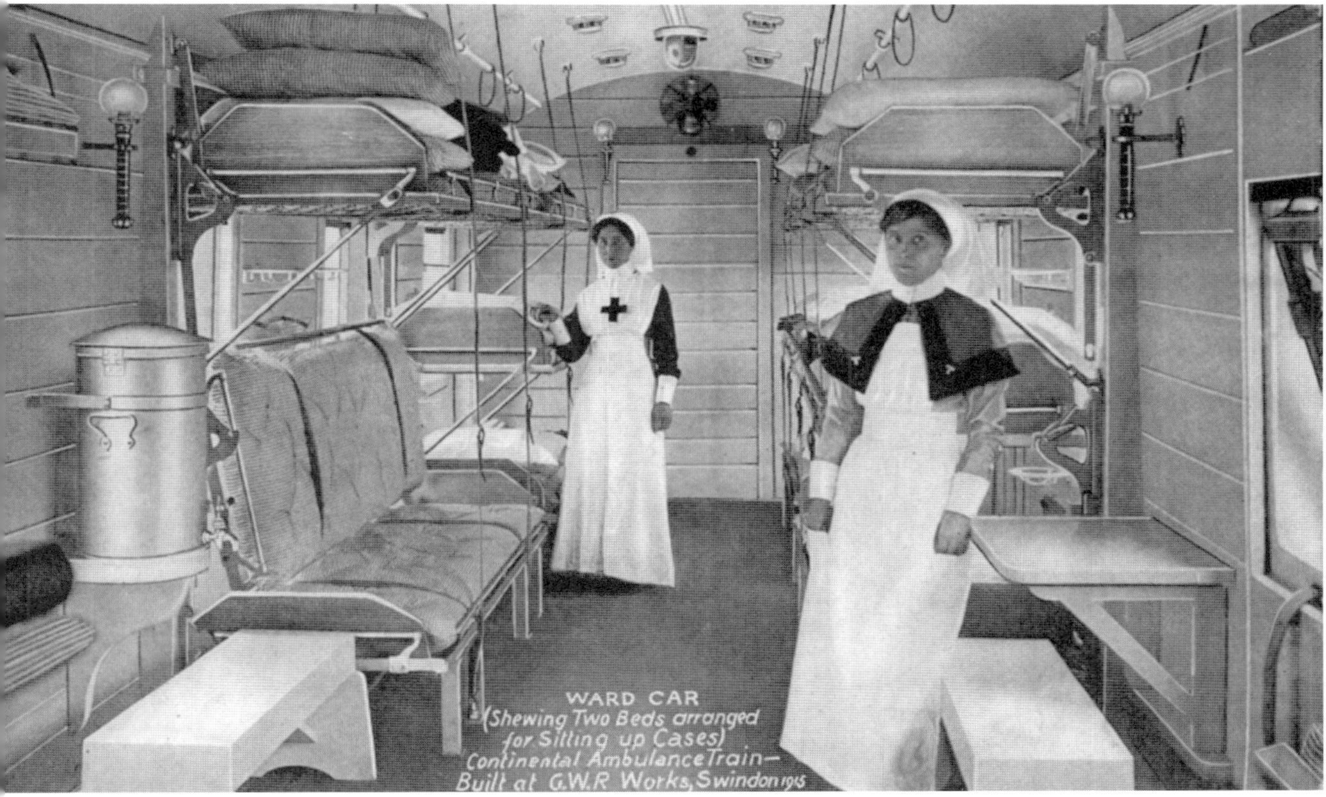

Beds arranged for seated patients in an ambulance train.

The treatment room in an ambulance train.

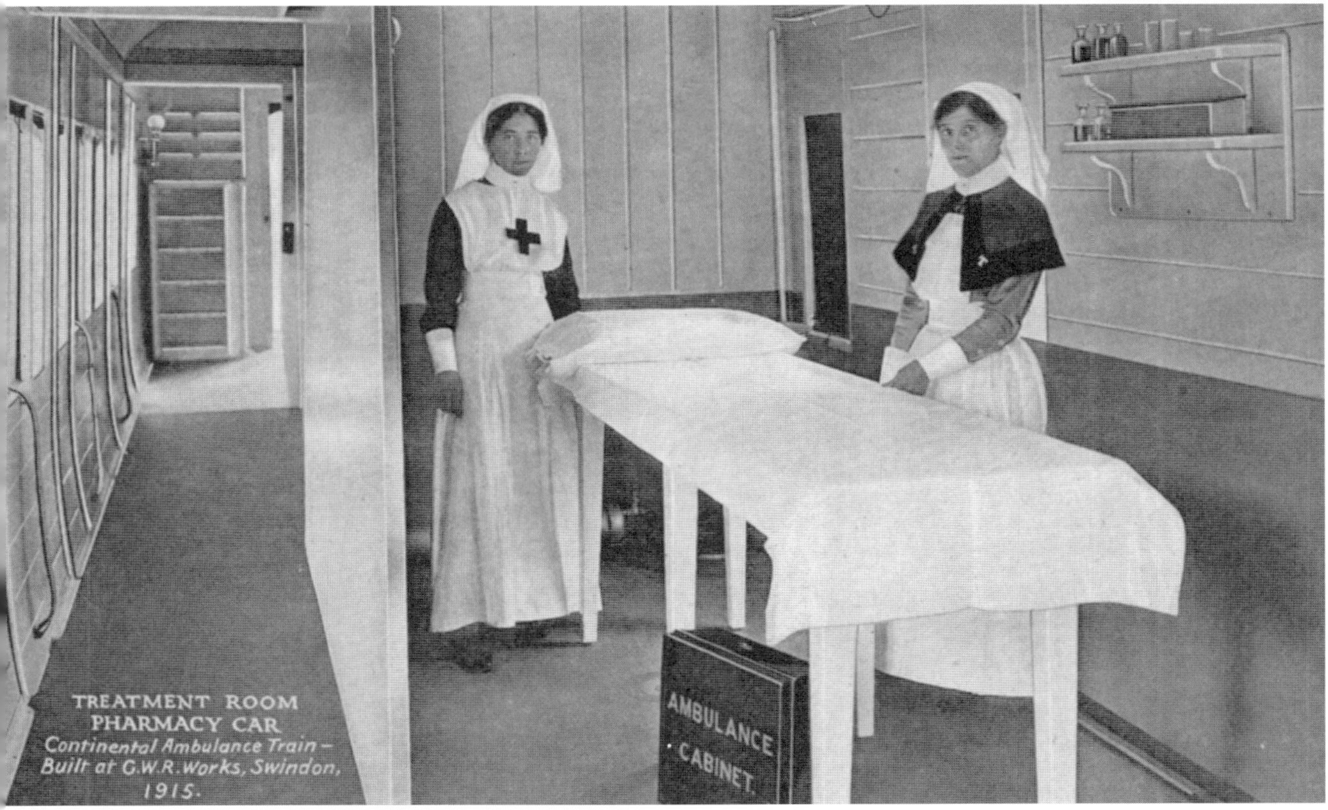

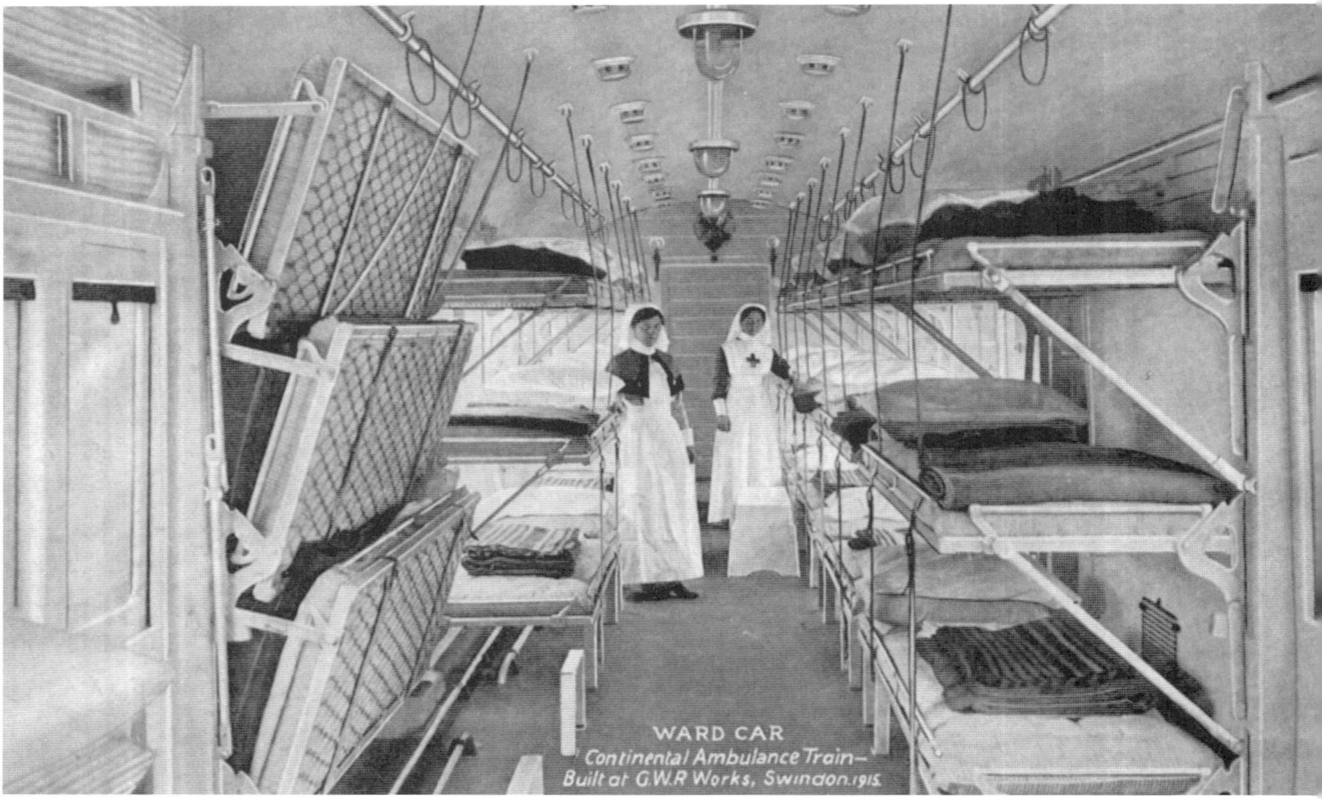

The interior of an ambulance train carriage, with some of the beds folded.

Personnel of 32nd Ambulance Train, RAMC, on the Western Front.

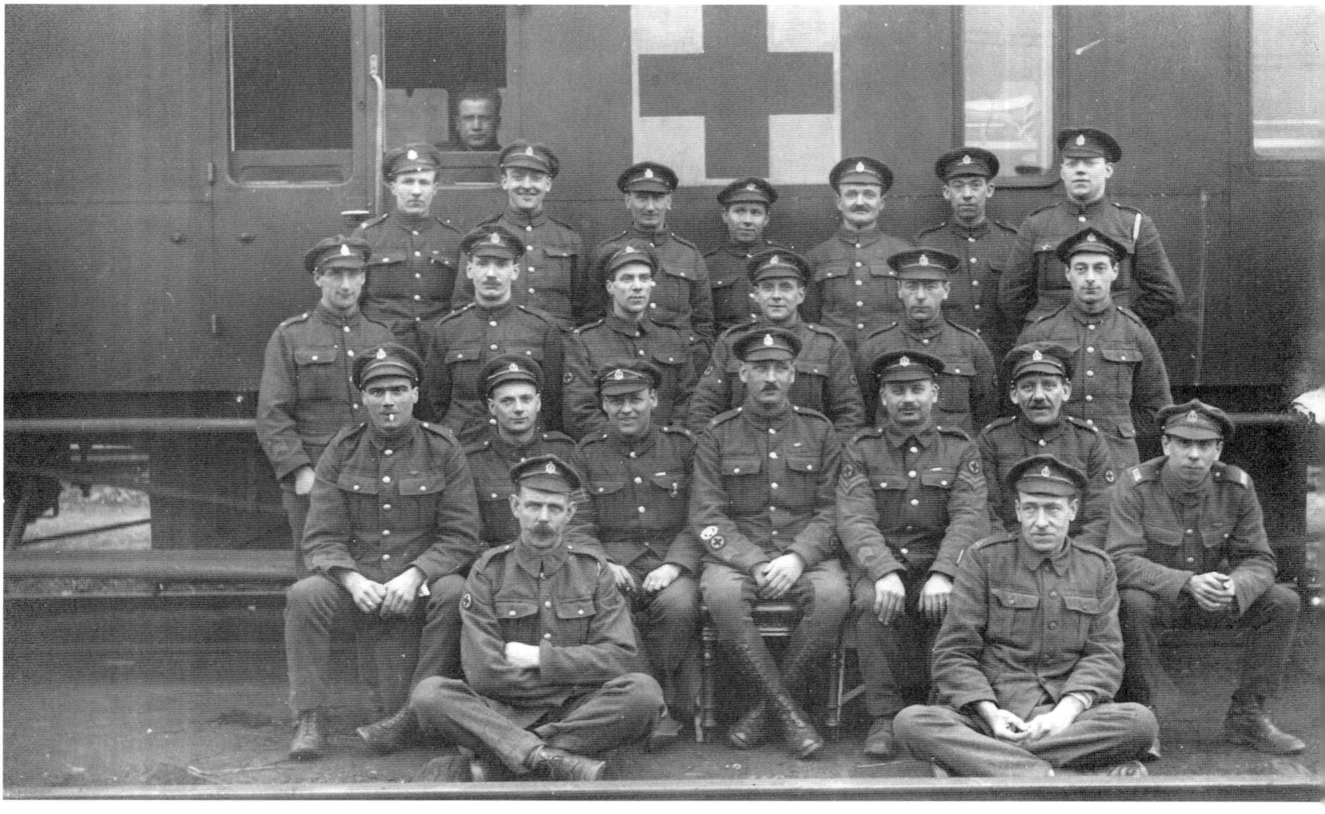

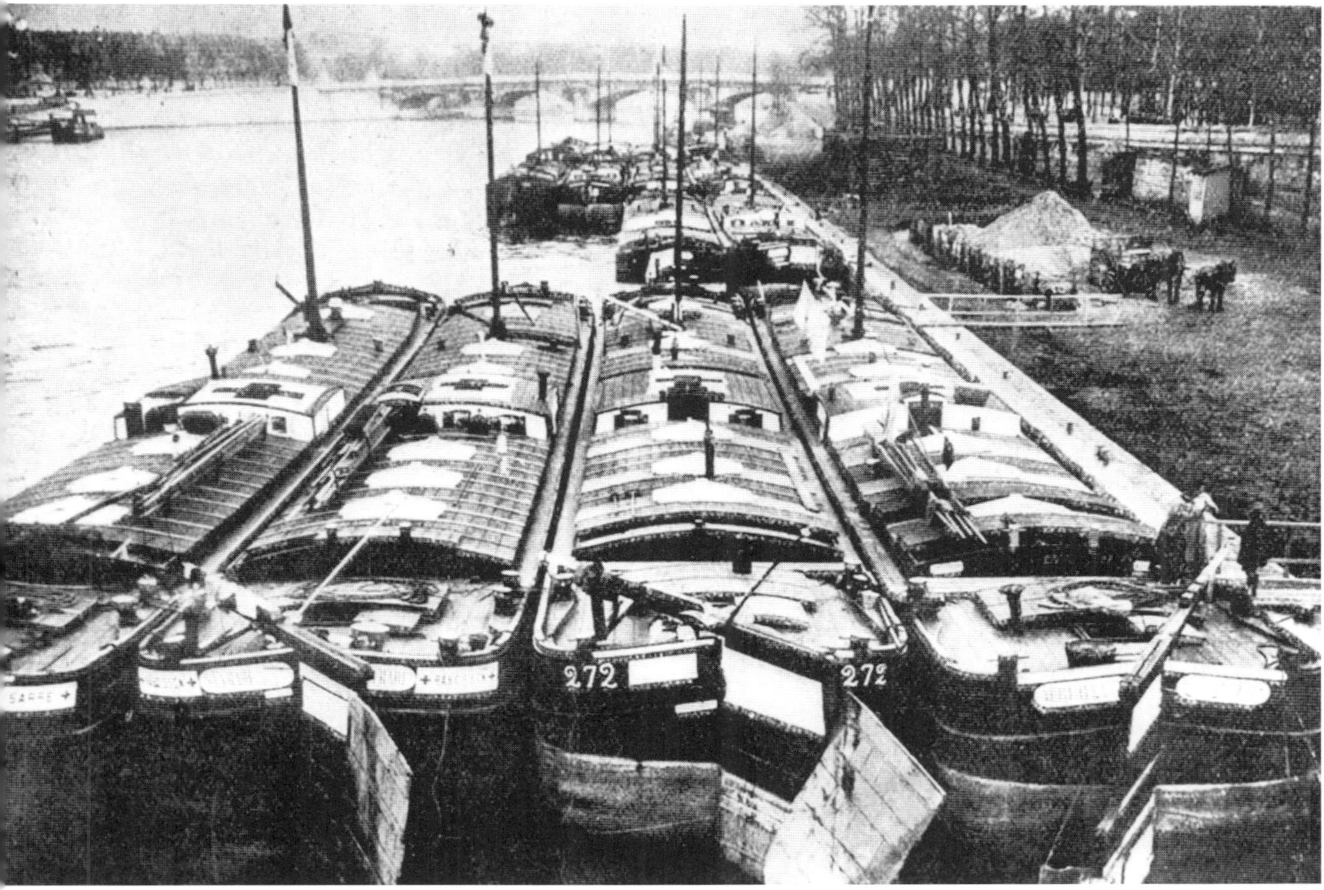

Four ambulance barges on the River Seine, France. The Red Cross emblem is visible on each barge. (*The British Red Cross Society*)

A nurse in the ward of an ambulance barge on the River Seine, France. (*The British Red Cross Society*)

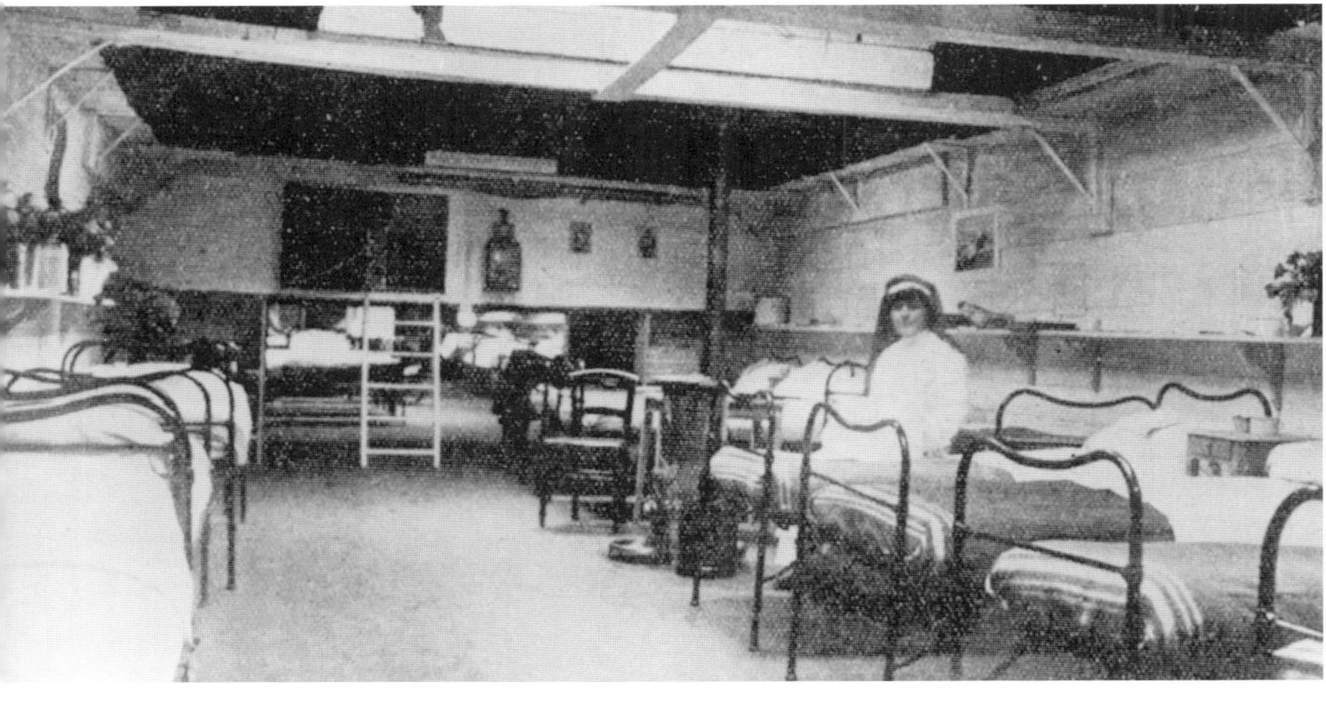

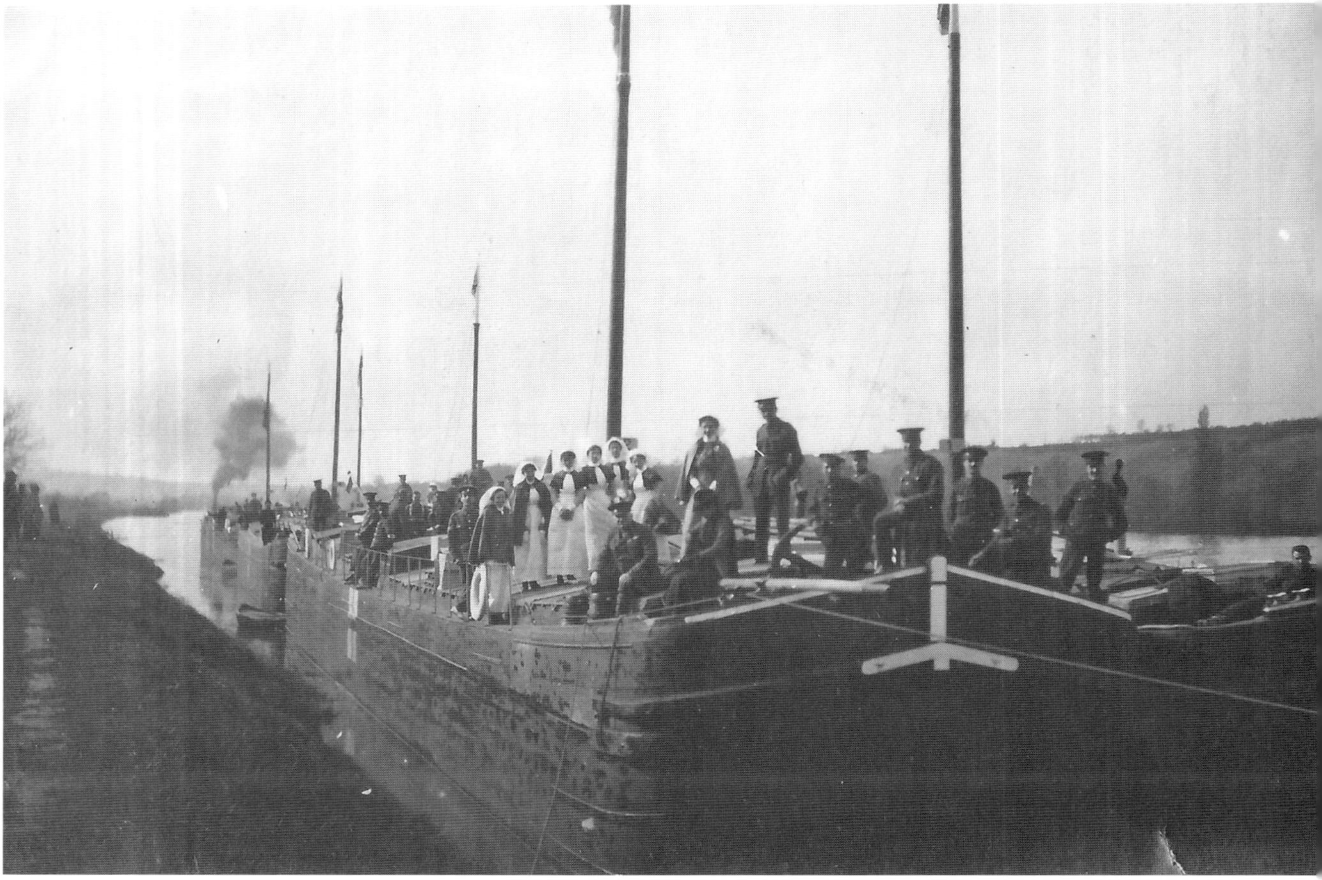

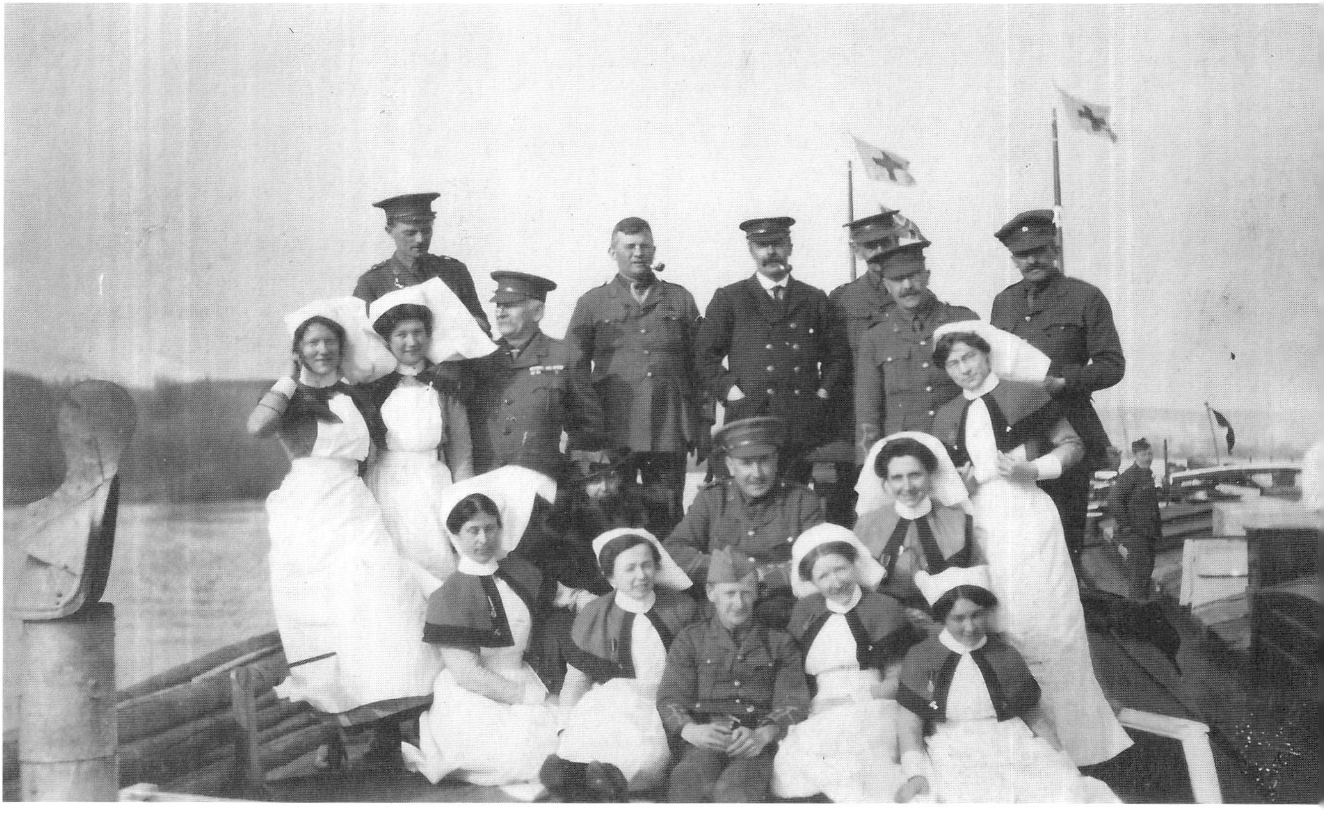

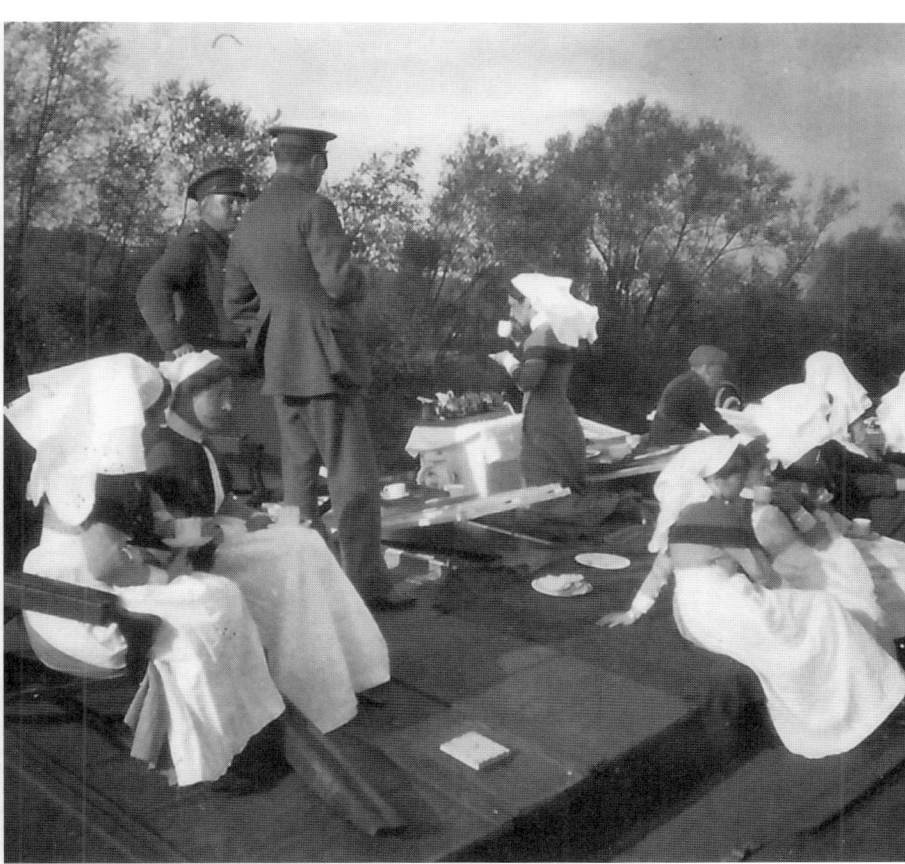

Afternoon tea on No. 1 Ambulance Flotilla, on the River Seine, Spring 1915. Acting Matron Kate Read is kneeling in the centre of the photo, by the tray of teapots. *(Army Medical Services Museum)*

(**Opposite, above**) No. 1 Ambulance Flotilla, on the River Seine, France, 1915. Nurses and RAMC personnel are standing on the decks of the barges. This, and the following six photographs, form part of the Kate Read Collection held at the Army Medical Services Museum. Sister Kate Read, A.R.R.C., Queen Alexandra's Imperial Military Nursing Service Reserve, served with No. 1 Ambulance Flotilla from April to October 1915. *(Army Medical Services Museum)*

(**Opposite, below**) Visitors and medical staff on board No. 1 Ambulance Flotilla; Red Cross flags can be seen flying from the barges. On the reverse of this photo Sister Read noted their names. Back row (left to right): Mr Gossip – Medical Officer; Colonel Yate – Medical Practitioner; Mr Greenfield – Medical Officer; Captain Bowes – The Skipper; Mr Boyle – Medical Practitioner; Mr Mulholland – Medical Officer; Mr Grant – Medical Practitioner. Middle row (left to right): Sister Coulson; Sister Mills; Mrs Yate; Captain O'Grady; Acting Matron Kate Read; Sister Bayly. Front row (left to right): Sister Cooke; Sister Draper; Mr Sainsbury; Sister Cameron; Sister Gibbens. The visitors included three volunteer Medical Practitioners, too old or unfit to join the army, who supported the medical services. *(Army Medical Services Museum)*

The ward in a barge of No. 1 Ambulance Flotilla, ready to receive casualties. A nursing sister and RAMC private are pictured. A bookcase, gramophone and plants help to make the ward more welcoming. (*Army Medical Services Museum*)

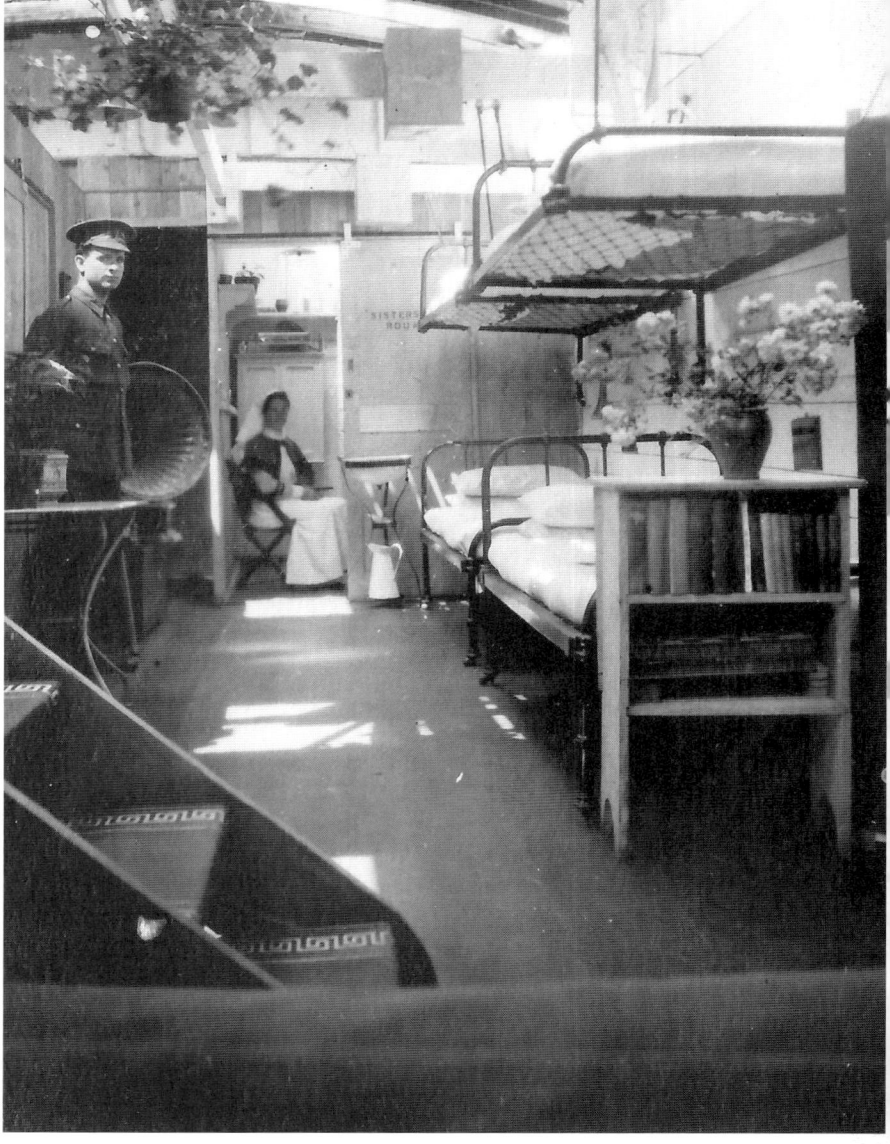

(**Opposite, above**) British Water Ambulance vehicles, with drivers and medical staff. They are waiting to be called to collect casualties from Ambulance Trains, who would then be transported to Rouen on the barges of the Ambulance Flotilla. (*Army Medical Services Museum*)

(**Opposite, below**) Sister Cooke and Sister Draper with patients of No. 1 Ambulance Flotilla. Awnings erected on the decks of the barges can be seen. (*Army Medical Services Museum*)

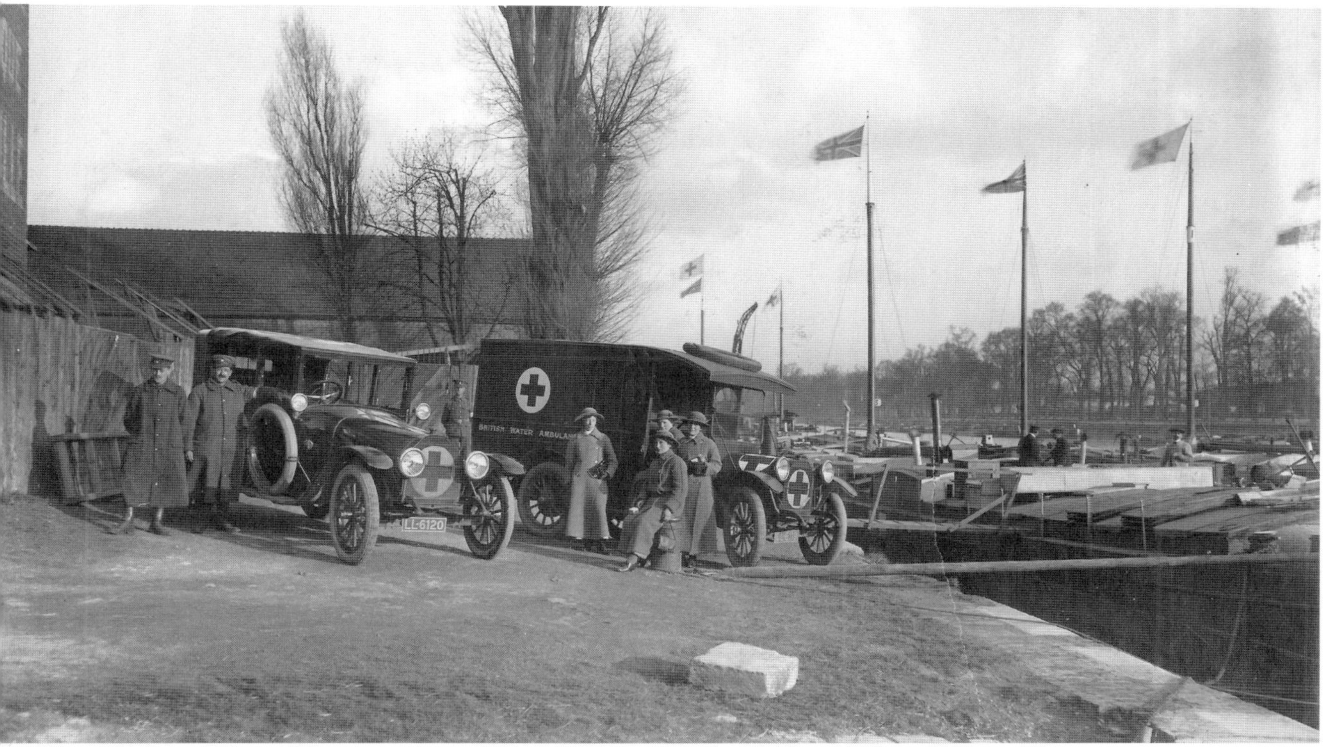

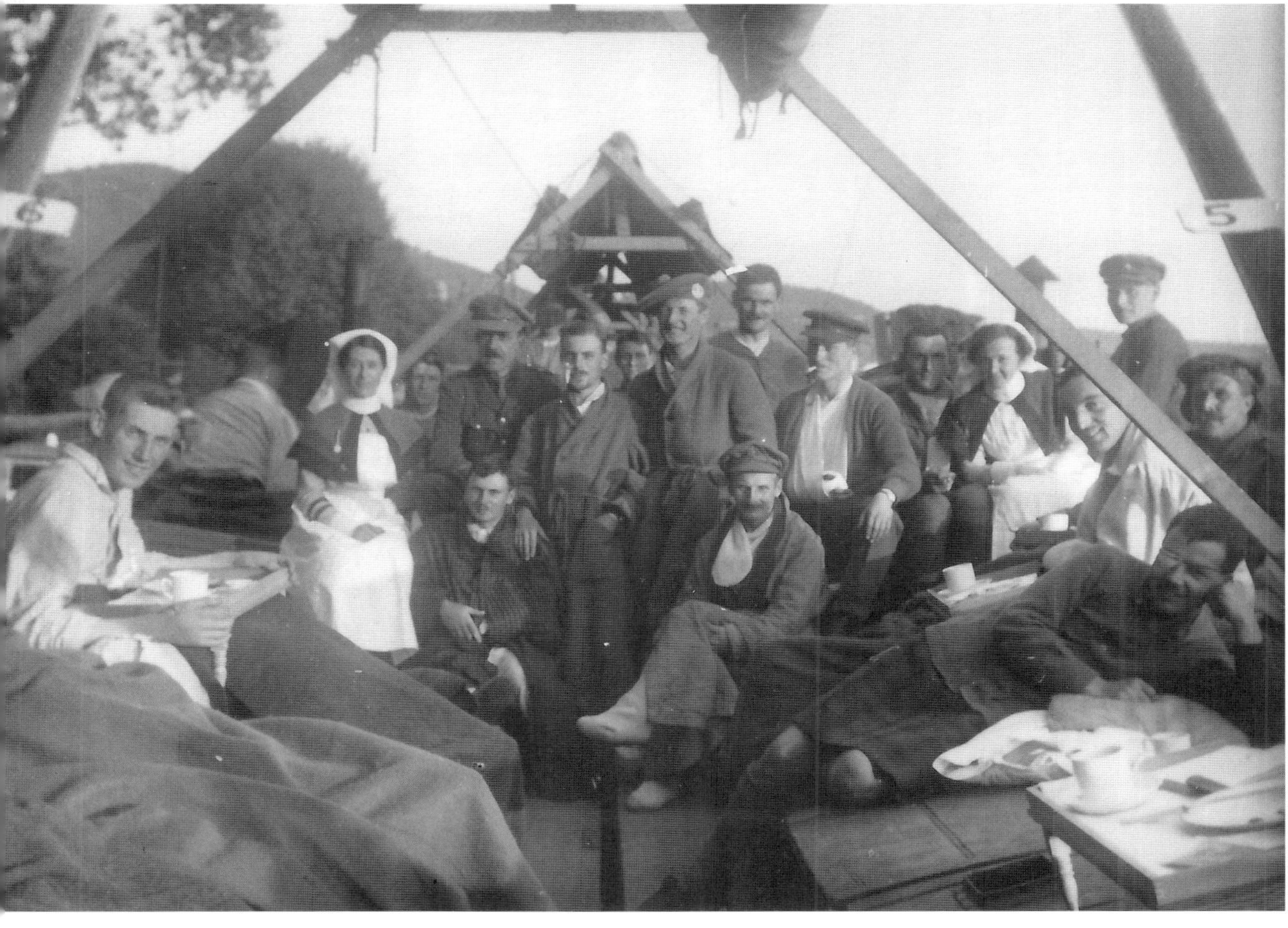

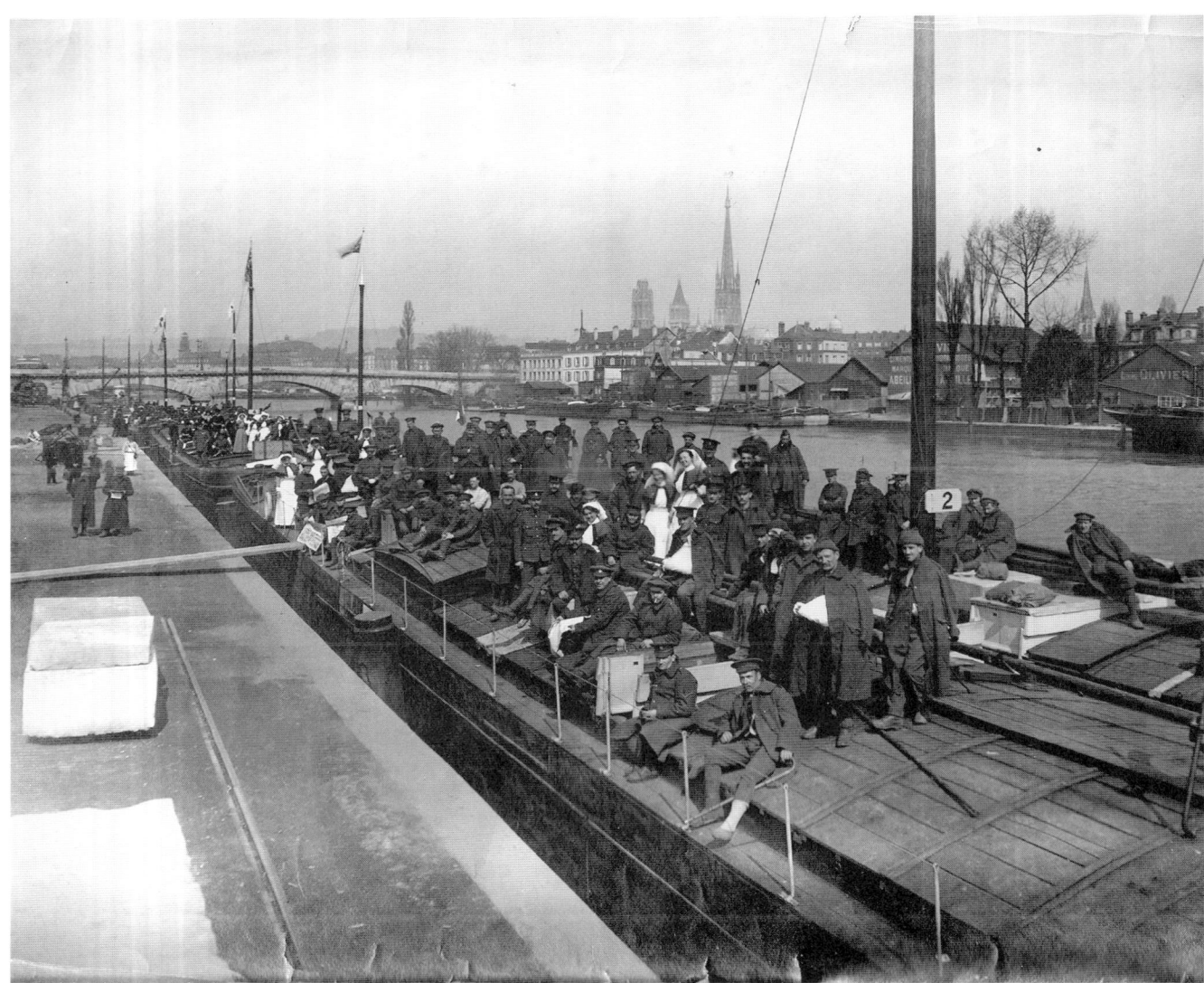

(**Above**) No. 1 Ambulance Flotilla moored at Rouen with staff and casualties still on board. The barges are moored at the quayside, Quai d'Elbeuf, now known as Quai Jacques Anquetil. The spires of Rouen Cathedral are visible in the distance. (*Army Medical Services Museum*)

(**Opposite, above**) A QAIMNS Reserve Staff Nurse and RAMC personnel on the Western Front.

(**Opposite, below**) RAMC officers and nursing staff of the QAIMNS and the QAIMNS Reserve. The photograph was taken on 17 April 1915, at No. 8 General Hospital, Rouen, France.

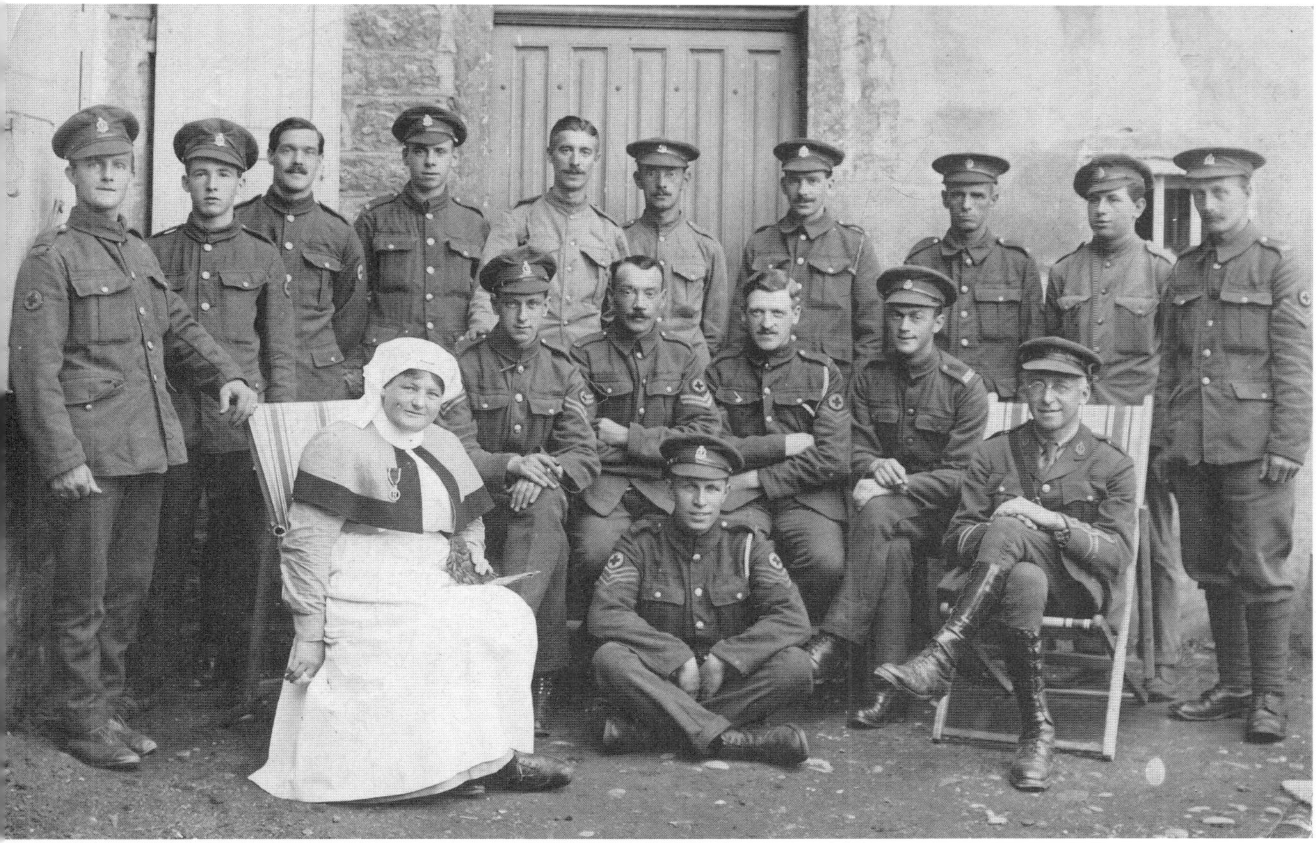

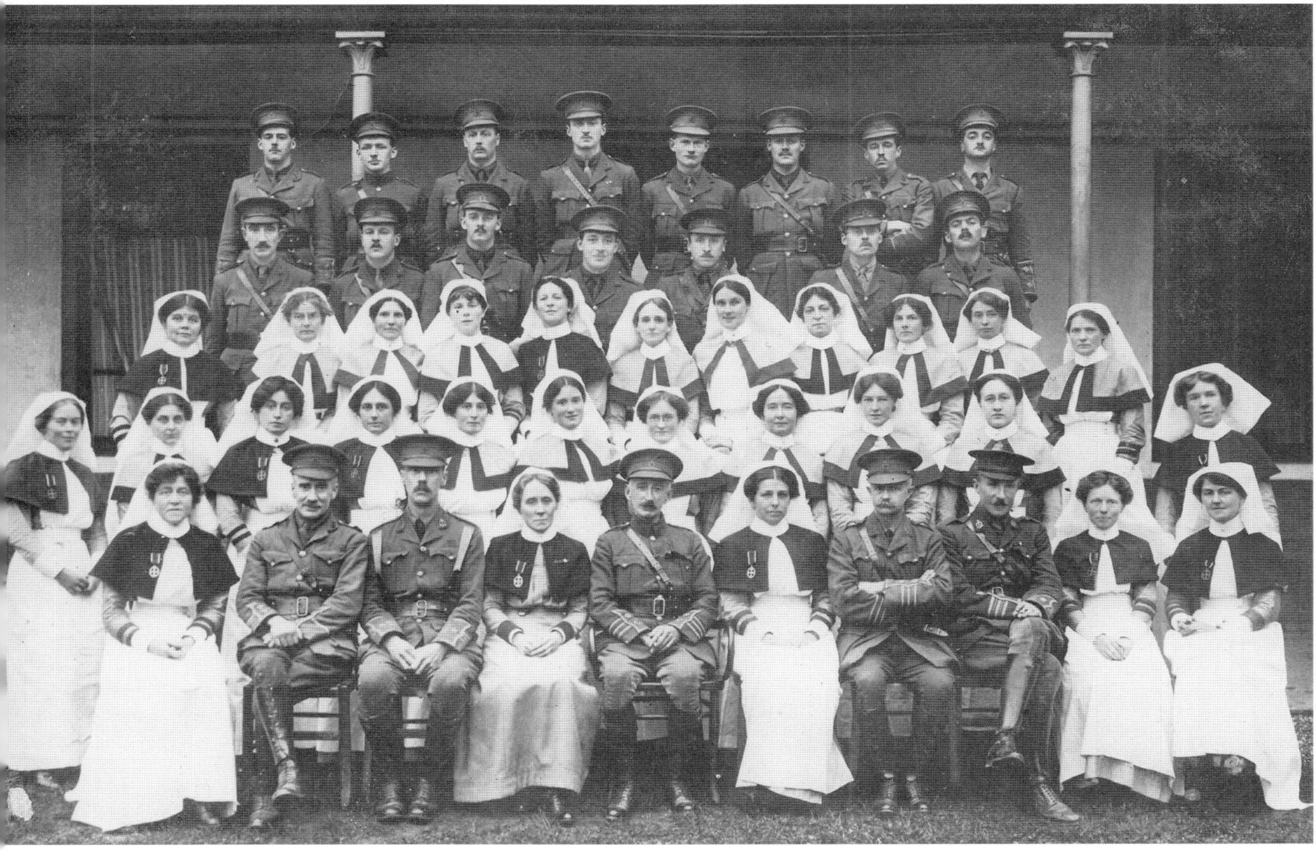

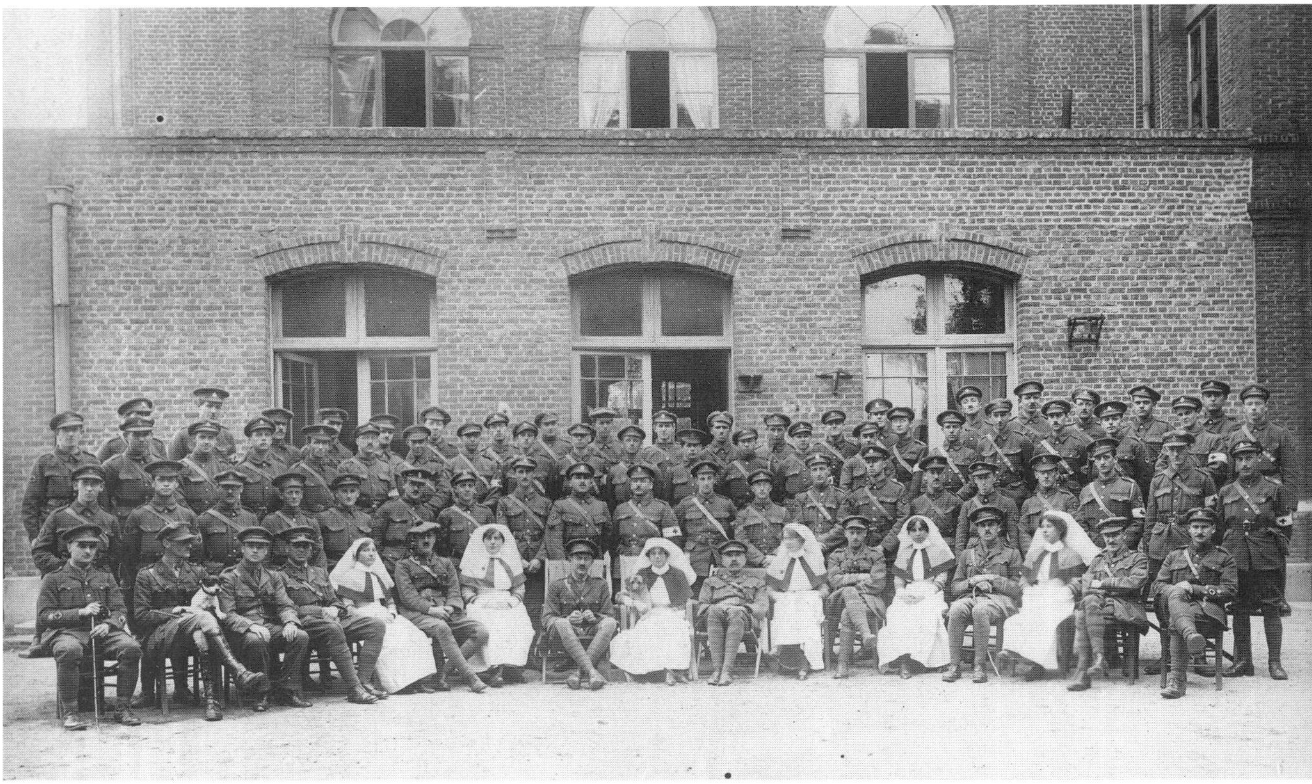

RAMC and Territorial Force Nursing Service (TFNS) personnel outside a military hospital on the Western Front.

RAMC and TFNS personnel inside a military hospital ward on the Western Front. The medical records of the patients can be seen hung behind their beds, below the row of photos and pictures.

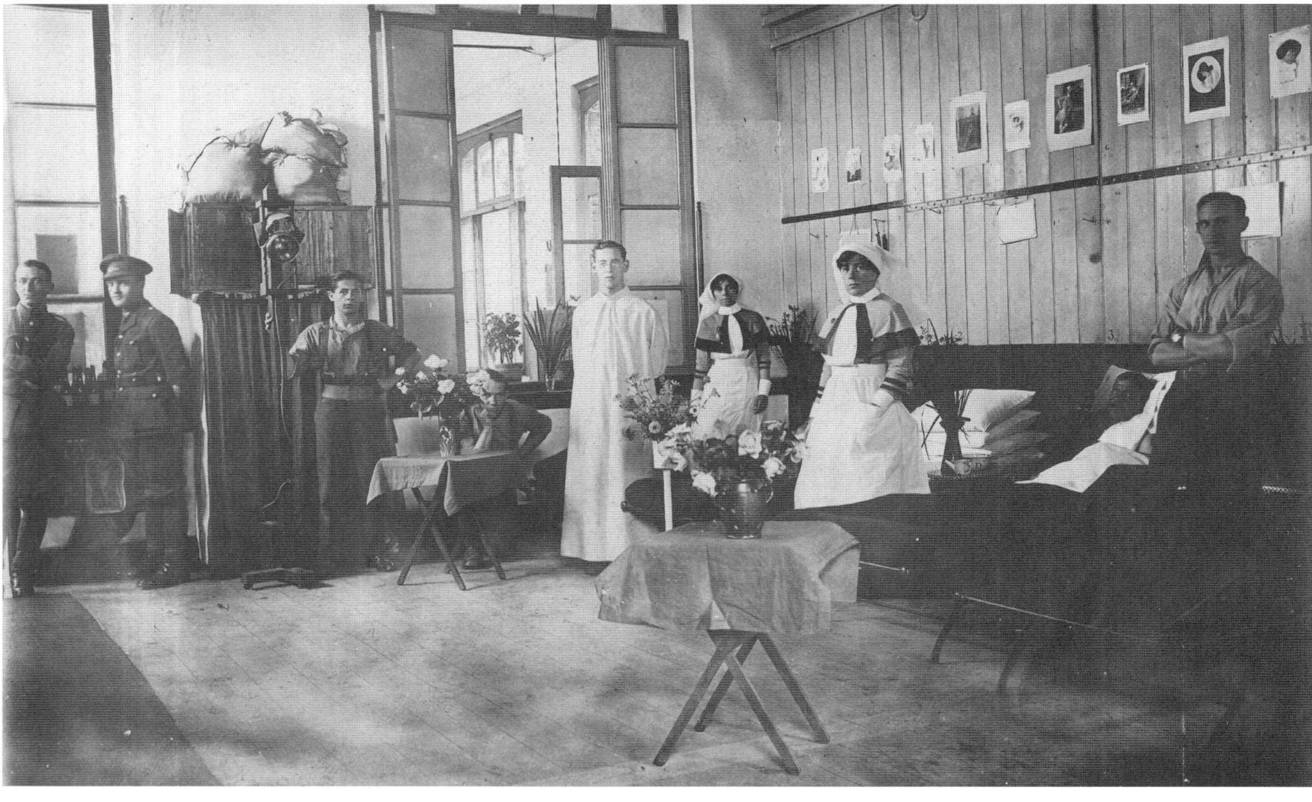

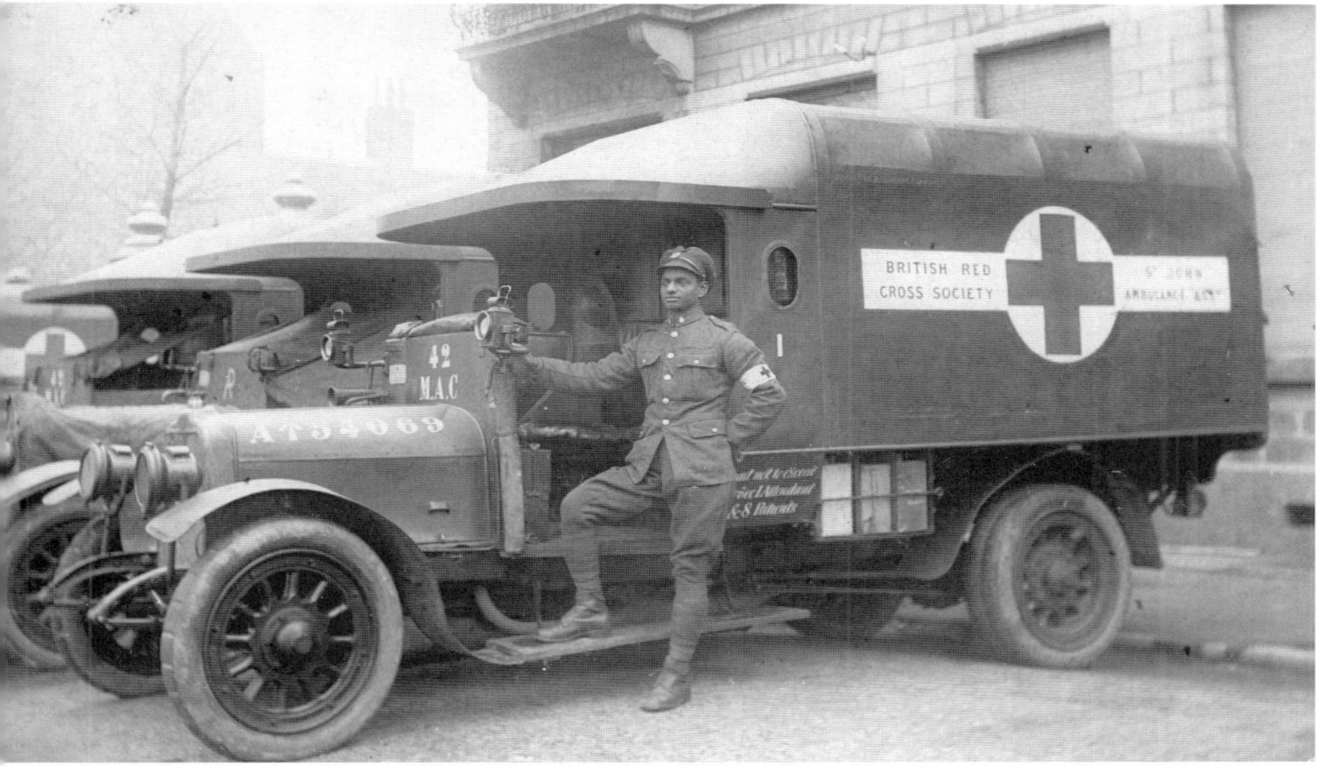

M/351407 George Robinson, Army Service Corps, serving with the 42nd Motor Ambulance Convoy. The photo is inscribed on the reverse '351407 George Robinson, 5 Station Street, Dumbarton, Glasgow'. *(Mr Andrew Read)*

Volunteer, lady ambulance drivers at Le Treport, France. The reverse is inscribed 'Drivers in Aunt May's Red X Ambulance Group at Le Treport 1916'. *(Mr Andrew Read)*

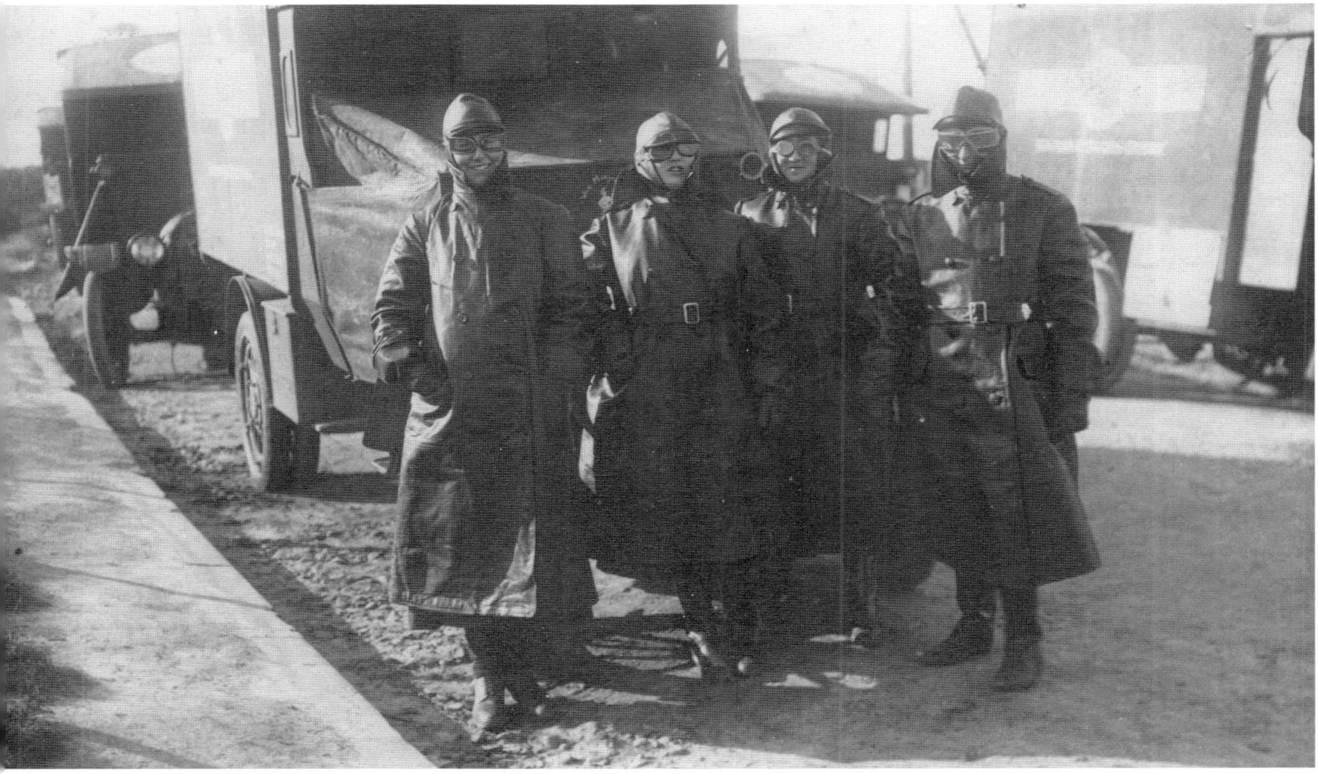

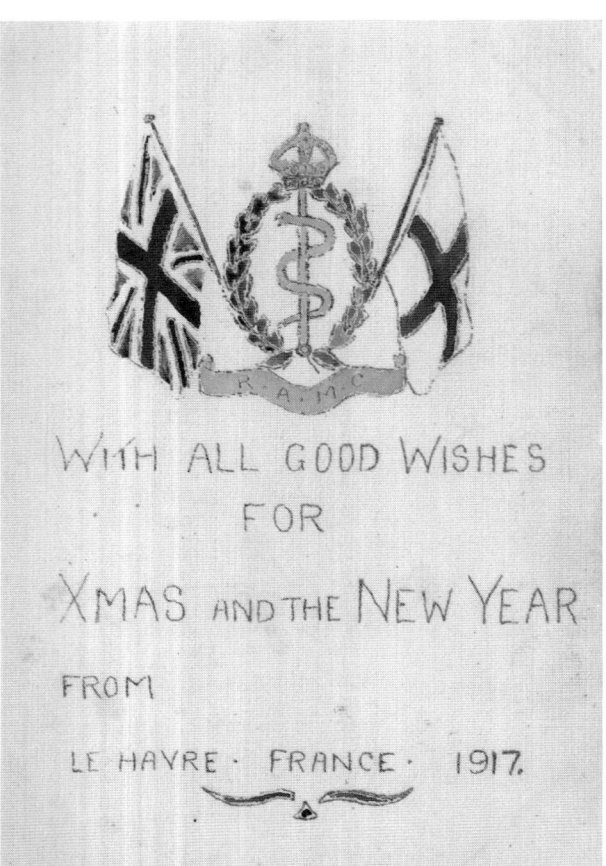

A greetings card, drawn by hand, which features the RAMC cap badge. A number of RAMC hospitals were located in the Le Havre area.

A postcard of the *Carisbrook Castle*, used as a hospital ship during the First World War. On the postcard a wounded soldier has noted his casualty evacuation route from Neuve Chapelle to hospital in St Helens, via a hospital in Boulogne and HMHS *Carisbrook Castle*. The reverse of the postcard is dated Sunday, 14 March 1915.

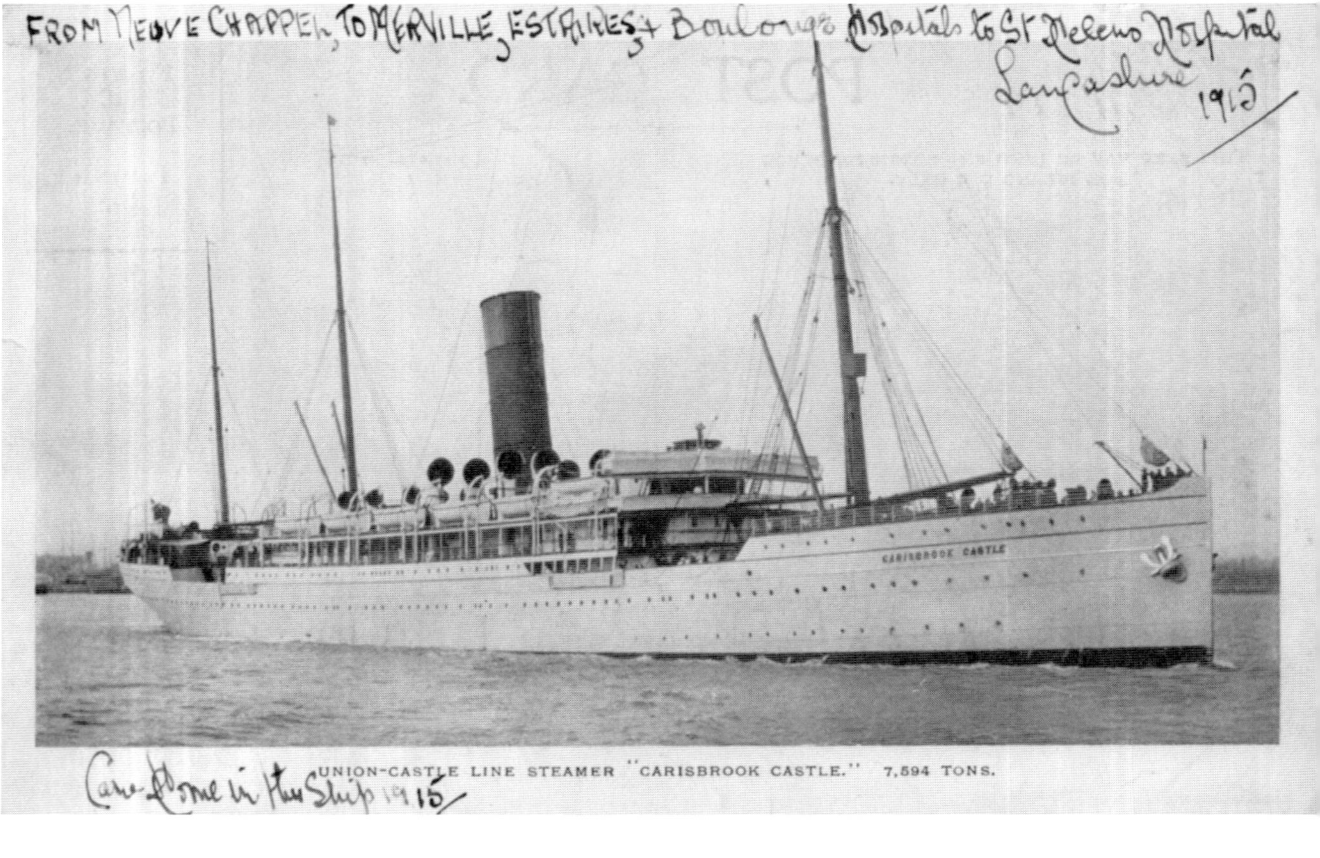

Chapter 4

A Global War

The global nature of the First World War created a number of challenges for the medical services. Campaigns in Gallipoli, Macedonia, Italy, Africa and the Middle East, all required solutions to be found to cope with extremes of climate and distance from the UK.

From 25 April 1915 British, ANZAC and French forces were involved in the Gallipoli campaign, until evacuation from the peninsula by 8 January 1916. After the initial landings, trench warfare developed and heavy casualties were sustained during attempts to break the deadlock. The numbers of casualties far outweighed the estimates prior to the start of the campaign and initial medical provision was inadequate. Difficulties were experienced in evacuating the sick and wounded under fire from beaches close to the front line and there was also a lack of ambulance launches, as all available boats were required to bring reinforcements ashore.

As the campaign continued, medical arrangements improved, but the Gallipoli Peninsula could not benefit from regular casualty evacuation routes from the front line to base area. Instead gullies and tracks were used as roads, on which casualties were transported to the beaches by stretcher and occasionally ambulance wagon. Small boats replaced ambulance convoys, and took casualties to hospital ships which took the sick and wounded to hospitals in Egypt or Mudros. From there casualties could be taken by hospital ships for further treatment in Malta, or the United Kingdom if appropriate.

In Mesopotamia the extreme temperature and diseases such as sand-fly fever, malaria and enteric fever were a constant problem for the medical services. During the campaign in Mesopotamia supplies of medical and sanitary materials were often in short supply.

The British Salonika Force was involved in conflict in Macedonia from October 1915 to the end of October 1918. Poor transportation infrastructure in the area created many difficulties and there were great climatic extremes. During the campaign the biggest threat came from malaria; the conditions of warfare intensified the disease which had been endemic in the area. In Macedonia non-battle casualties exceeded battle casualties in the proportion of twenty to one for all ranks.

The global nature of the First World War is reflected in the photographs taken overseas and those of medical personnel. Colonial and Dominion medical units worked closely with the RAMC throughout the First World War and contributed greatly to the treatment of casualties.

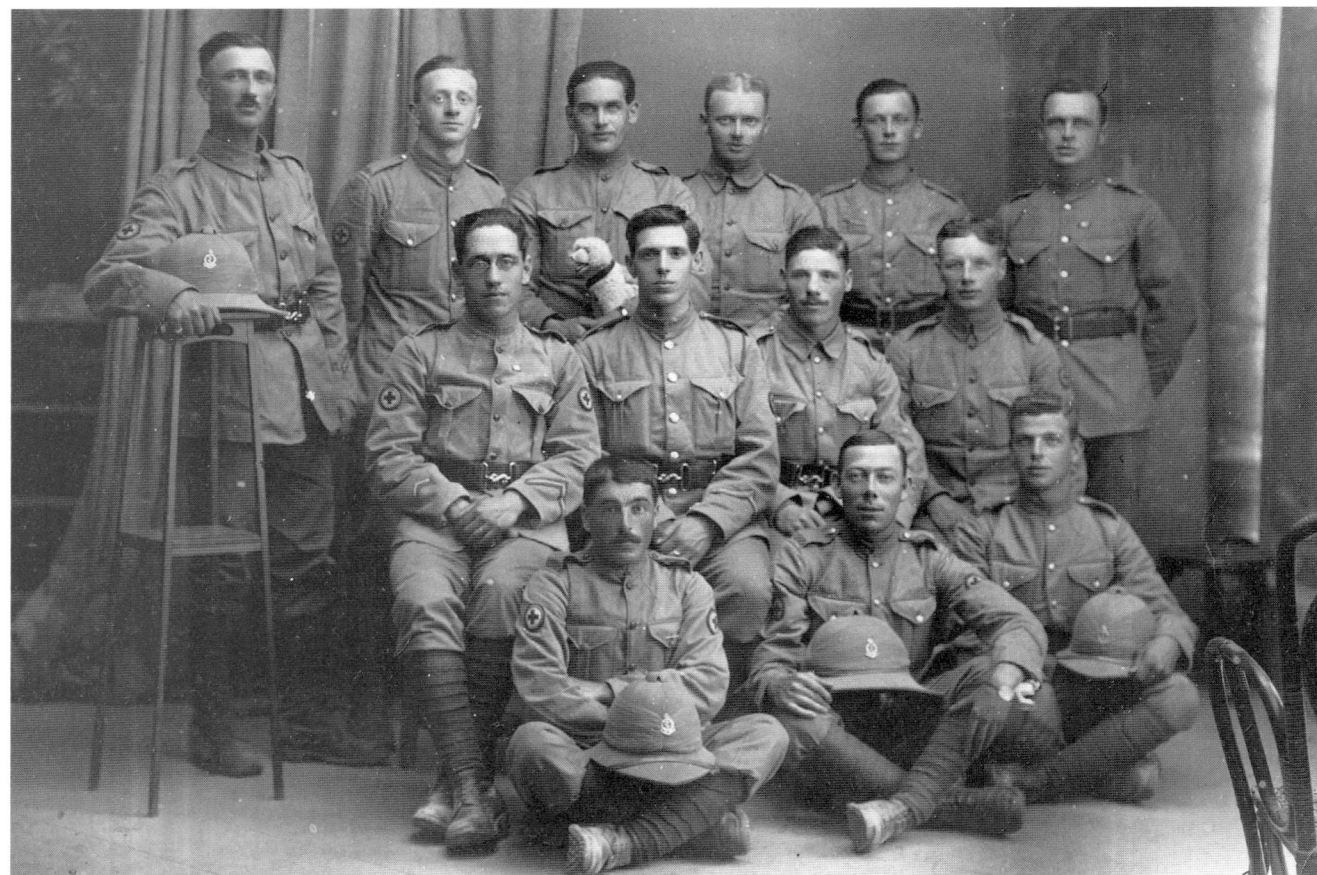

(**Above**) Personnel of the 41st Field Ambulance RAMC. The unit served overseas with the 13th (Western) Division in Gallipoli, Egypt and Mesopotamia. The division suffered over 12,000 casualties during its time in the Middle East.

(**Opposite, above**) The photo is signed on the reverse 'W. H. Taylor, 1st City of London Field Ambulance, RAMC TF. 1917'; from 1916 the unit was in Salonika.

(**Opposite, below**) The 3rd Welsh Field Ambulance, RAMC (TF) photographed at Northampton in August 1914. The unit served overseas from July 1915 with the 53rd (Welsh) Division in the Gallipoli campaign and subsequently in Egypt and Palestine.

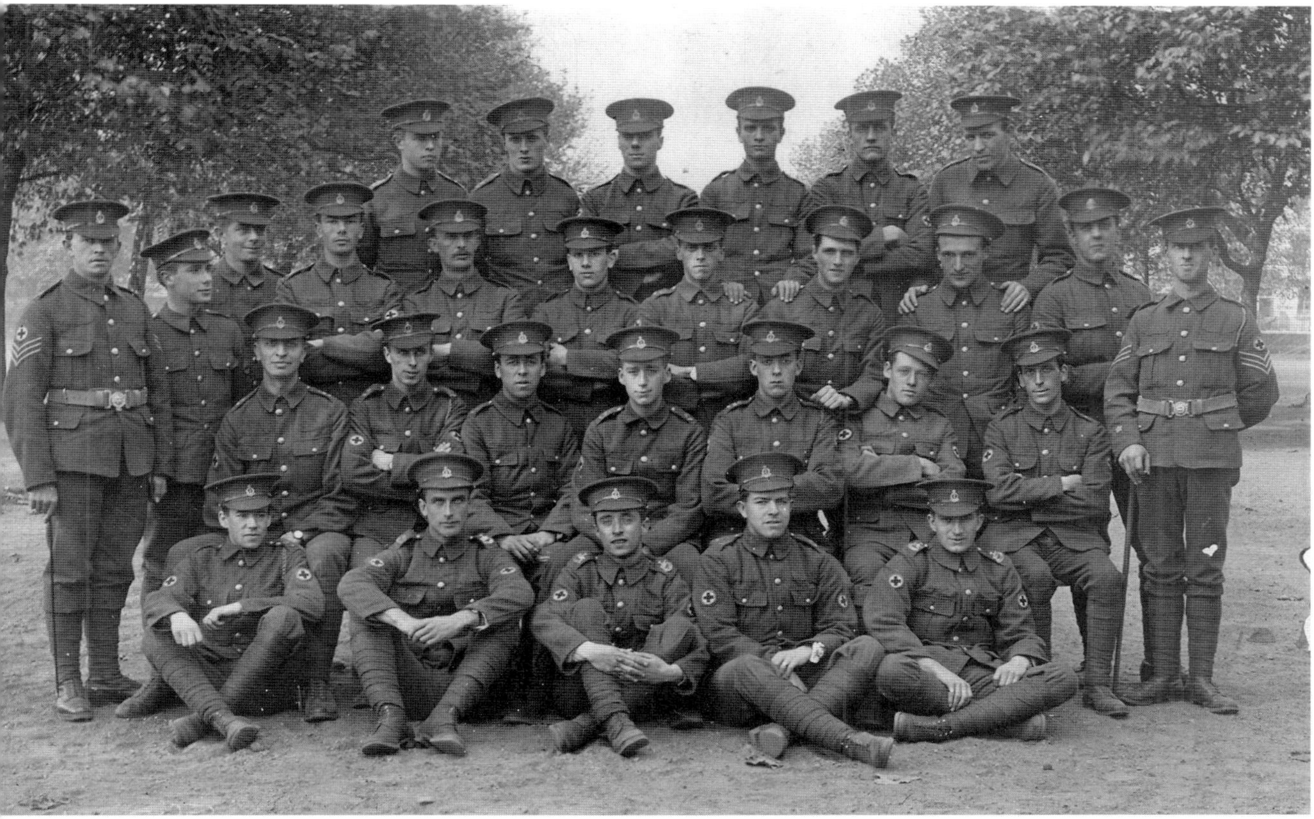

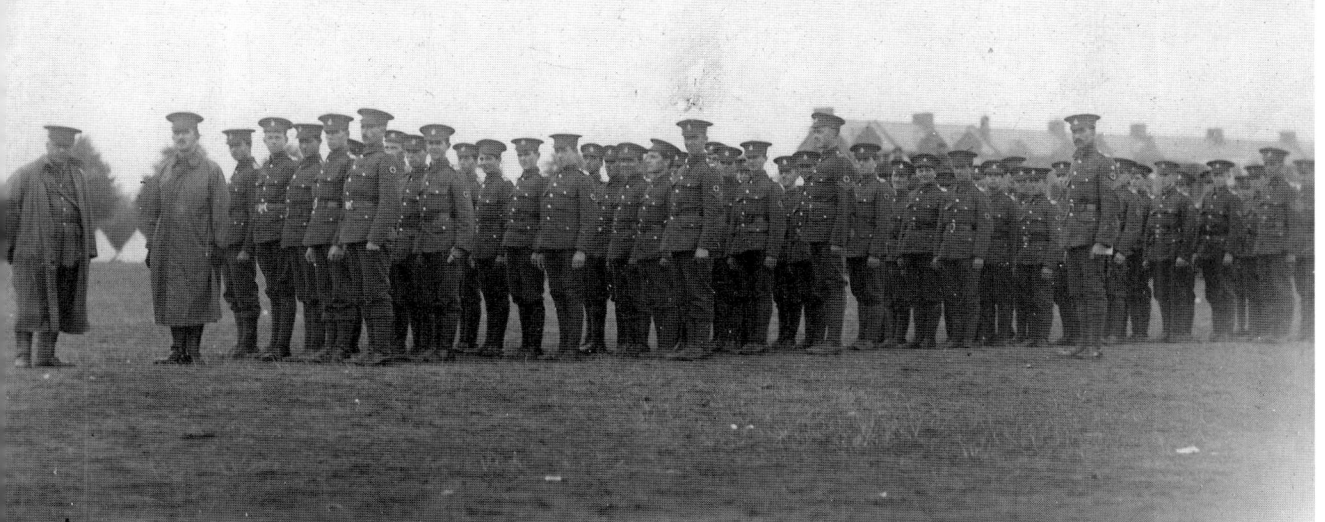

N. 110.   3RD. WELSH. R.A.M.C.

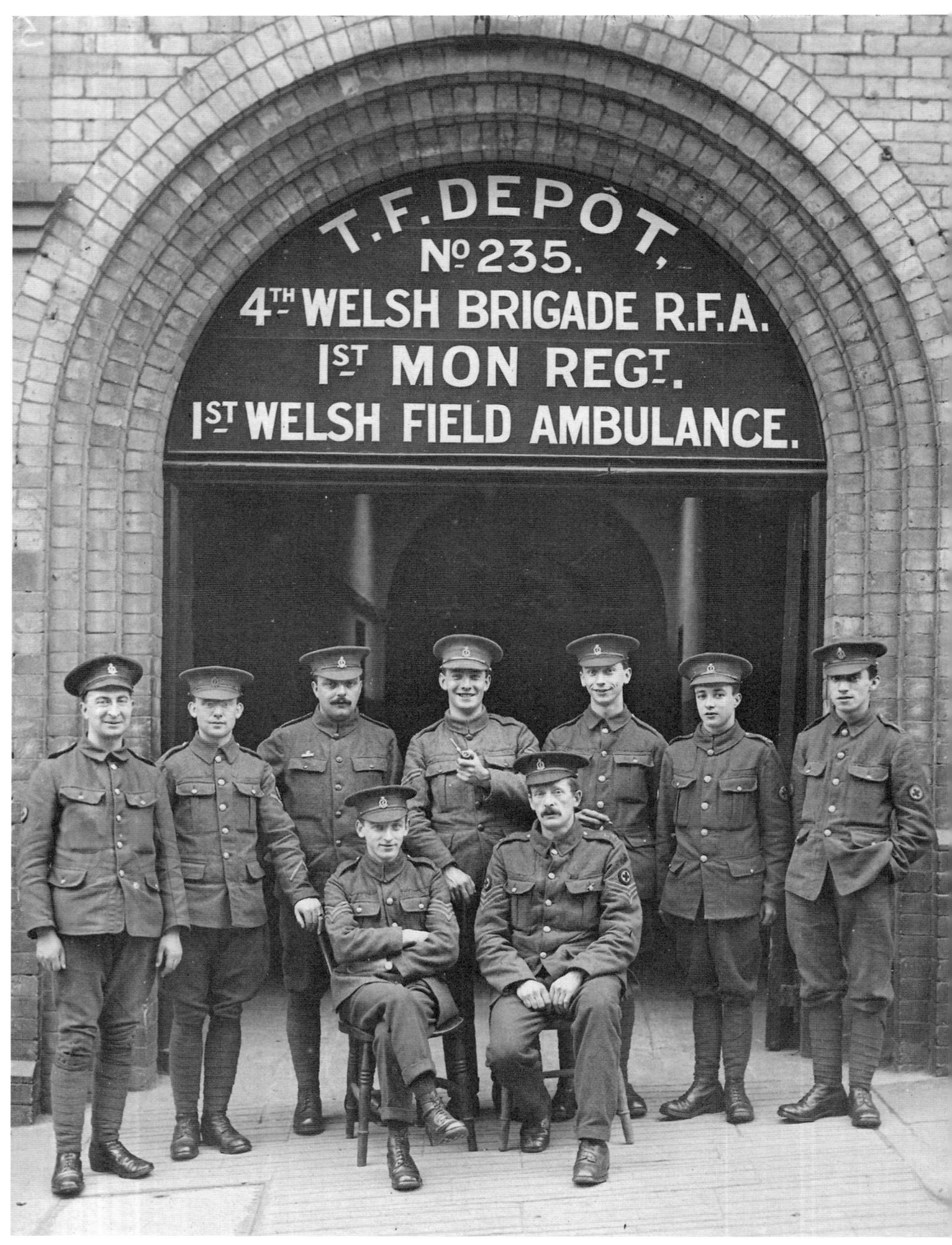

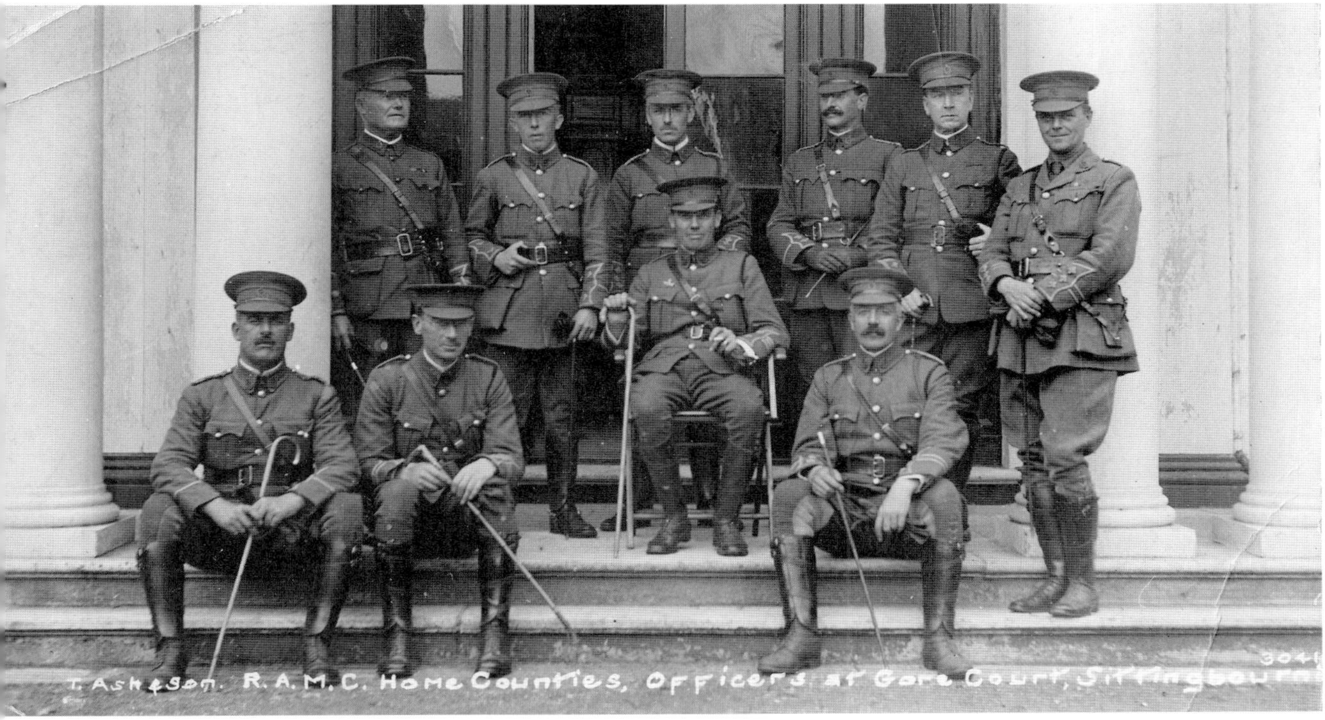

(**Above**) Home Counties RAMC (TF) officers, photographed at Gore Court, Sittingbourne. Home Counties Field Ambulance units served with the 27th Division on the Western Front in 1915 and from 1916 in Salonika.

(**Opposite**) Personnel of the 1st Welsh Field Ambulance, RAMC (TF) photographed outside the Territorial Force Depot at Newport. The unit served with the 53rd (Welsh) Division.

(**Below**) Orderly Room staff of the South Western Mounted Brigade Field Ambulance, RAMC. The unit served in the Middle East.

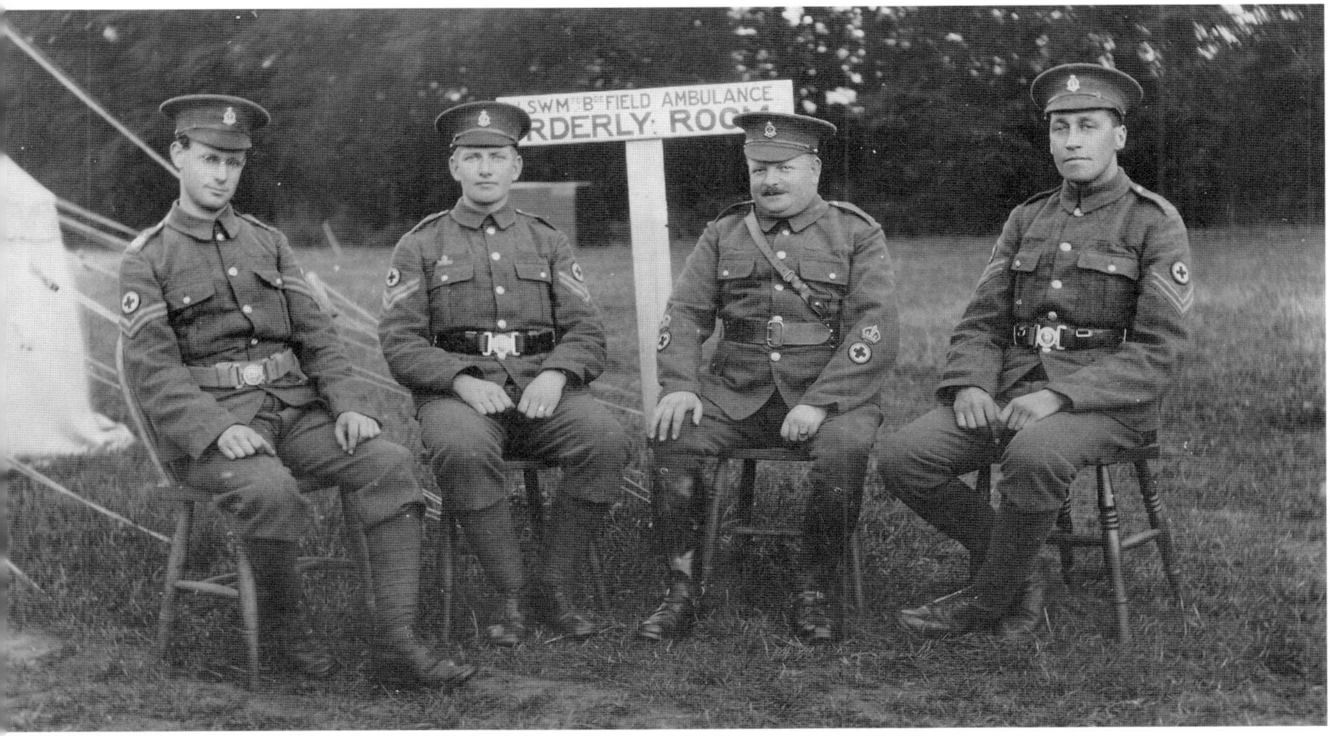

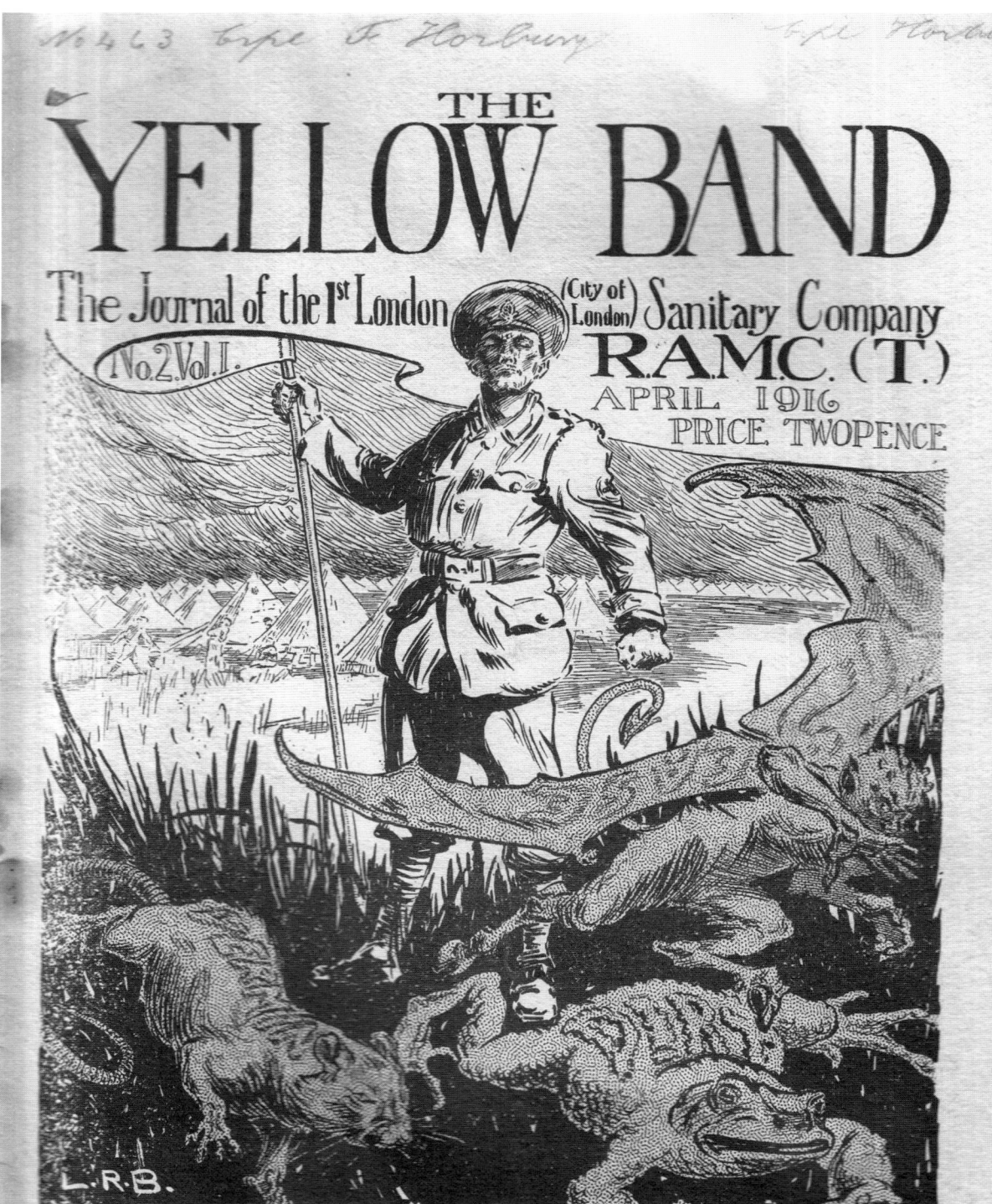

Cover of the April 1916 journal of the 1st (City of London) Sanitary Company, RAMC (TF). The cover is signed by a member of the unit, 463 Corporal Frank Horbury who enlisted on 12 October 1914 and was discharged, due to sickness, on 13 May 1916. The cover illustrates the problems faced by RAMC Sanitary units around the world during the First World War, including diseases, dirt and vermin.

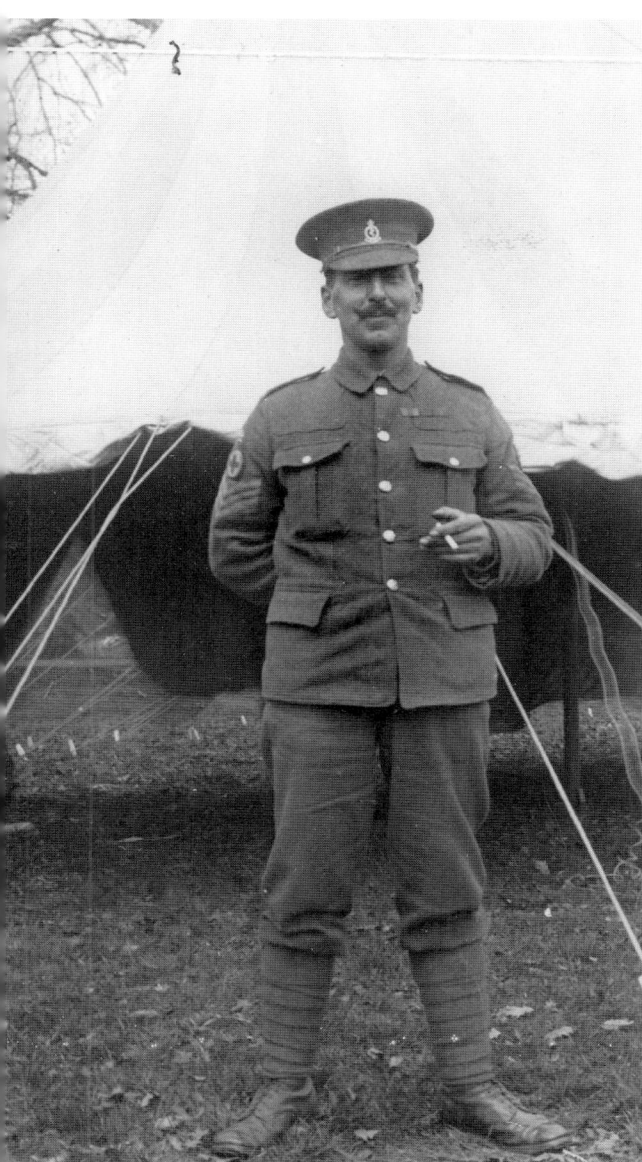 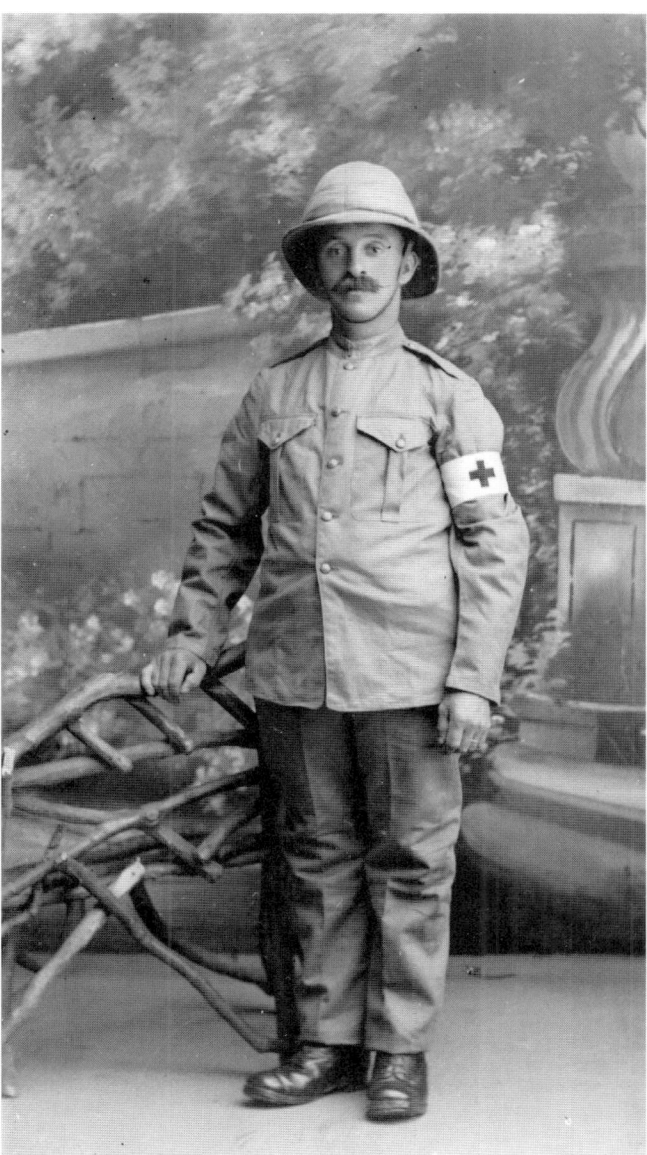

(**Left**) 186 / 437011 Staff Sergeant George Augustus Steventon, 2nd South Midland Field Ambulance, RAMC (TF). George Augustus Steventon was born in Sutton Coldfield, the son of Richard and Eliza Steventon, and baptized on 27 April 1879. He enlisted on 3 February 1900 and served in the 1st Volunteer Battalion, South Staffordshire Regiment during the South African War from 10 March 1900 to 20 May 1901. He joined the 2nd South Midland Field Ambulance, RAMC on 9 April 1908. In 1911 he was working as a plumber and living with his wife in Sutton Coldfield. During the First World War he served with the unit on the Western Front and on the Italian Front. He died in Sutton Coldfield on 13 October 1946.

(**Right**) A RAMC recruit photographed wearing a sun helmet at the RAMC training centre, Blackpool.

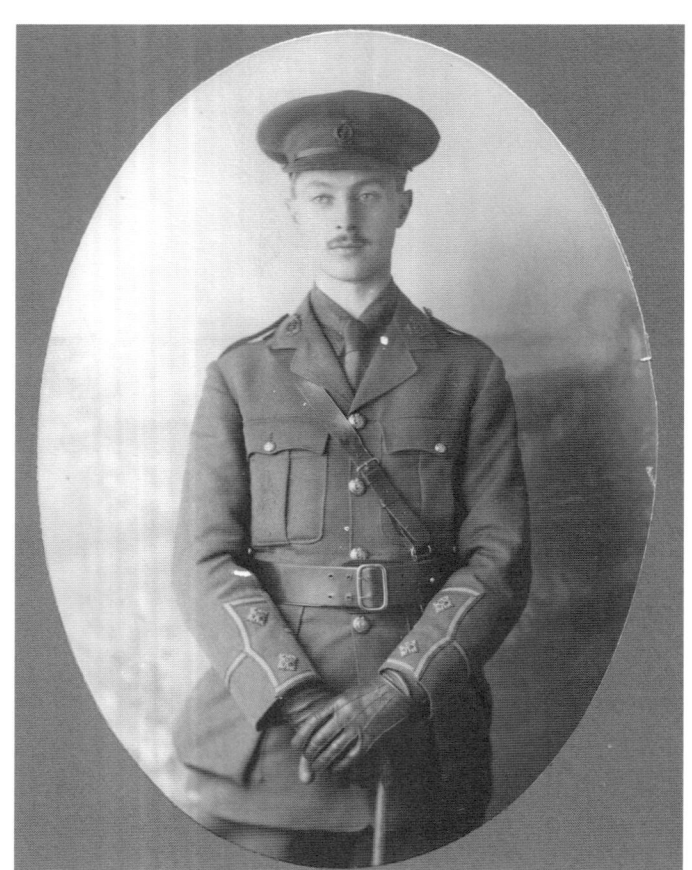

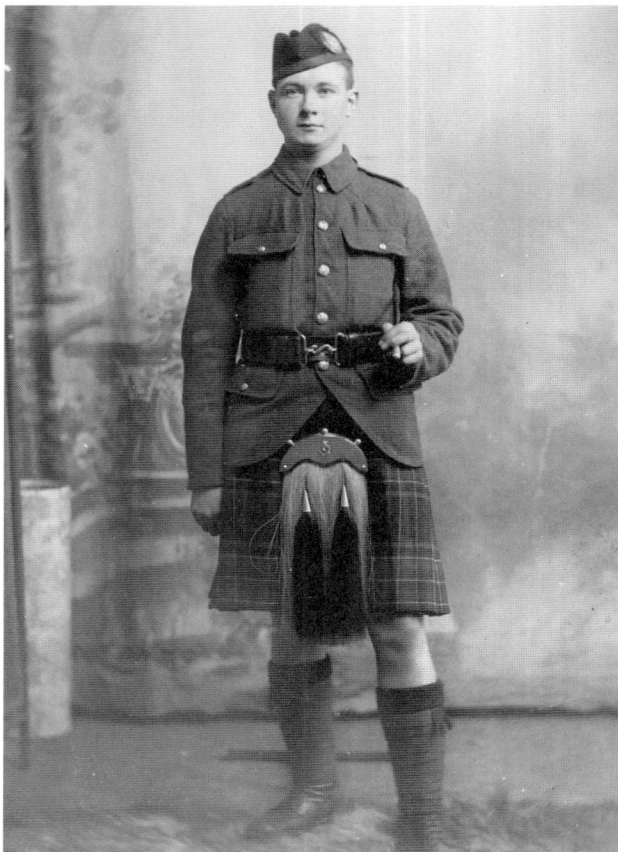

(**Above, left**) Lieutenant (later Captain) Harold Heathcote, RAMC. In 1911 when a medical student, aged 22, he was living with his brother and sister at South View, Buxton Road, Disley, Cheshire. He qualified as a Bachelor of Medicine and Bachelor of Surgery in 1911 and Doctor of Medicine in 1913 at the Victoria University of Manchester and served with the RAMC in Salonika from 26 November 1916. After the First World War he lived at Brookfield, Northenden Road, Sale, Manchester and worked in a range of medical roles in the area including at the Manchester Royal Infirmary, as an Assistant Medical Officer at the Monsall Fever Hospital and as an Assistant Medical Officer in Salford.

(**Above, right**) 2000 Private H. Bell, 2/1st Lowland Field Ambulance, RAMC (TF). Note the RAMC badge on his sporran. Units of the Lowland Field Ambulance were with the 52nd (Lowland) Division overseas at Gallipoli, Palestine and, during 1918, on the Western Front.

(**Right**) Sergeant J. Cameron, Highland Mounted Brigade Field Ambulance, RAMC. During the war the unit was in Gallipoli and the Middle East.

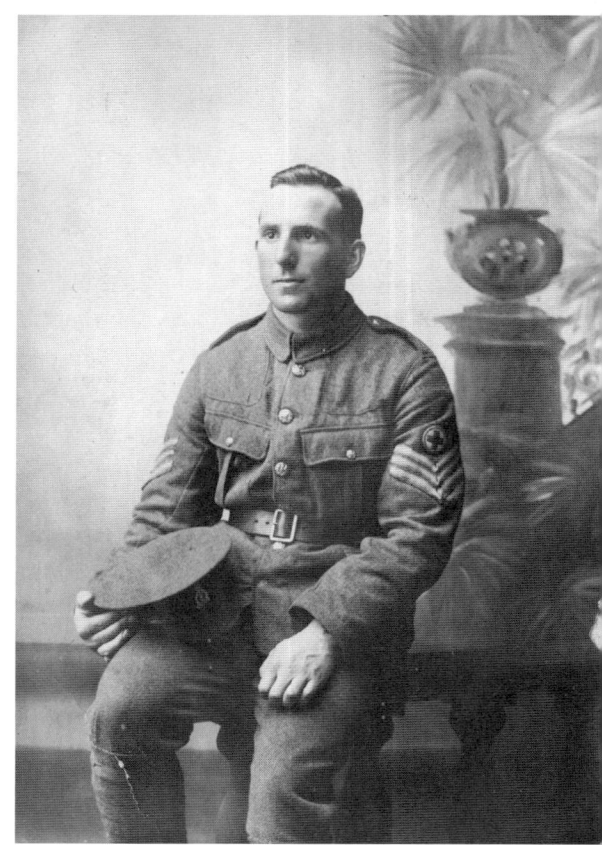

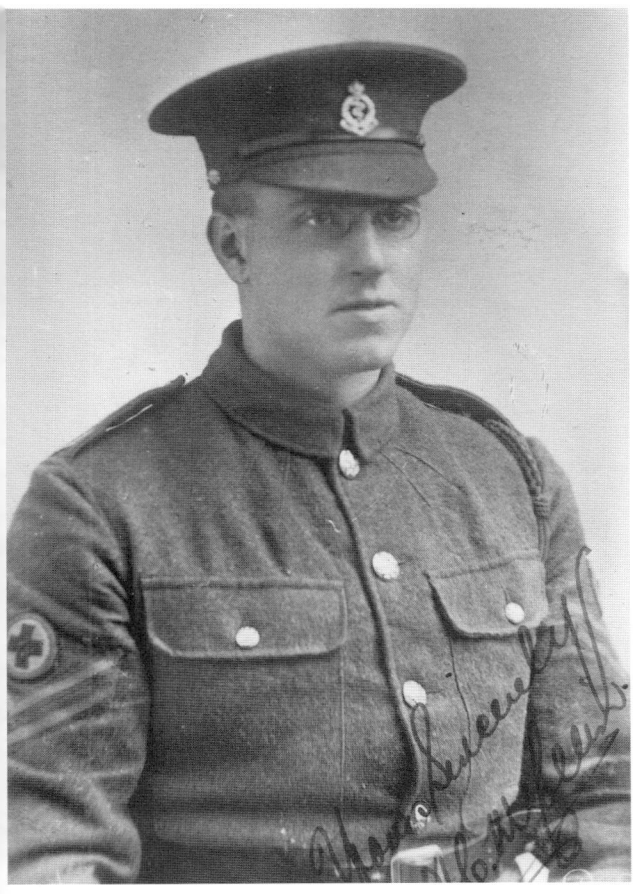
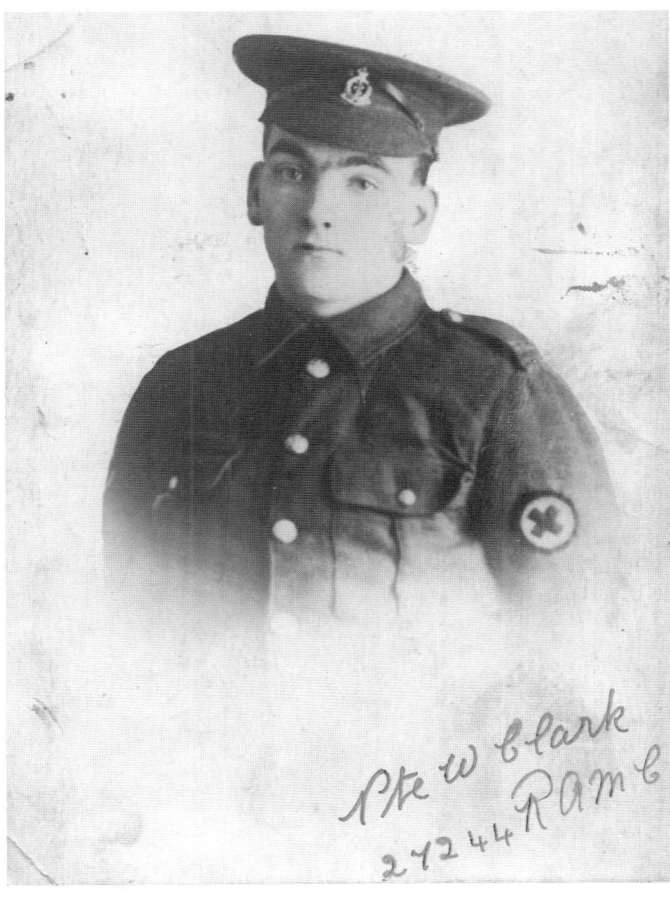
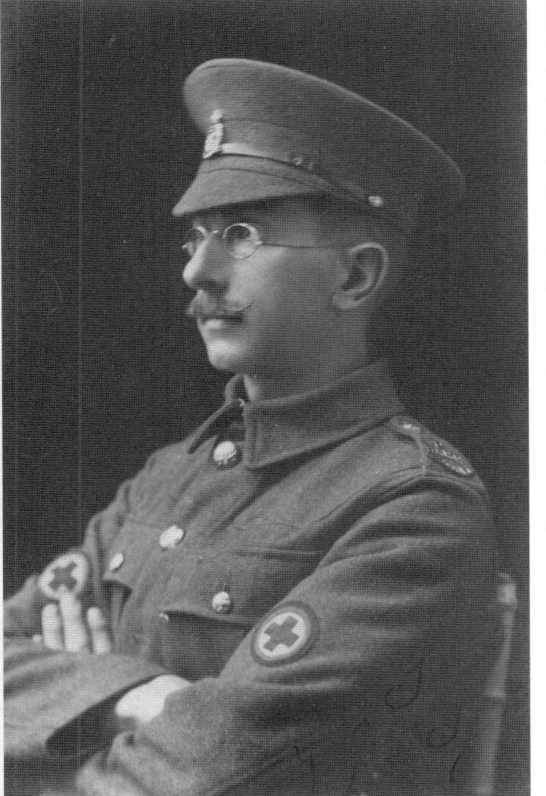

(**Above, left**) 1836 Corporal (later Acting Sergeant) Henry Charles McCollin, RAMC. Born in Poplar in 1888, in 1911 he was residing with his parents at 167 Byron Avenue, London where he was a clerk working for the National Society of the Prevention of Cruelty to Children. He served overseas with the RAMC after 1915, receiving the British War Medal and Victory Medal. He married Ethel A. Burnham in 1919 and died in London on 19 January 1965.

(**Above, right**) 27244 Private William Richardson Clark, 40th Field Ambulance RAMC. This unit served overseas with the 13th (Western) Division in Gallipoli, Egypt and Mesopotamia. In 1911 William Clark was living with his parents, four brothers and two sisters at 10 Rockwood Gardens, Greenside, Ryton, County Durham where he was working as coal miner. He served overseas from 20 October 1915, including the Gallipoli campaign. On 3 May 1916 he died from enteric fever in Mesopotamia, aged 23, and is buried in Amara War Cemetery, Iraq. William Richardson Clark was the son of Thomas and Annie Clark, of Greenside Old House, Greenside, Ryton, County Durham.

(**Left**) 2373 Private Llewellyn F. Thomas RAMC. Private Thomas served overseas with the RAMC after 1915, and received the British War Medal and Victory Medal.

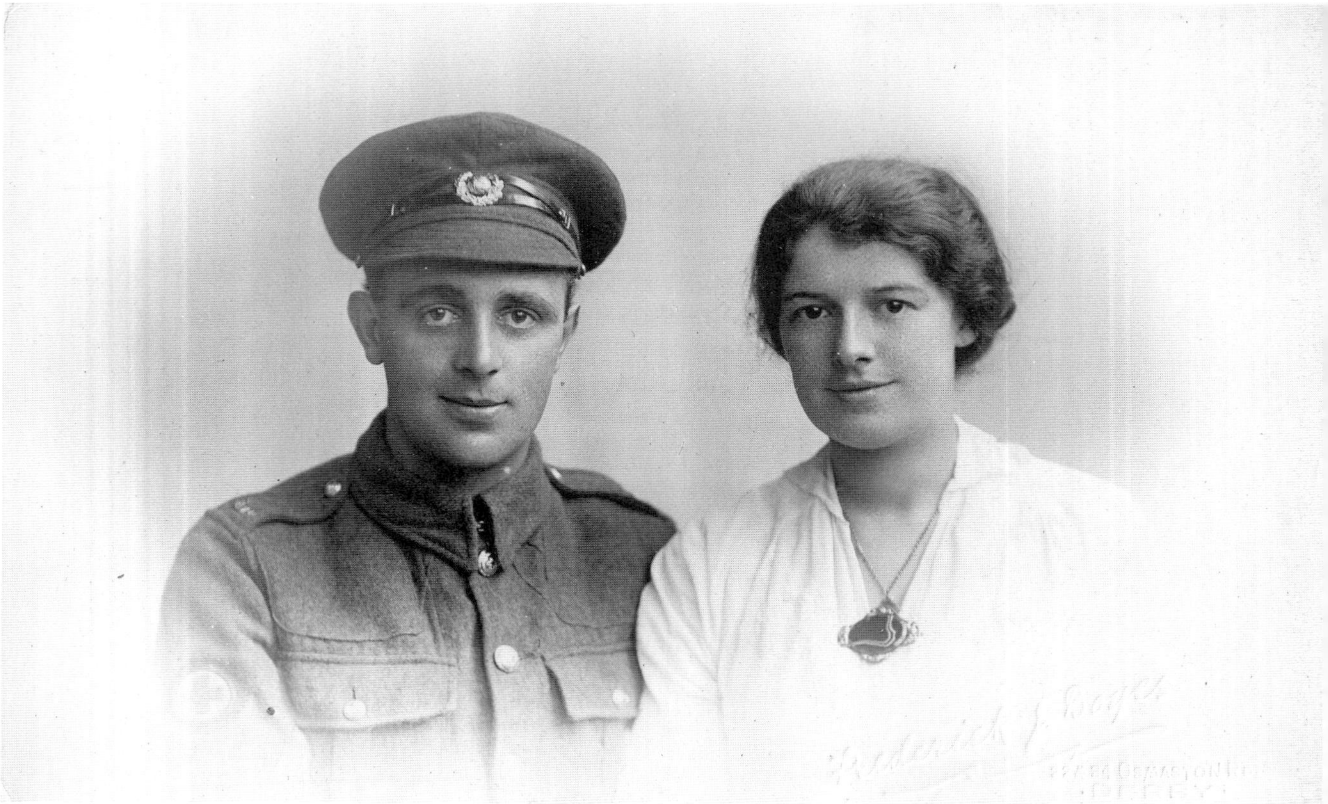

A medic serving with the 63rd (Royal Naval) Division, photographed with a family member. The 63rd Division served in the Gallipoli Campaign and on the Western Front.

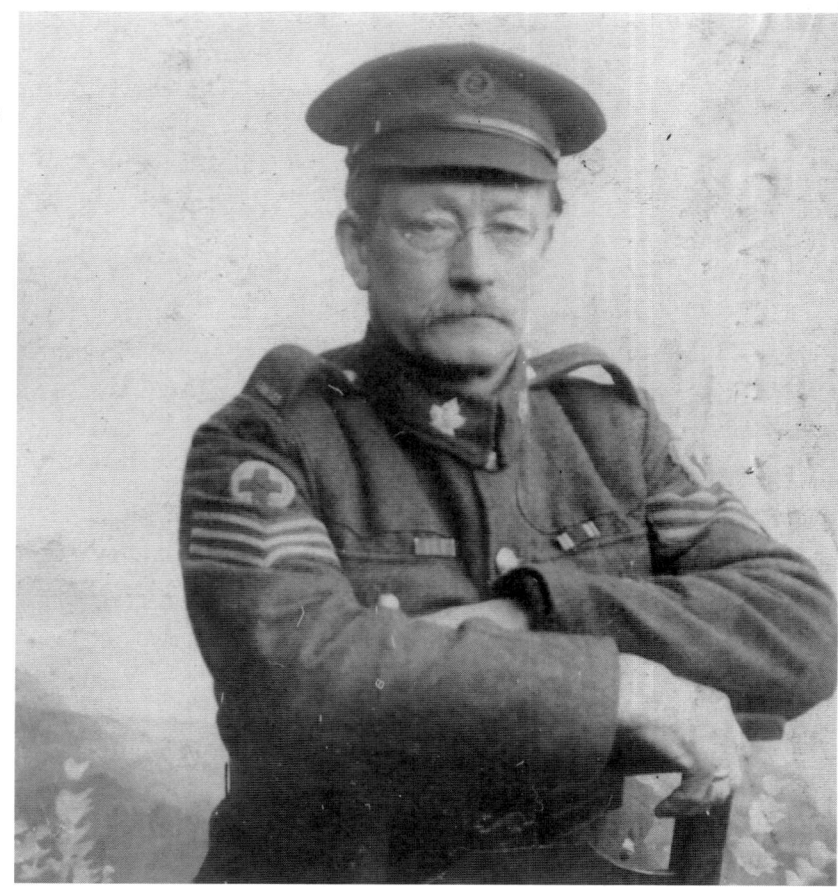

A sergeant of the Canadian Army Medical Corps (CAMC) which served with the Canadian Expeditionary Force on the Western Front from 1915. By the Armistice in November 1918, the Canadian Corps had enlarged to include four infantry divisions and supporting units.

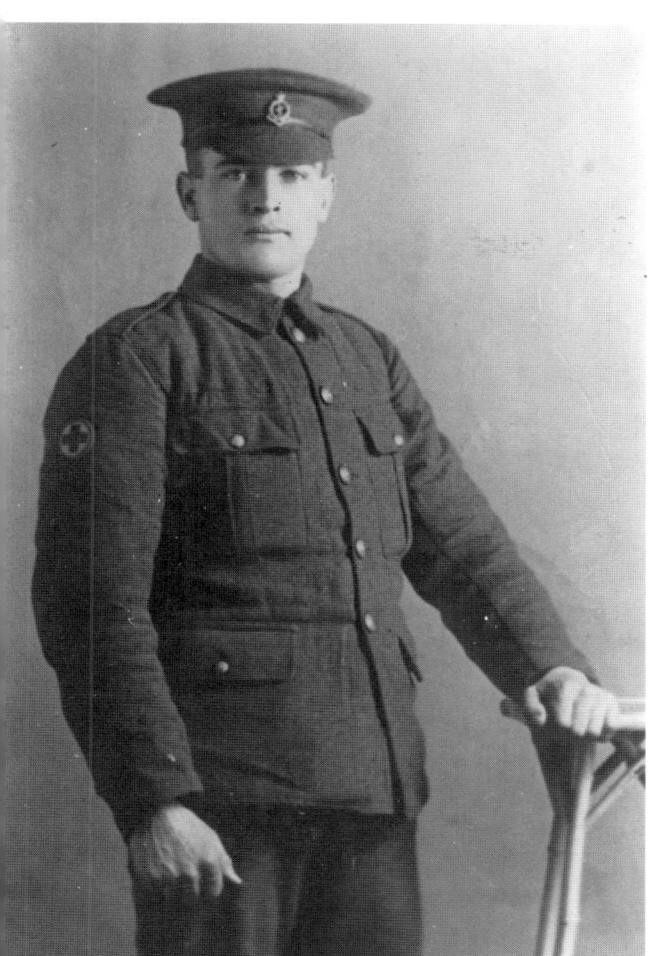
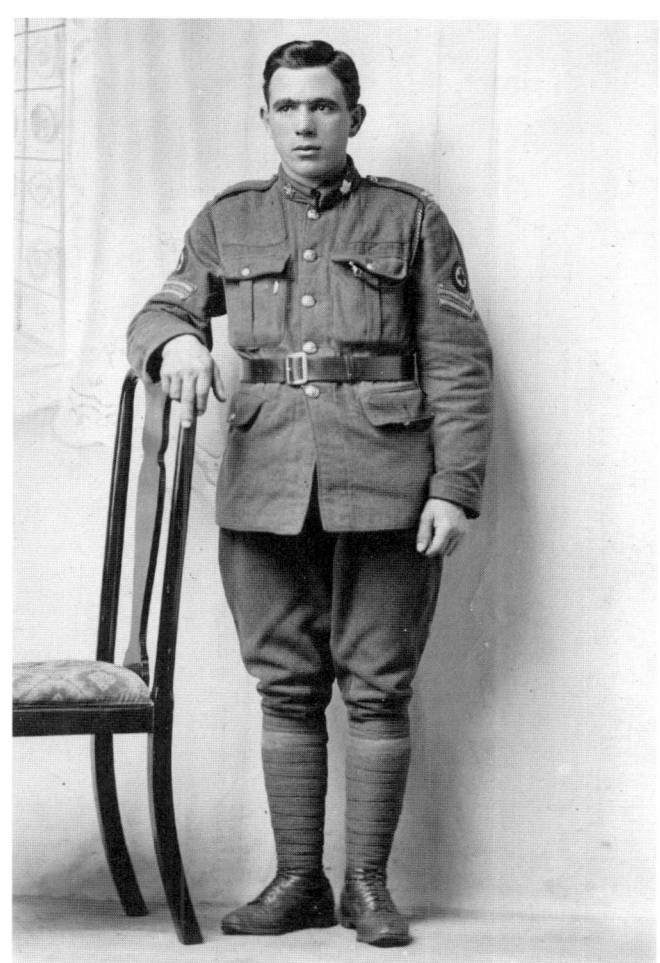
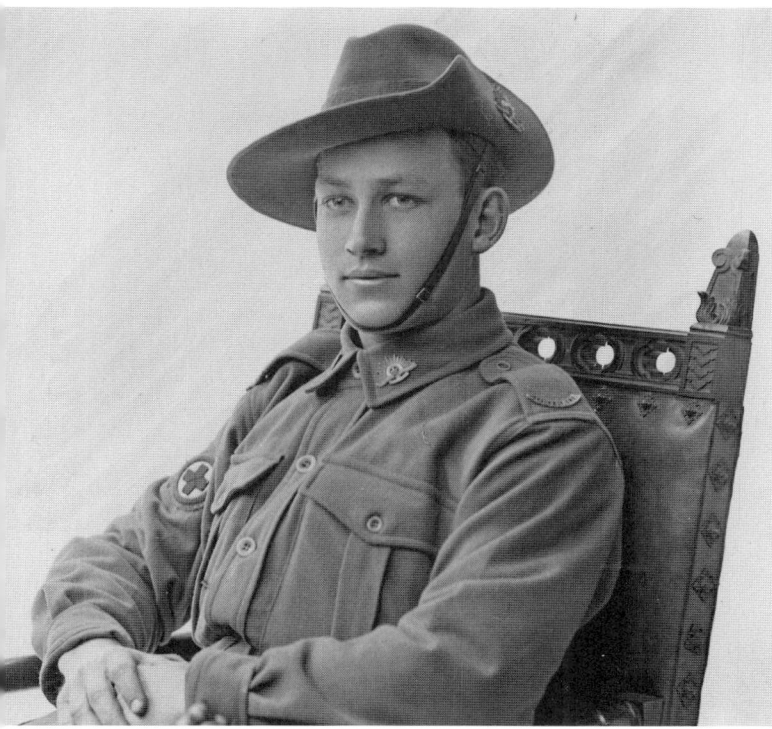

(**Above, left**) 68784 Private Henry G. Morley, RAMC. He worked on hospital ships from 16 August 1915 and was discharged on 7 April 1919.

(**Above, right**) A corporal of the Canadian Army Medical Corps (CAMC). Maple leaf badges are visible on his collar. The CAMC worked closely with the RAMC on the Western Front.

(**Left**) A private of the Australian Army Medical Corps (AAMC). The AAMC supported Australian forces at Gallipoli, in the Middle East and on the Western Front. During the First World War the AAMC grew in size and capability, working closely with the RAMC.

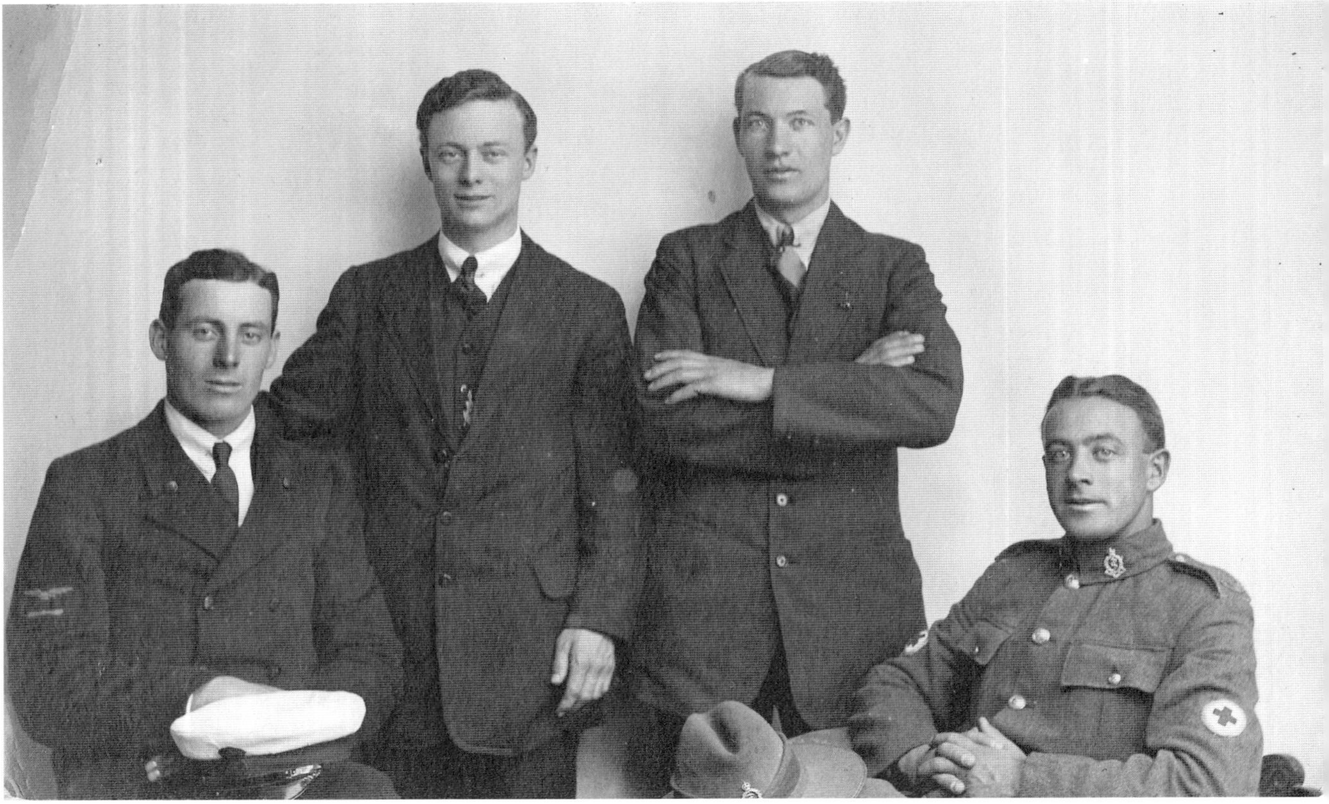

A private of the New Zealand Medical Corps (seated on the right) photographed with family members. The New Zealand Medical Corps supported the New Zealand Division in the Middle East and on the Western Front.

A corporal and a private from an Australian Light Horse Field Ambulance unit; their emu plumes were traditionally worn by units of the Australian Light Horse which saw service at Gallipoli and in the Middle East.

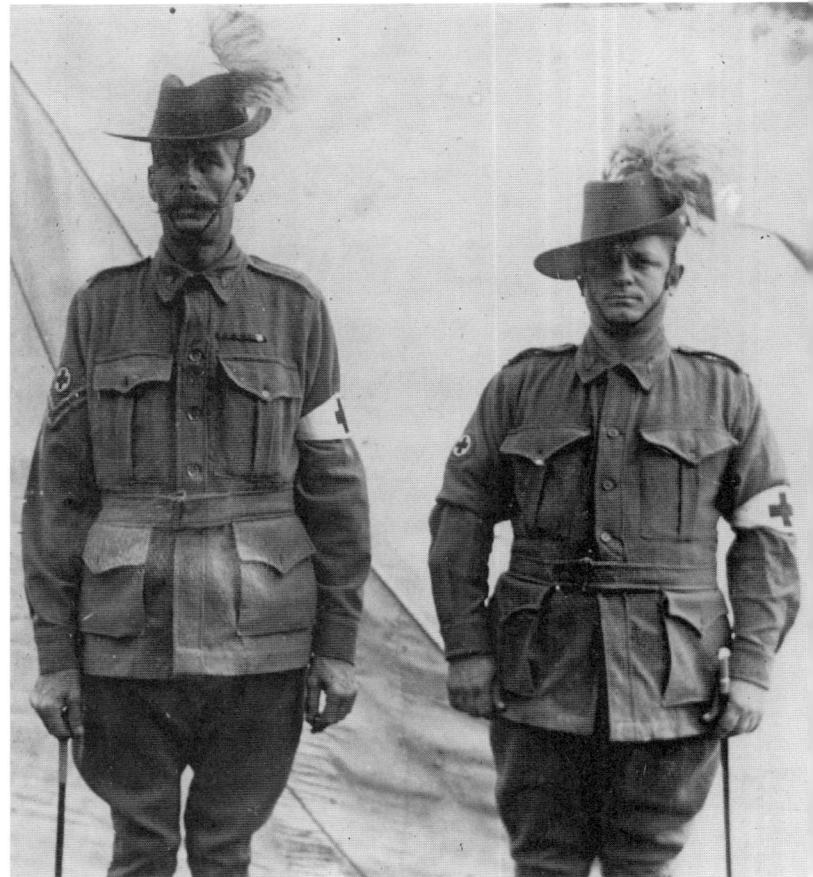

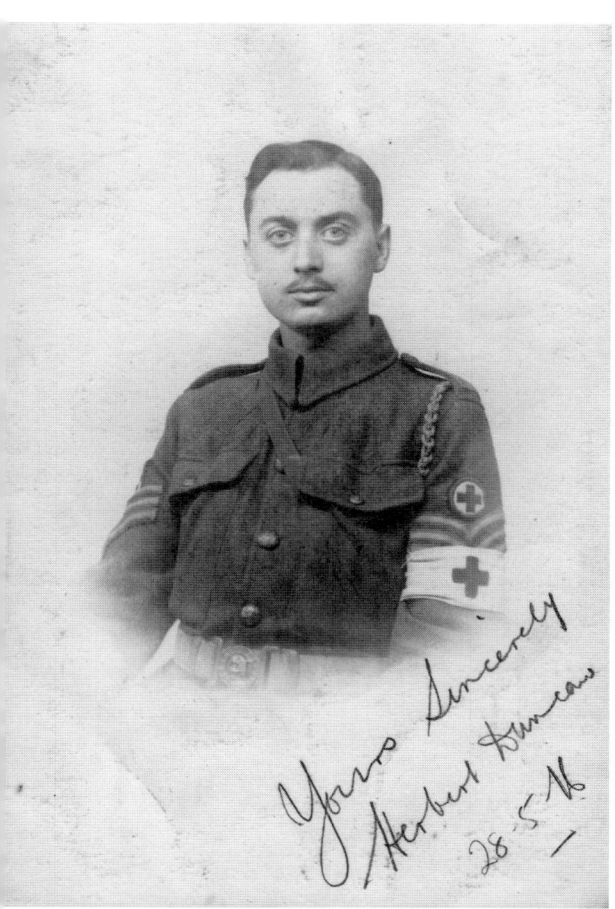
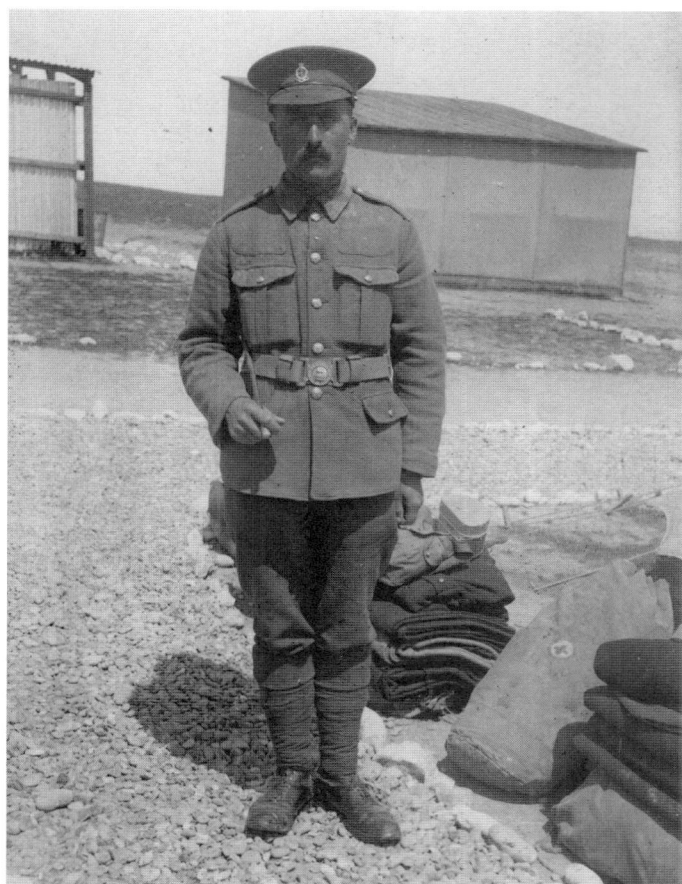

(**Left**) 589/493018 Sergeant Herbert Duncan, 81st (1st Home Counties) Field Ambulance RAMC (TF). The 81st (1st Home Counties) Field Ambulance served with the 27th Division. Whilst with the RAMC (TF), Herbert Duncan worked as fitter's mate, employed by the Admiralty at Chatham. He enlisted in the RAMC (TF) at Chatham on 21 May 1909 and arrived on the Western Front on 22 December 1914. In November 1915 he moved with his unit to the Salonika Front. Whilst in Salonika, he was Mentioned in Despatches, awarded the Meritorious Service Medal and the Serbian *Croix de la Misericorde* for gallantry and devotion to duty in the field. He was discharged from the Territorial Force on 31 July 1919 and awarded the Territorial Efficiency Medal, his character noted as exemplary.

(**Right**) 63144 Private Reginald Leggett, RAMC. He served on HM Hospital Ship *Britannic* from 22 December 1915 to 7 April 1916. From 18 April 1916 he was in Mesopotamia and South Russia. Private Leggett enlisted at Chesterfield, Derbyshire on 21 August 1915, aged 19 years. Prior to enlistment he worked as a clerk. He kept a diary during his service overseas with the RAMC, describing his time on HMHS *Britannic* and in Mesopotamia. In his diary, on 13 December 1915 he noted: 'Detailed for duty on board the Hospital Ship "*Britannic*". Had never thought that I should have the luck to serve on the sea and especially on the largest British ship afloat'.

On 23 December 1915: 'We are right out at sea – I shall be glad when I get over this awful seasickness'.

On 24 December 1915: 'Feeling better today. Passed Cape Finisterre about 5.30pm – had to work pretty hard all afternoon getting beds ready'.

On 25 December 1915: 'Christmas Day, but how different to what I had expected a few weeks before. Feeling absolutely A1 this morning and very hungry. All seasickness gone now. Went to the service in the lounge. The dinner provided for us was absolutely excellent. Had a view of Cape St. Vincent shortly after dinner. After tea a concert was given in our mess. It was very fine, but how I longed to be home for this special time. Watches to be put forward 36 minutes at midnight'.

Six days later, on 31 December 1915, after sailing through the Strait of Gibraltar and docking at Naples Harbour, HMHS *Britannic* arrived at Mudros Harbour, from 6.15pm to 10.30pm patients were brought on board.

On 1 January 1916: 'Loading patients all day. My ward was filled soon after breakfast'.

On 3 January 1916: 'More patients came on board during morning, and we weighed anchor and left Mudros for home at about 3.30pm'.

On 9 January 1916: 'At daybreak we were travelling dead slow within sight of the Isle of Wight. We stopped in the Solent waiting for high tide. It was 3.30pm before we were docked in Southampton. The "*Aquitania*" was lying alongside us in the dock. My patients were very lucky and I was too; I was thankful for they were all off the ship by tea time – 5.00pm'.

His diary describes further journeys to the Mediterranean to bring back casualties and his following service in Mesopotamia from April 1916. During late 1918 Reginald Leggett was admitted to hospital in Mesopotamia suffering from malaria and dysentery. In his diary, on 6 December 1918 he noted: 'Was marked for evacuation home. A few days later the evacuation was cancelled as I was discharged to duty in the main office because it was a light job.'

On 11 May 1919 'Left today to go to Baku. We are on a small paddle steamer and the Caspian Sea is very rough'.

On 12 May 1919: 'Reached Baku at dinner time and was posted to the 25 Casualty Clearing Station. This is a nice building and hospital. Baku is a very nice place indeed. It is quite European and quite different to what we have seen this long while'.

On 6 August 1919: 'Today we have embarked on-board the Hospital Ship "*Glengorm Castle*" for home. I am jolly glad too. It was getting very monotonous'.

After arriving at Marseilles on 18 August 18 1919, he arrived at Le Havre, via Rouen, by No. 34 Ambulance Train on 22 August 1919. The final entry was made in his diary on 23 August 1919: 'Into dock this morning and left by Ambulance Train to Paddington Station. We had a char-a-banc to take us all across London. Hyde Park Corner, Vauxhall Bridge to Bermondsey Military Hospital, Ladywell Road, Lewisham, London, SE13, and a very nice hospital too'.

Captain R. Steele, RAMC, speaking with a mounted RAMC sergeant in Macedonia. A soldier is being treated at the roadside by RAMC orderlies.

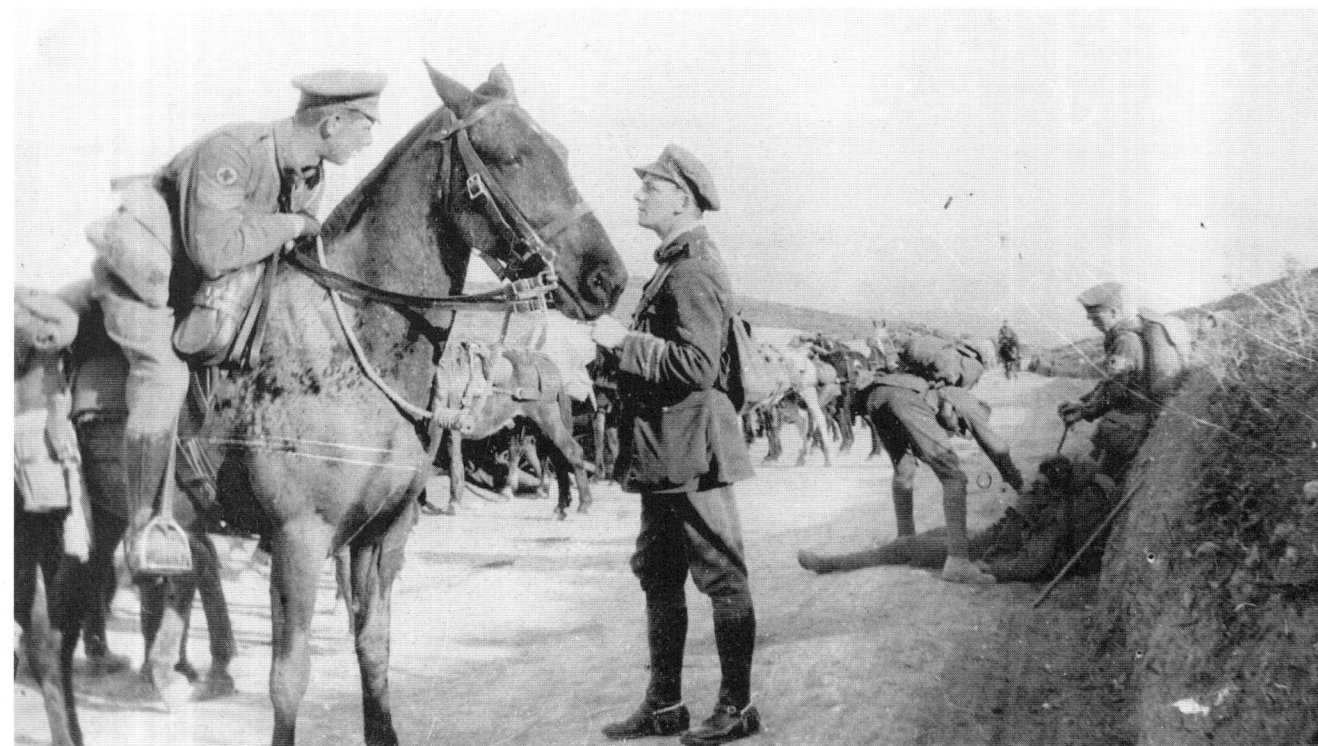

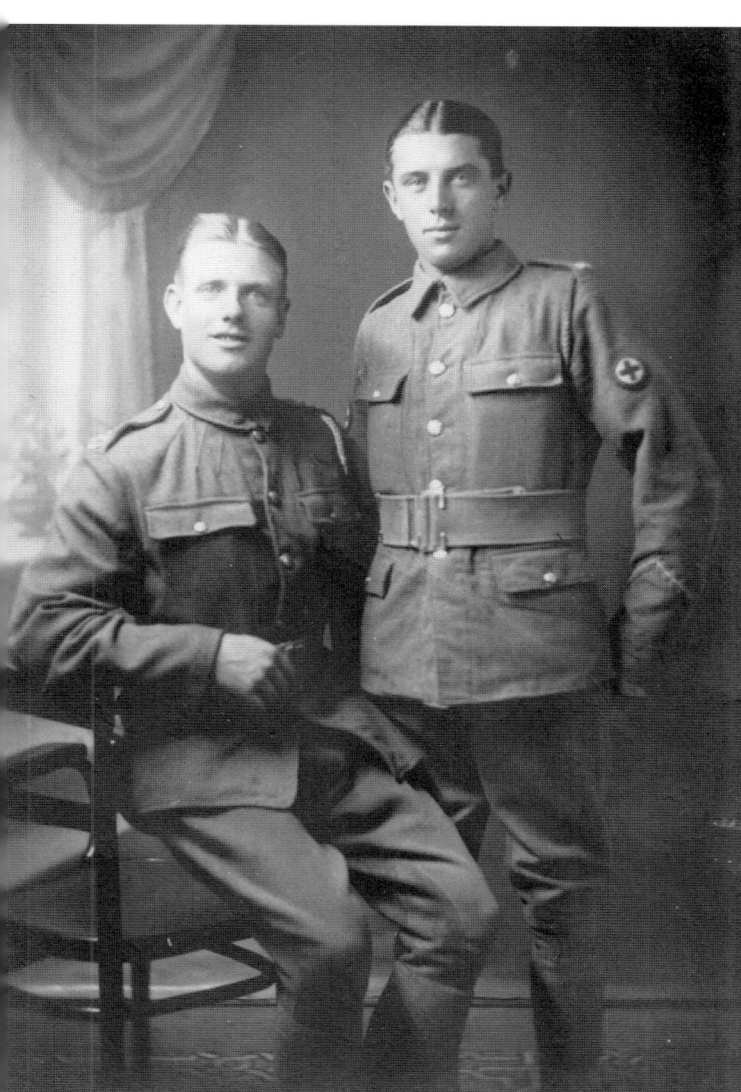

391/492044 Private Jack Albury Edward Jarman, RAMC and 393/492045 Private Leonard Richard Hurrell, RAMC. They were photographed in Alexandria, Egypt, 26 March 1917. They enlisted in the South Eastern Mounted Brigade RAMC on the same day, 15 September 1914.

Jack Albury Edward Jarman was born in Margate in 1897. Prior to enlisting he worked as a golf caddy and his home address was 2 Hill View, Twenties, Margate. He served in the Gallipoli area from 8 October 1915 to 1 February 1916; Egypt from 6 February 1916 to 29 April 1918 and on the Western Front from 8 May 1918 with 230th Field Ambulance, RAMC. In 1919 he was living in Garlinge, Margate.

Leonard Richard Hurrell was born in Margate in 1896. Prior to enlisting he worked as a golf caddy and his home address was 8 Lawn Cottage, Garlinge, Westgate-on-Sea. He served in Gallipoli, 8 October 1915 to 3 December 1915; Egypt 9 December 1915 to 29 April 1918 and on the Western Front from 8 May 1918 with 230th Field Ambulance, RAMC. In 1920, living in Westgate-on-Sea, he requested a military character certificate in support of his application to join the Metropolitan Police Force.

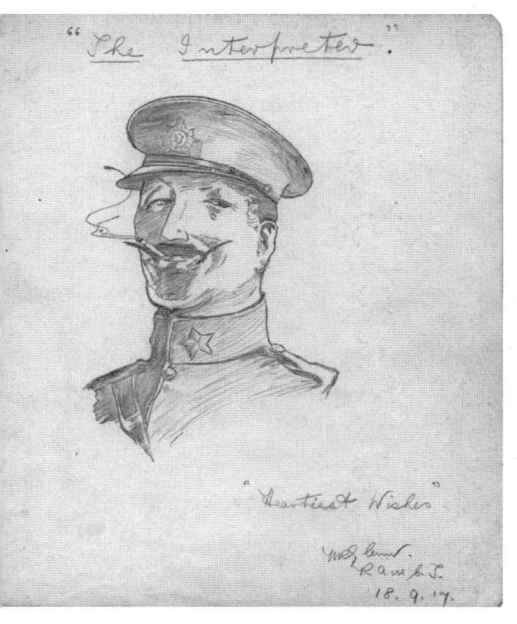

A pencil sketch of an interpreter, drawn by an RAMC Territorial Force soldier, 18 September 1917.

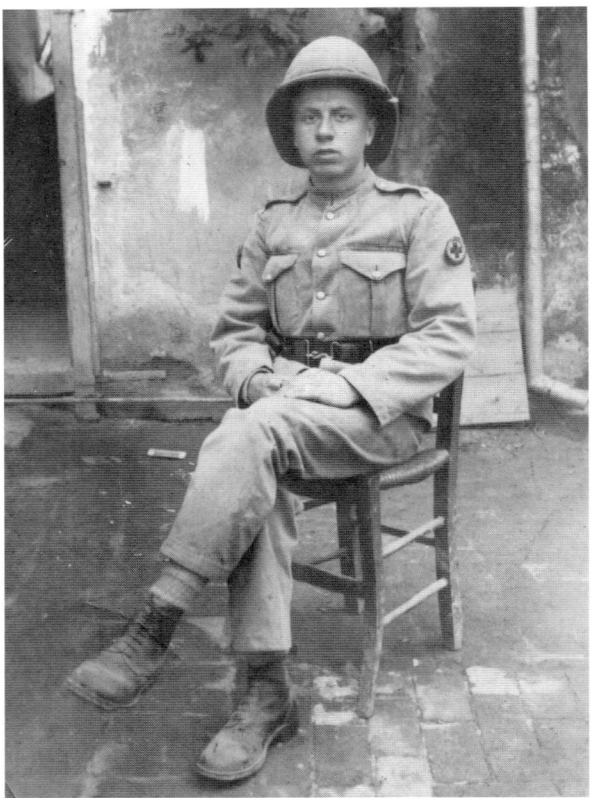

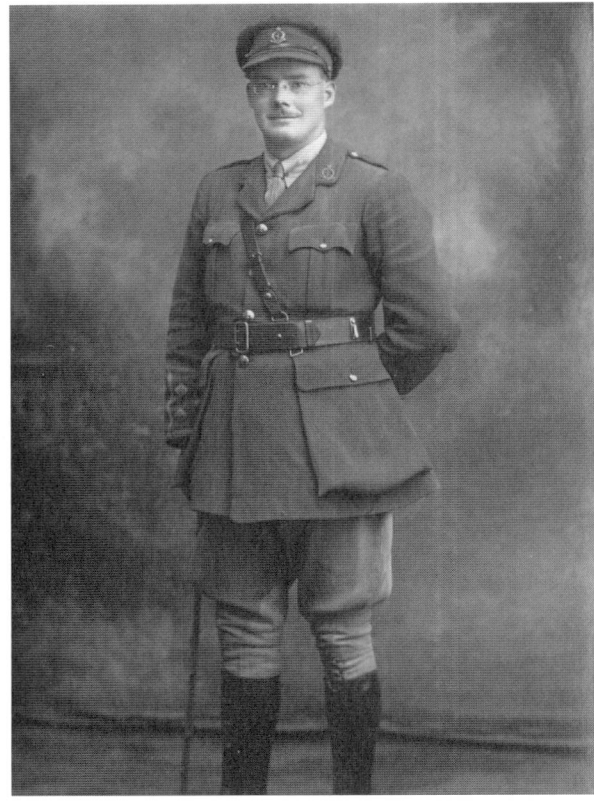

A RAMC private in Salonika.

A RAMC lieutenant in Salonika.

A RAMC lance corporal in warm weather uniform.

A RAMC private in Italy.

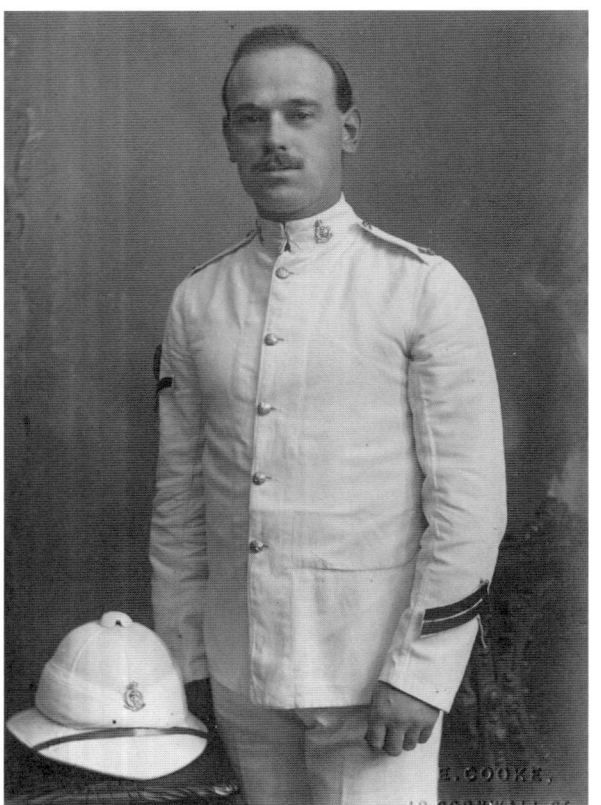

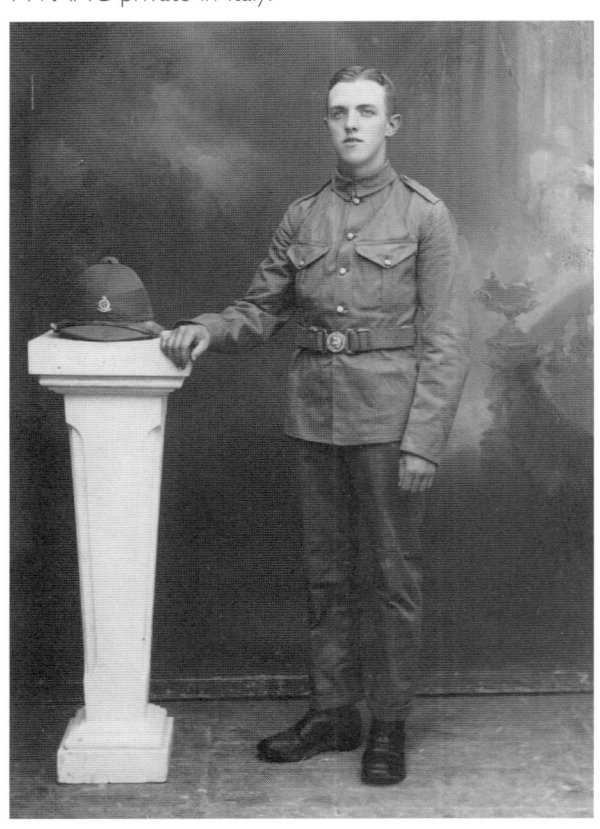

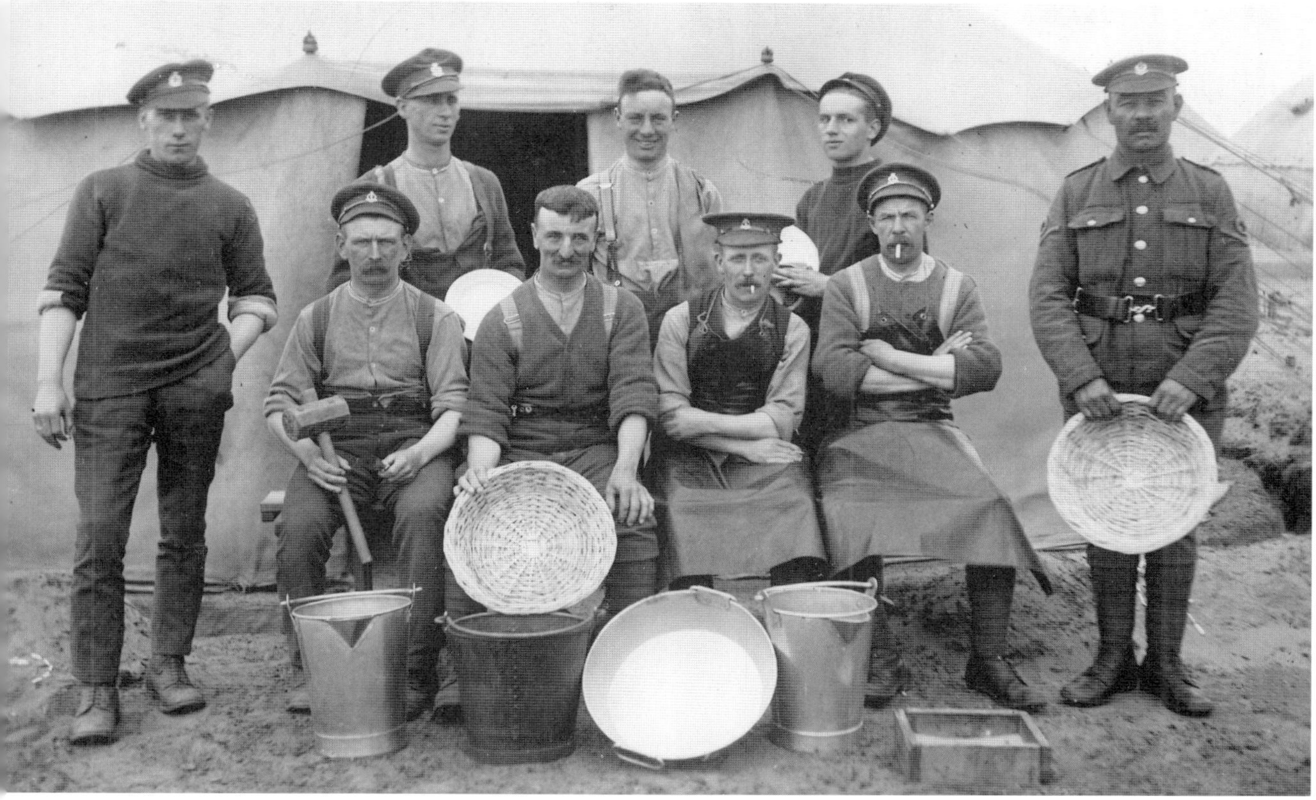

RAMC personnel in Italy.

Two RAMC warrant officers and a sergeant in Egypt.

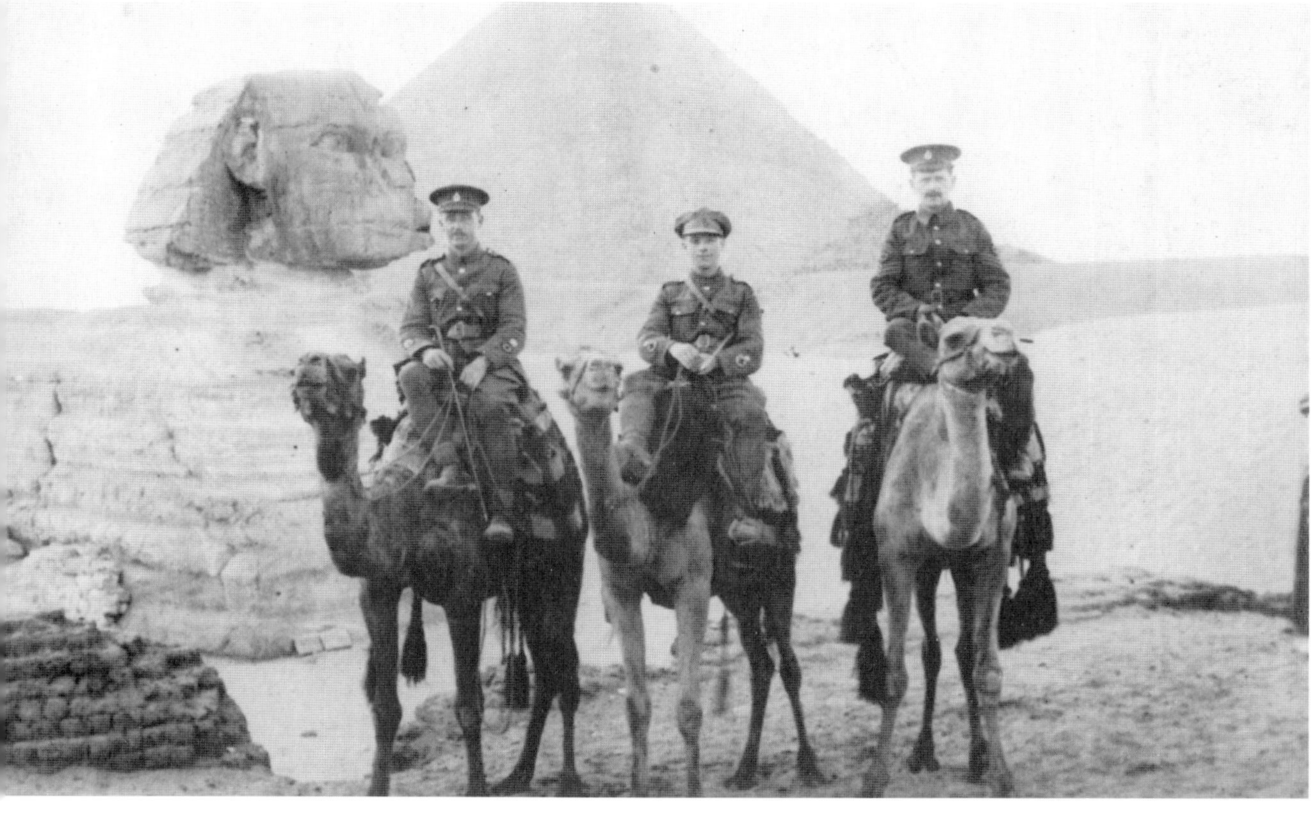

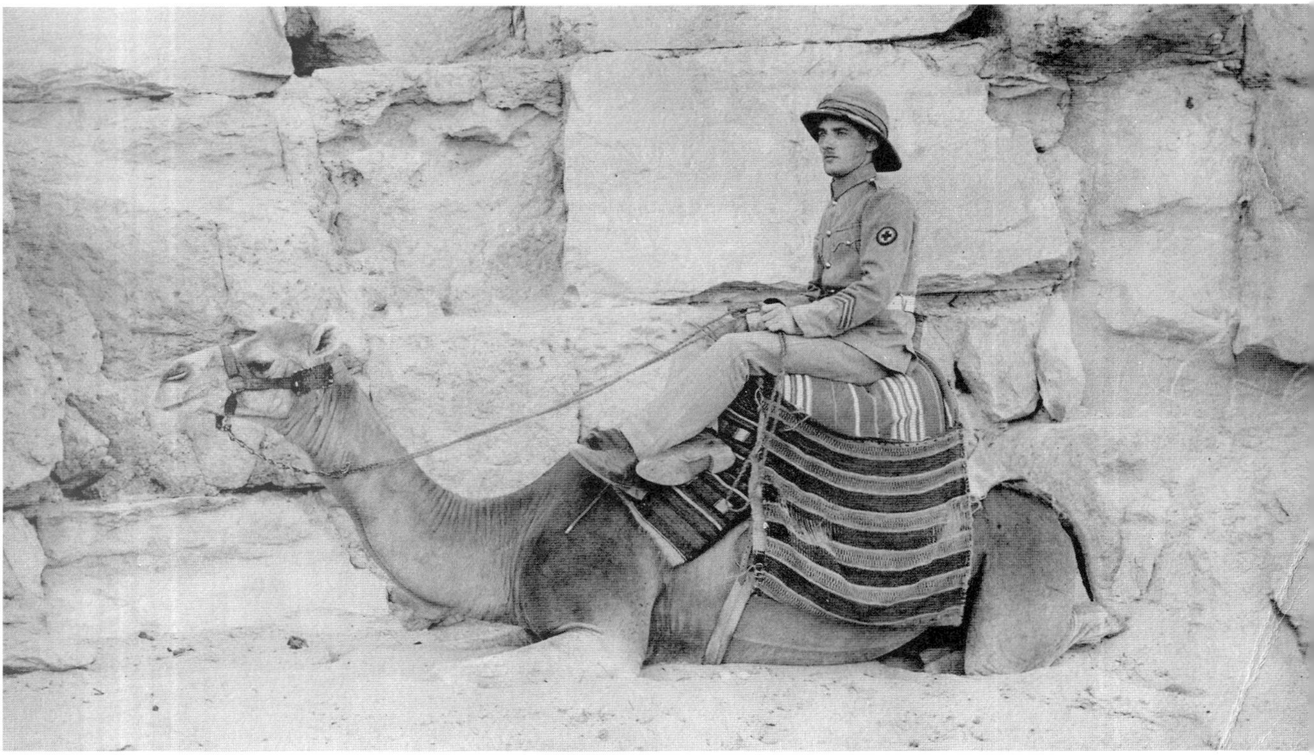

(**Above**) A RAMC private in the Middle East.

(**Opposite**) RAMC personnel in Palestine.

(**Below**) A RAMC field ambulance section camp in Macedonia. On the reverse of the photograph is noted: 'Todorovo – Field Ambulance 'C' section camp, Winter 1916/17 – photo 8/3/1917.'

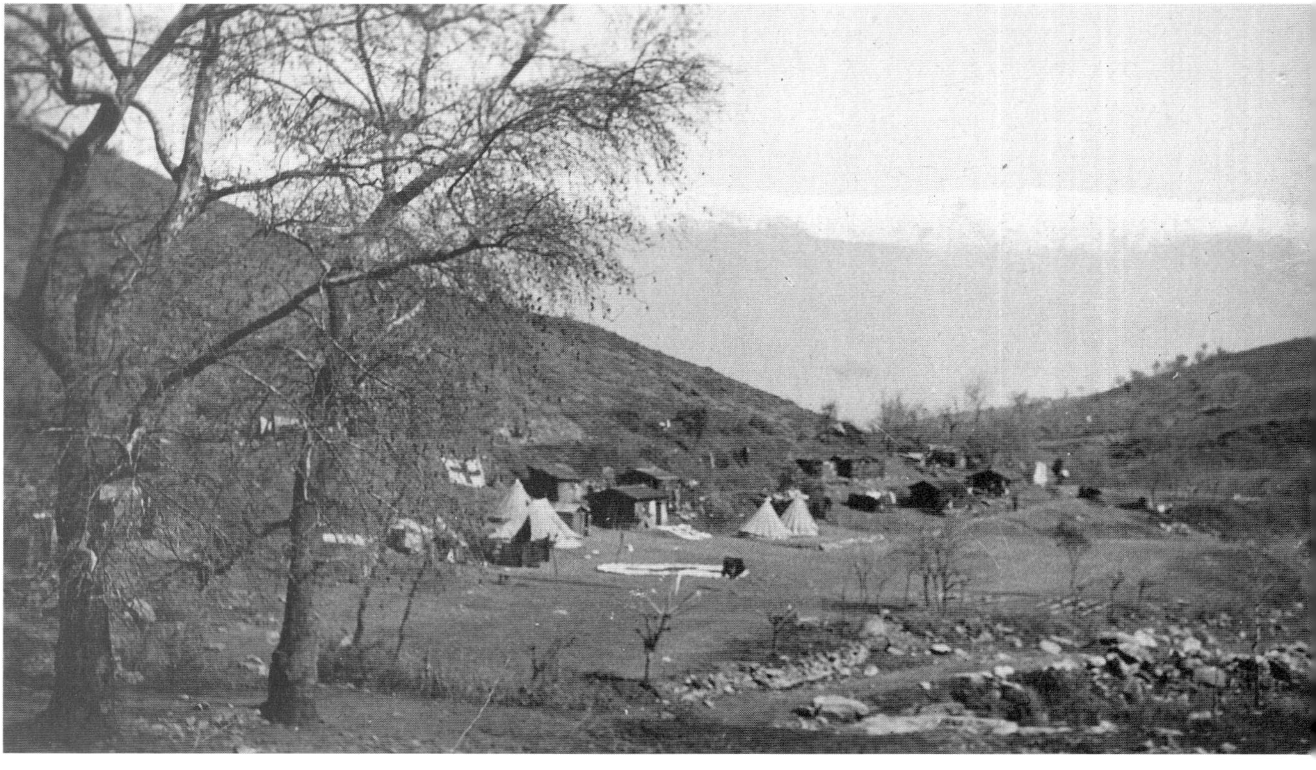

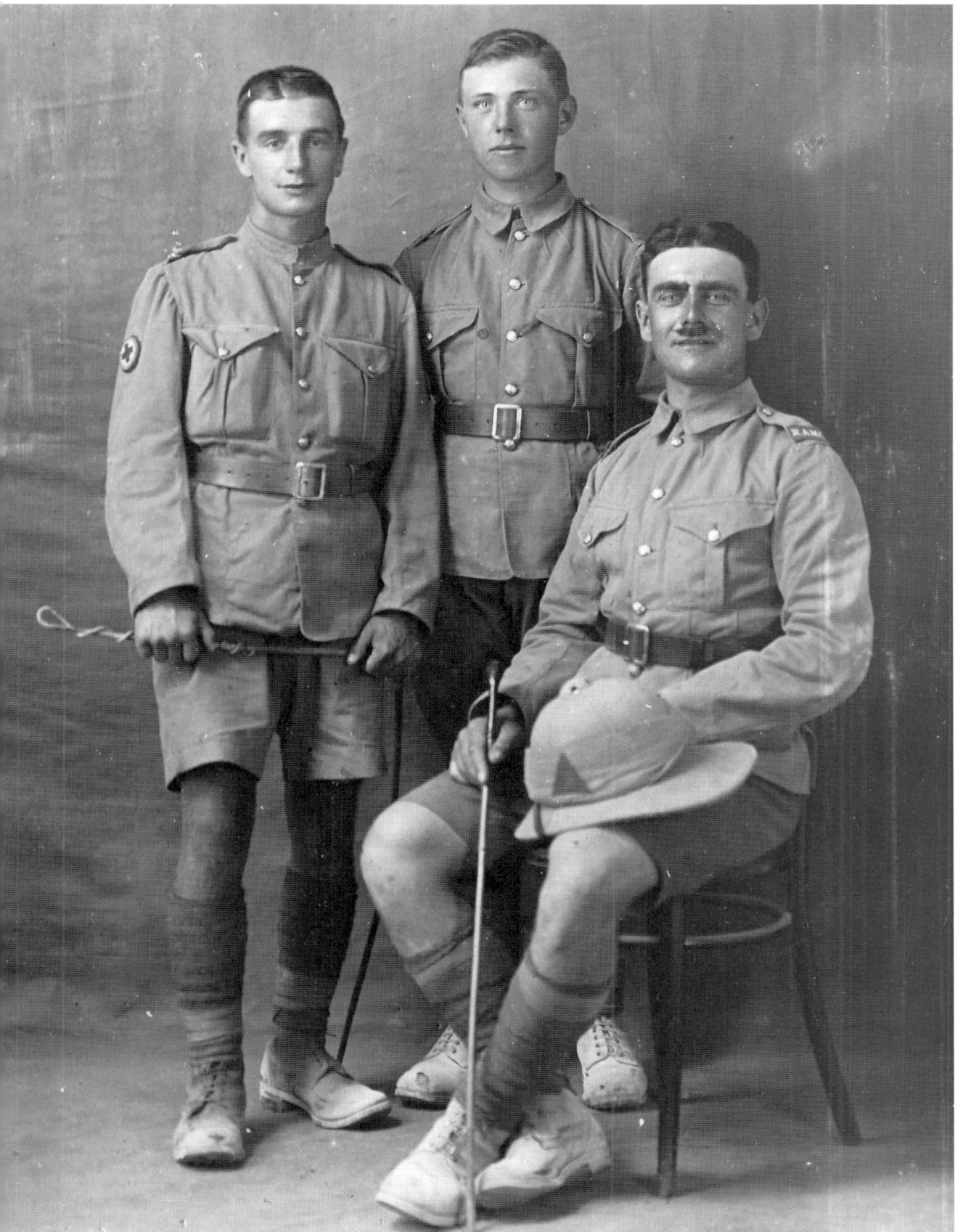

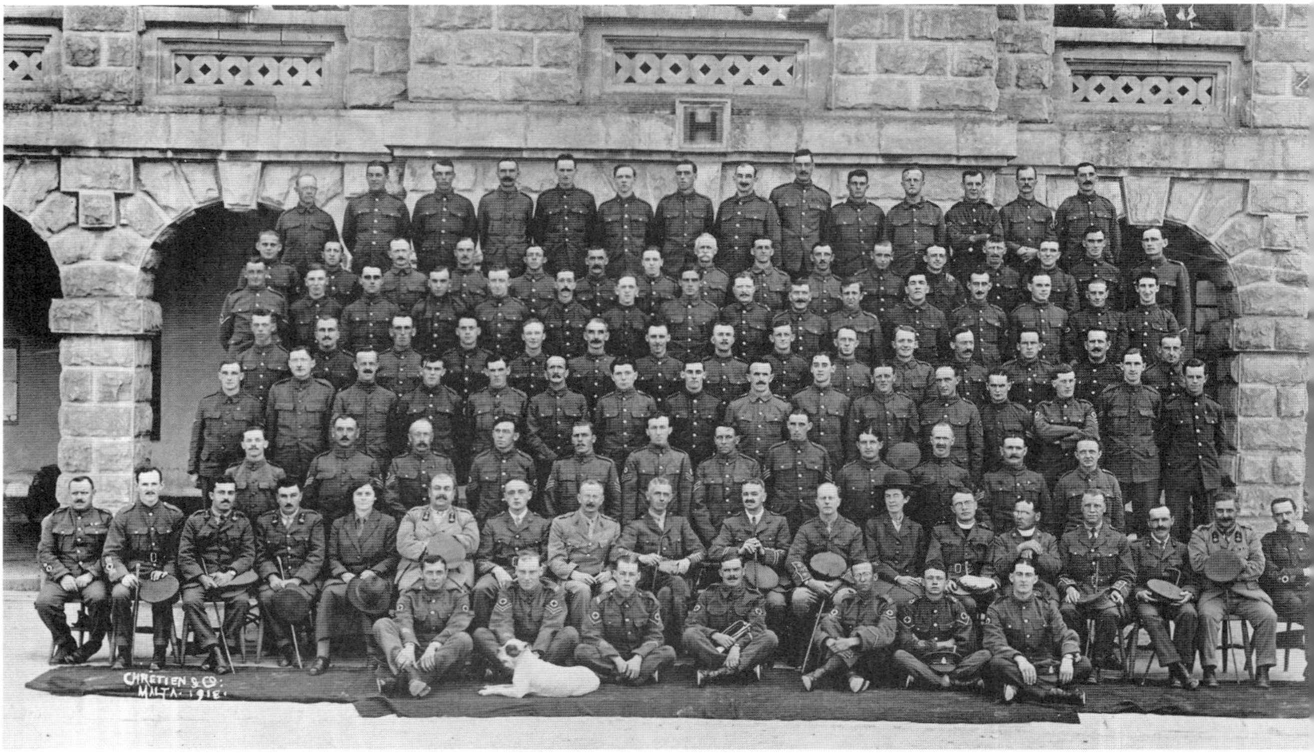

RAMC personnel at St Andrews Military Hospital, Malta, 1918.

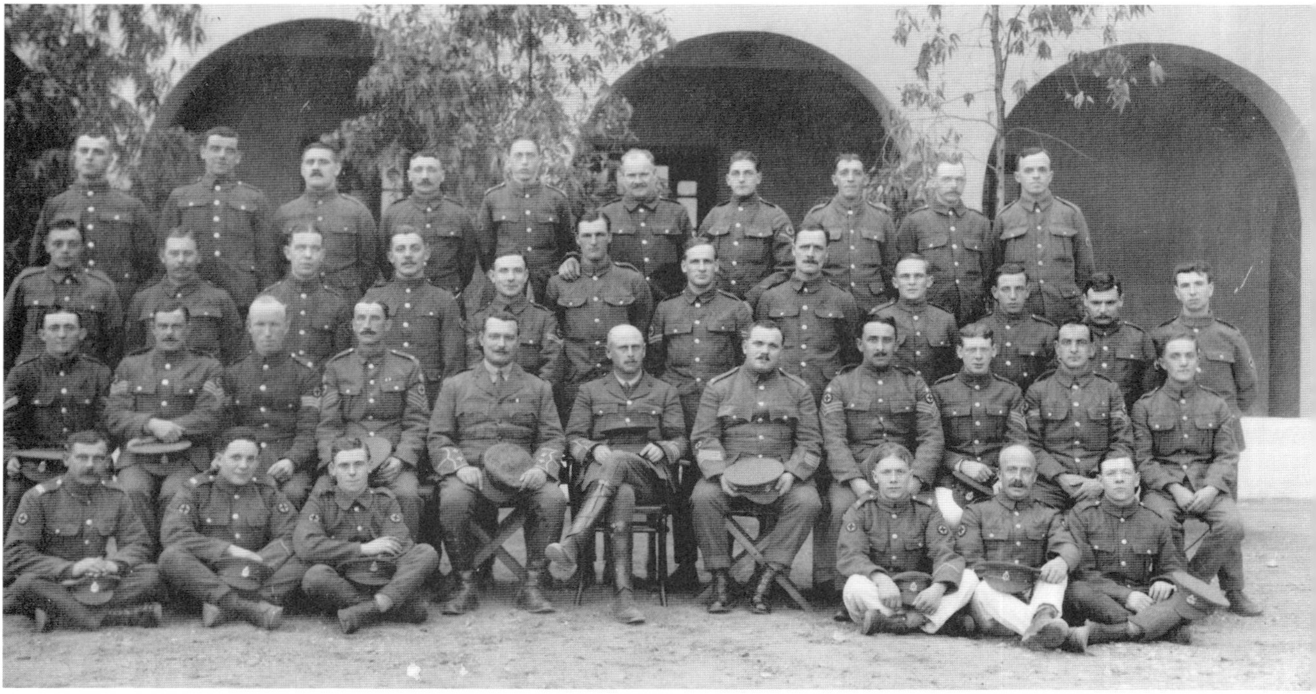

RAMC personnel outside a hospital in the Middle East.

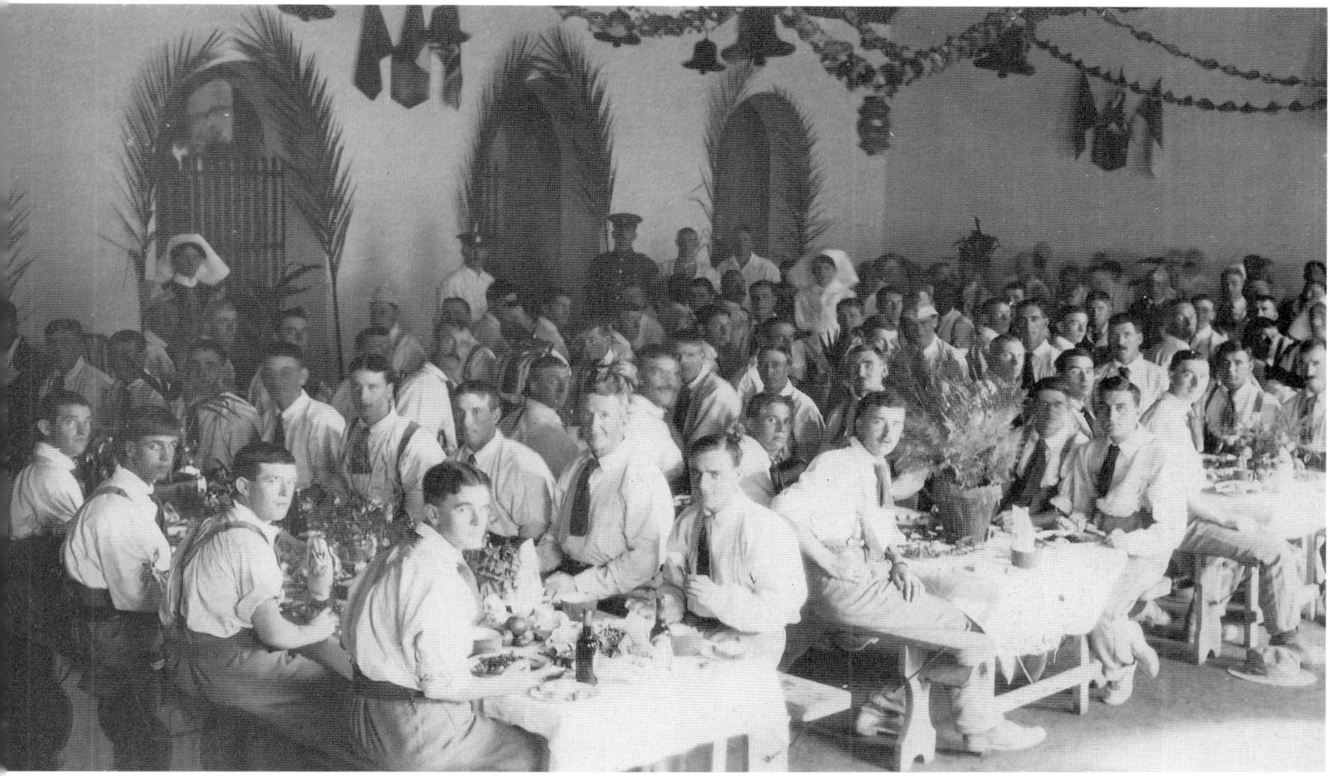

Patients with RAMC personnel and nurses, on Christmas Day at 27th General Hospital, Egypt.

A nurse serving at an overseas British Army medical facility.

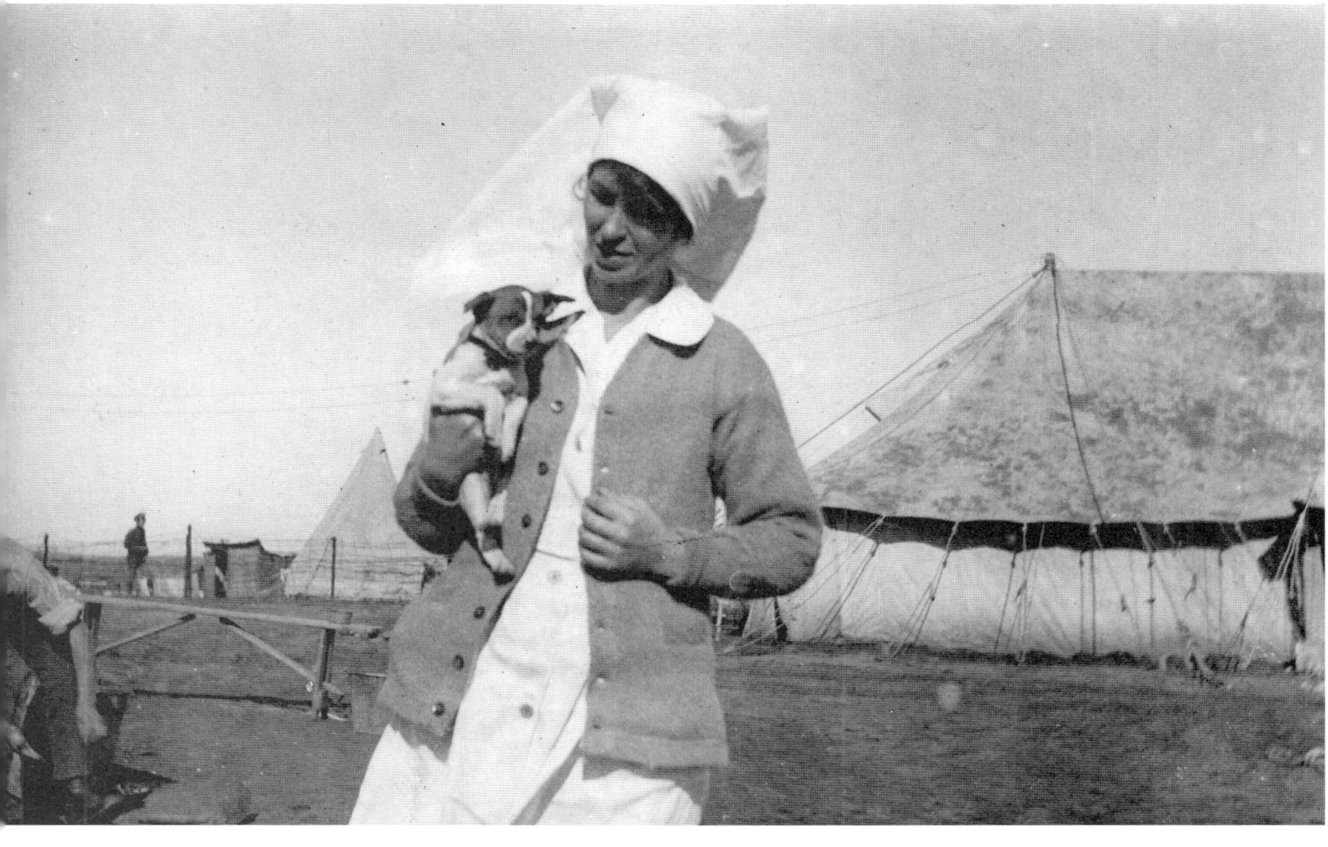

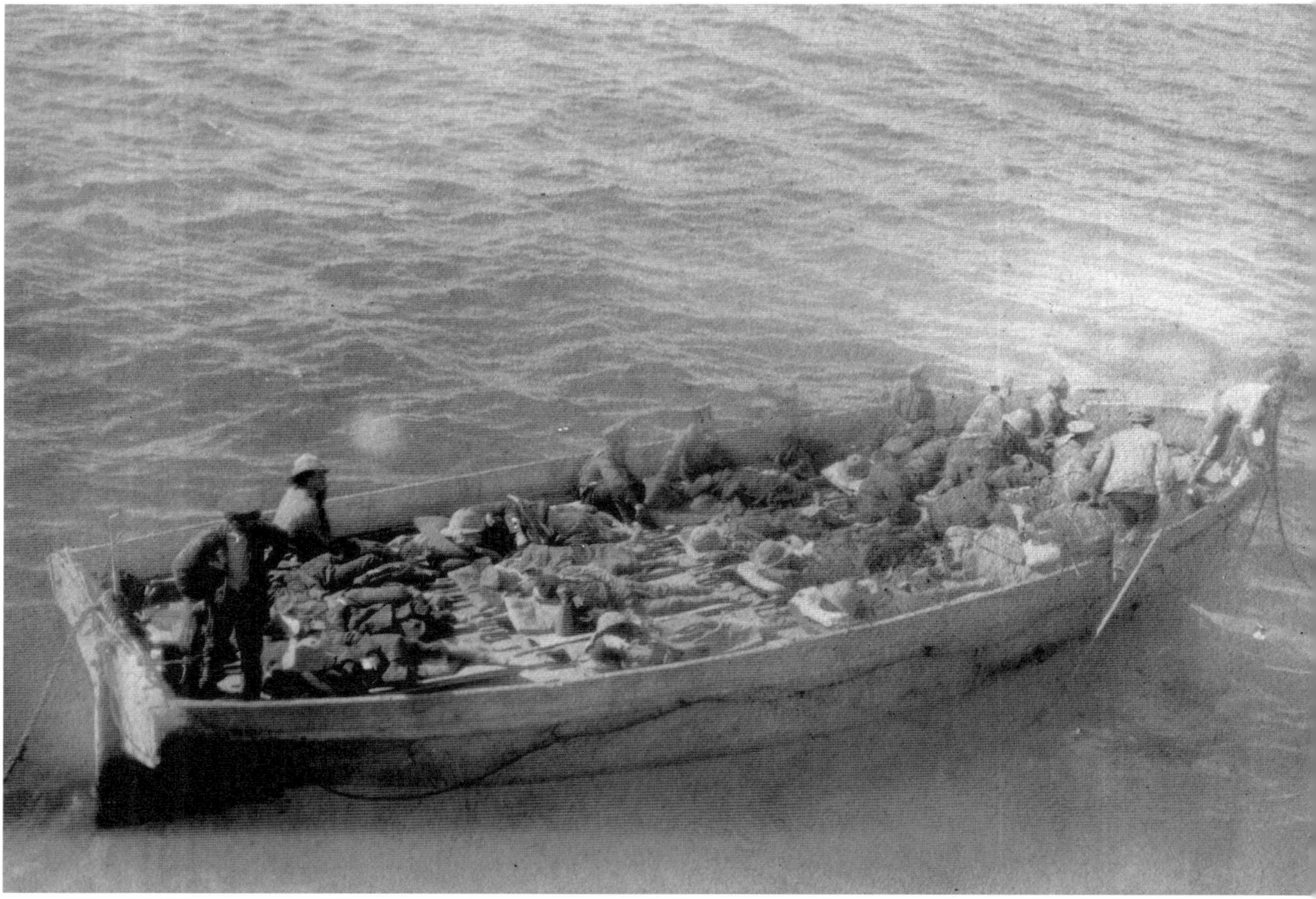

Casualties on a barge approaching a hospital ship during the Gallipoli Campaign. The lack of shade on deck is evident.

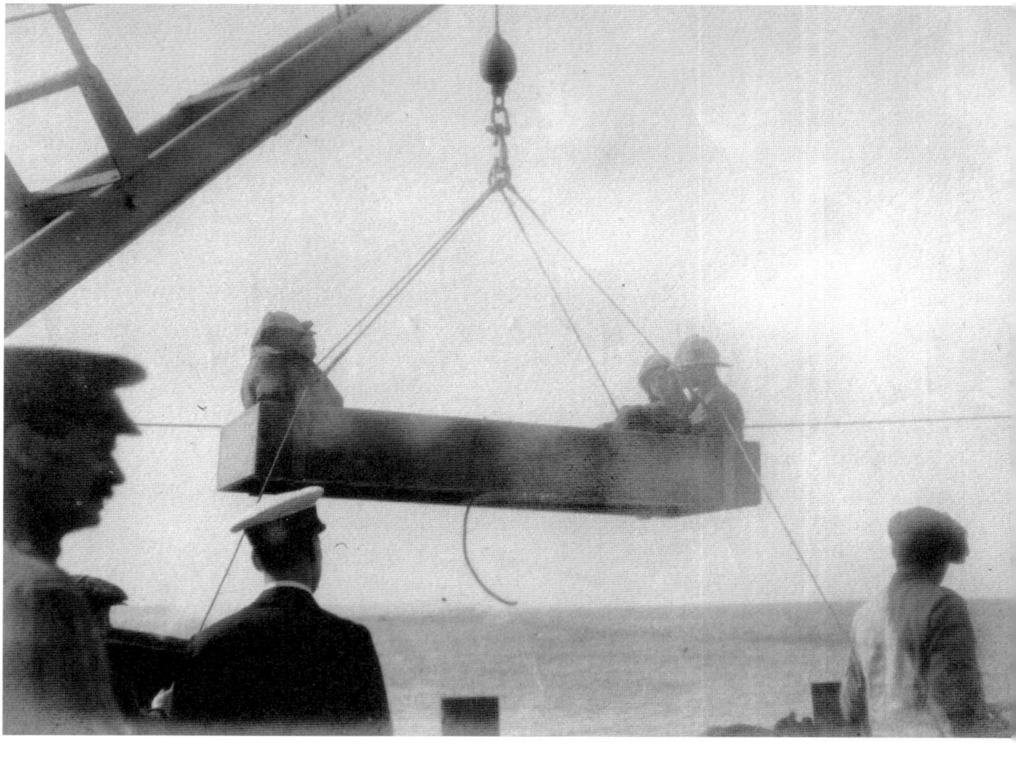

Bringing wounded on board a hospital ship during the Gallipoli Campaign.

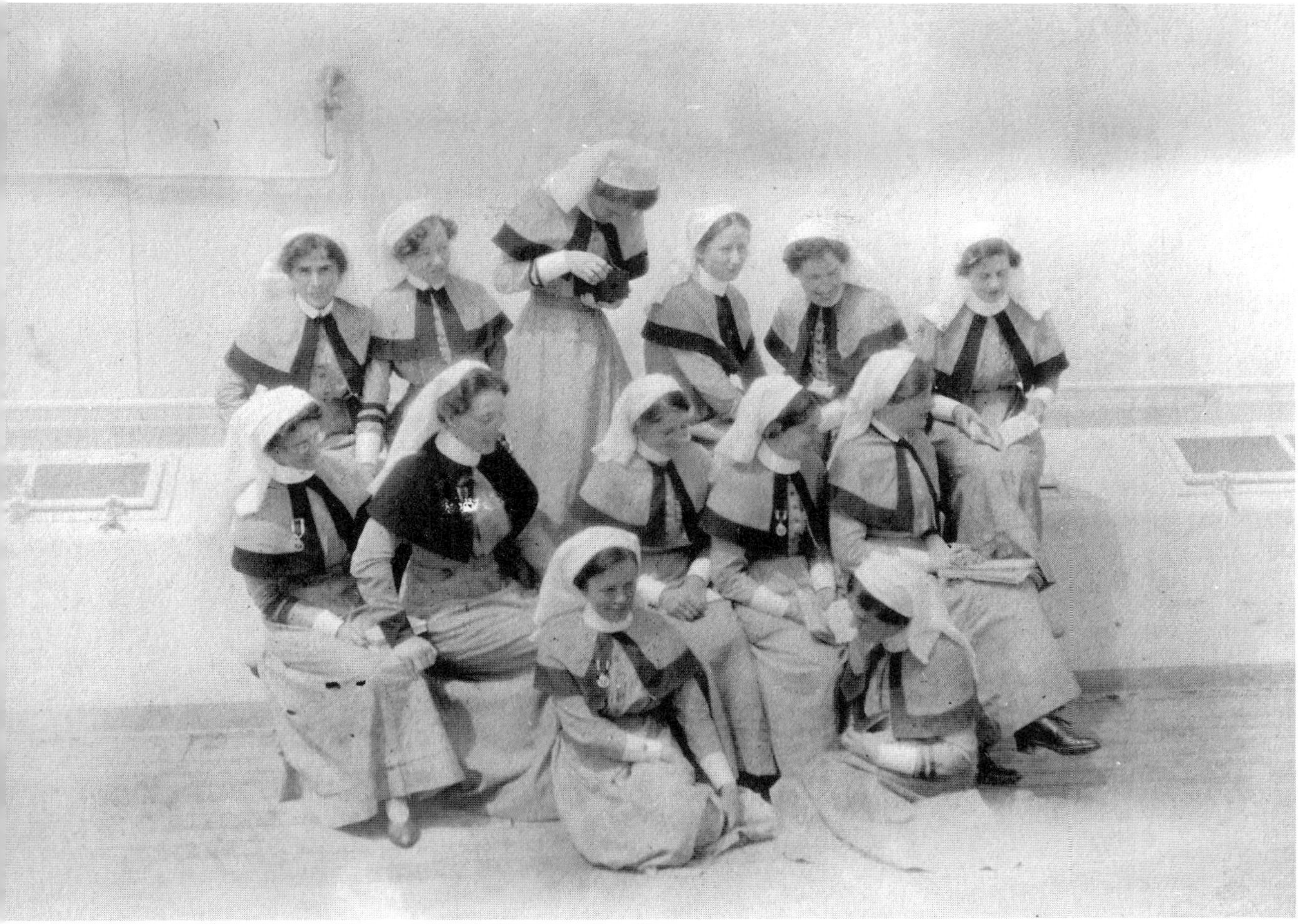

Nursing staff on a hospital ship during the Gallipoli Campaign.

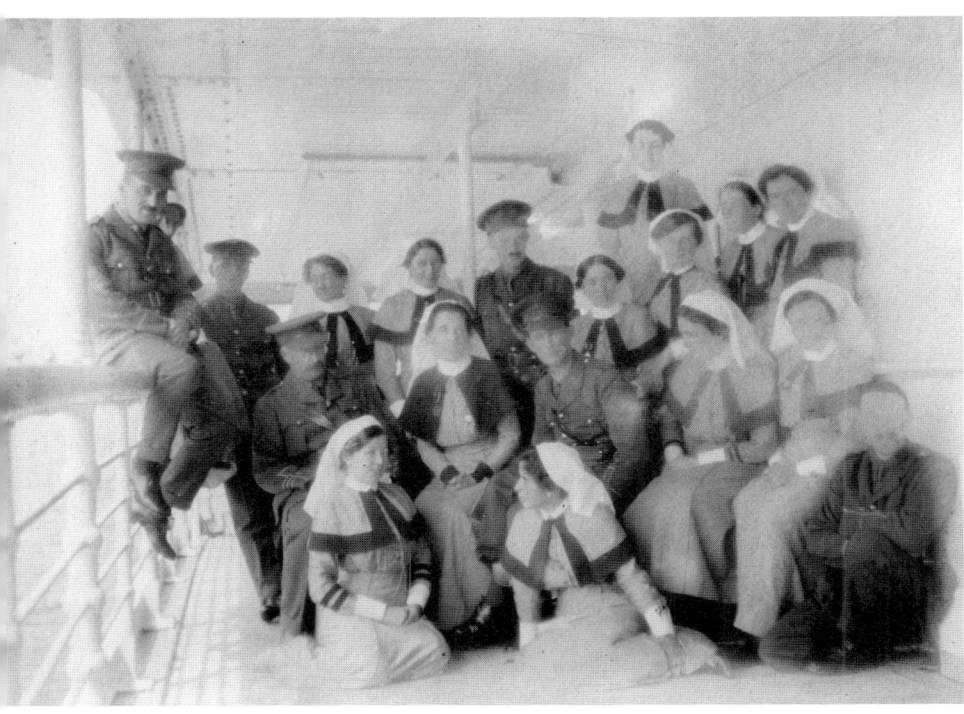

RAMC officers and nursing staff on a hospital ship during the Gallipoli Campaign.

A Christmas card sent from Private Thomas A. Smith RAMC, whilst serving on HM Hospital Ship *Oxfordshire* in 1914.

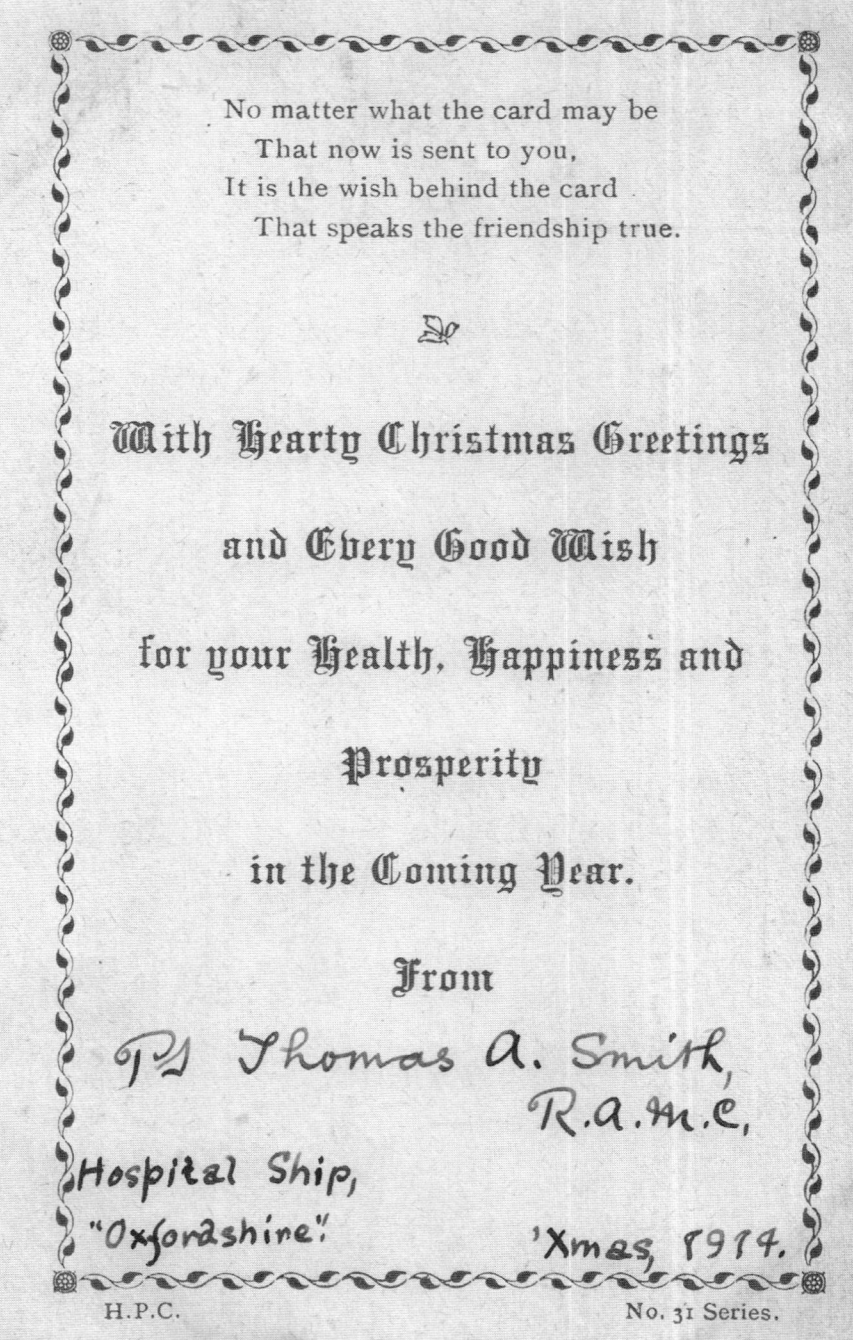

(**Opposite, above**) RAMC personnel on board a hospital ship.

(**Opposite, below**) Royal Mail Steam Ship *Carisbrook Castle* which was requisitioned for use as a hospital ship during the First World War.

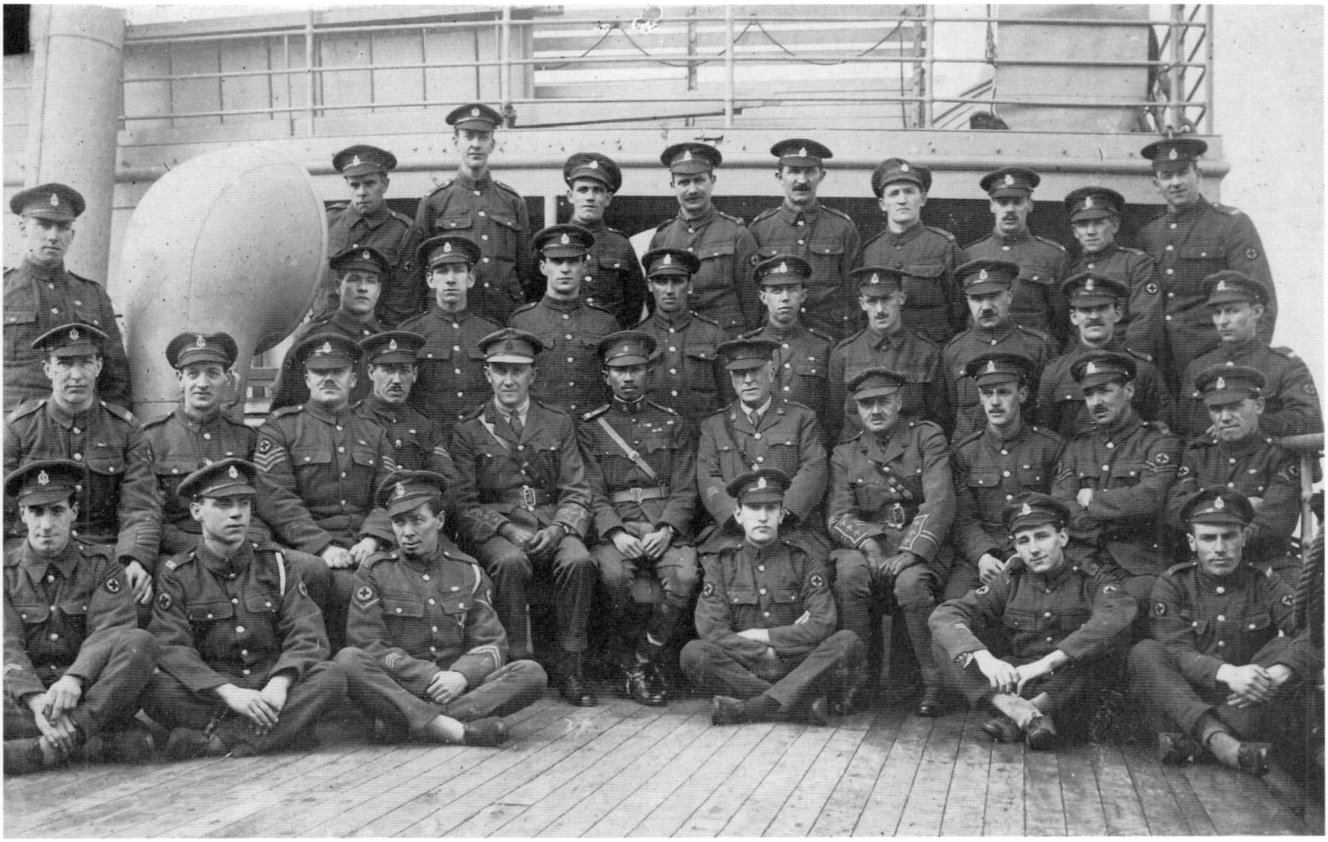

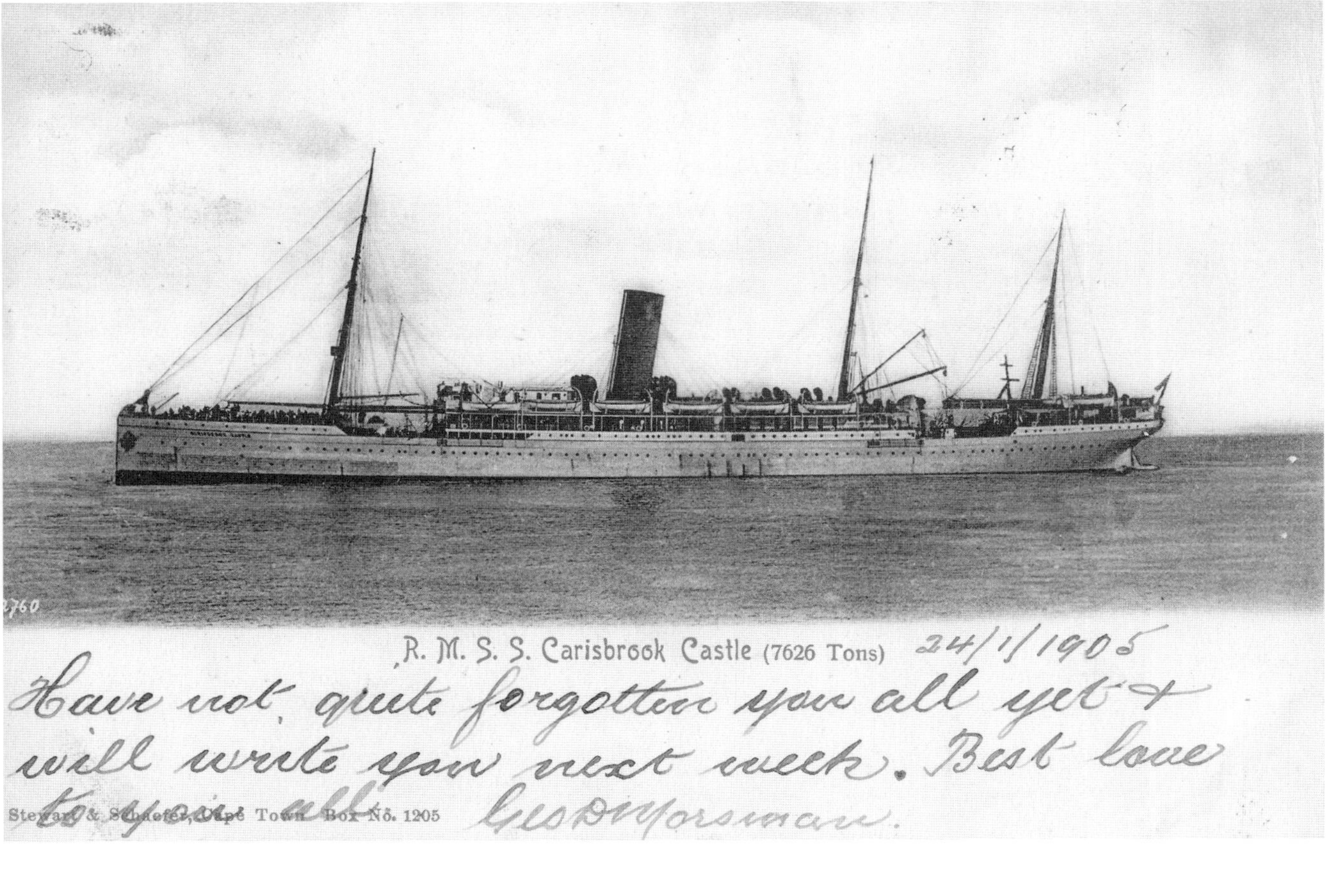

R.M.S.S. Carisbrook Castle (7626 Tons) 24/1/1905

Have not quite forgotten you all yet & will write you next week. Best love to you all
Geo D Morsman.

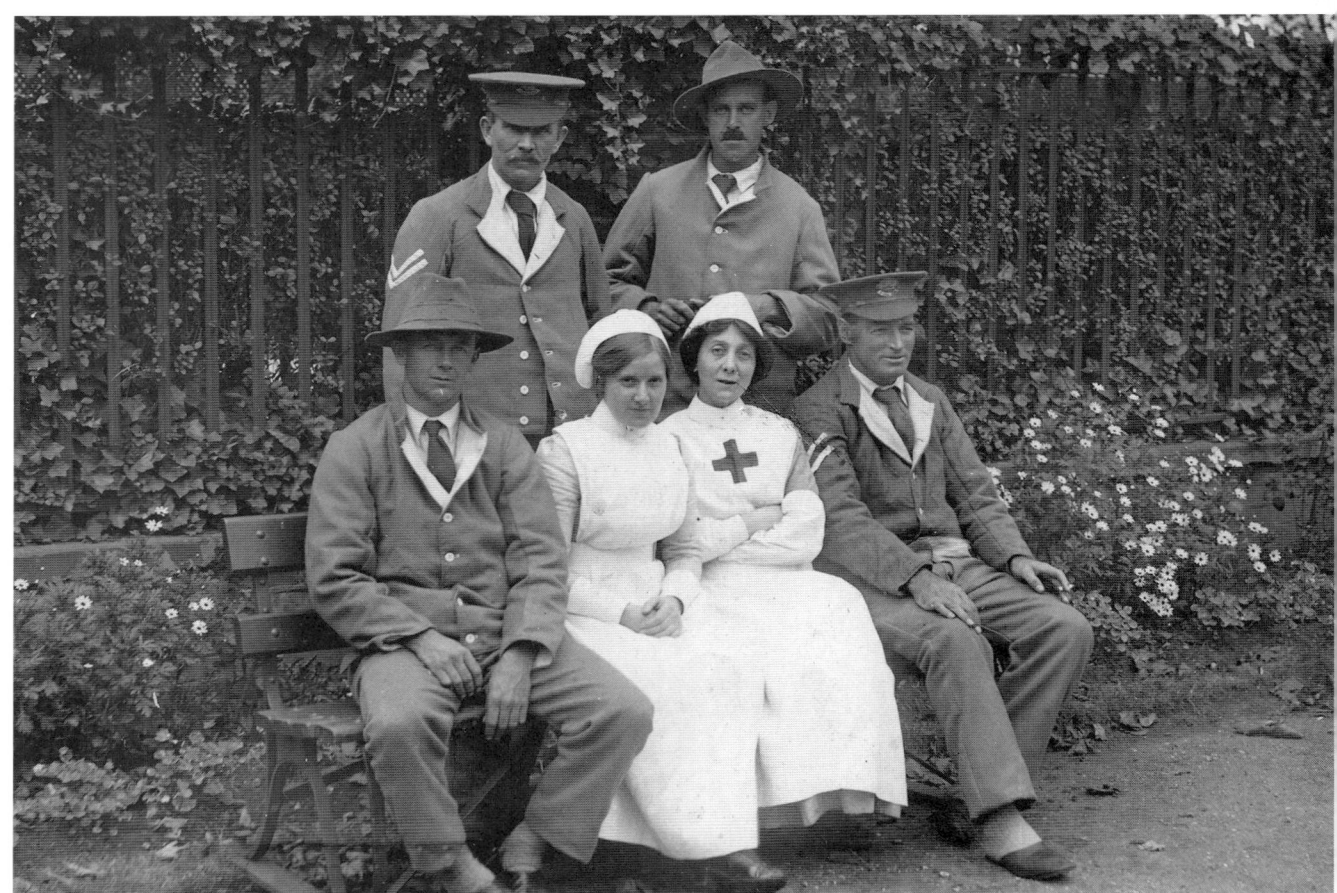

A group of wounded Australian personnel evacuated from Gallipoli by hospital ship, via Malta, recovering at Fulham Military Hospital with nursing staff. The photo is signed on the reverse 'A Few Colonials. W.T. Liddle Eltis; P.J. Lynch; Parkinson; Howarth. Hammersmith 2.10.1915.'

297 Peter John Lynch enlisted on 21 October 1914 at Guildford, Western Australia, aged 30. He was born at Maryborough, Victoria and worked as a labourer. He lived at Clyde Street, Cottesloe Beach, Western Australia, with his wife Annie Lynch. He served with the 10th Australian Light Horse and was promoted lance corporal on 15 May 1915. He suffered a gunshot wound to his right cheek on 31 May 1915 and was again wounded on 7 August 1915 at Walkers Ridge, this time a shell wound to his thigh which resulted in his being evacuated to the UK where he arrived in Fulham on 14 September 1915. On 1 August 1916 he was posted to the 3rd Australian Light Horse Brigade Machine Gun Squadron and later served with the 3rd Australian Light Horse Training Regiment. On 19 September 1917 he was posted back to the 10th Australian Light Horse. Promoted to sergeant, he embarked at Suez to return to Australia on 5 February 1919.

2026 William Thomas Liddle Eltis enlisted on 21 September 1914 at Albert Park, Melbourne. He was born at Glenferrie, Victoria and worked as a storeman. He had previously served with the Australian Light Horse and the Victorian Mounted Rifles and later with the mechanical transport, Divisional Supply Column in the 9th Australian Army Service Corps. His wife was Heather Marion Eltis of 7 St Johns Avenue, Mont Albert, Victoria. William Eltis was evacuated from Gallipoli with fibrositis and rheumatism. He was also blown 12 feet by an exploding shell, suffering concussion. Evacuated to the UK and admitted to hospital in Fulham on 14 September 1915, he remained there until 18 January 1916 and was discharged at Melbourne on 30 October 1916, age 33.

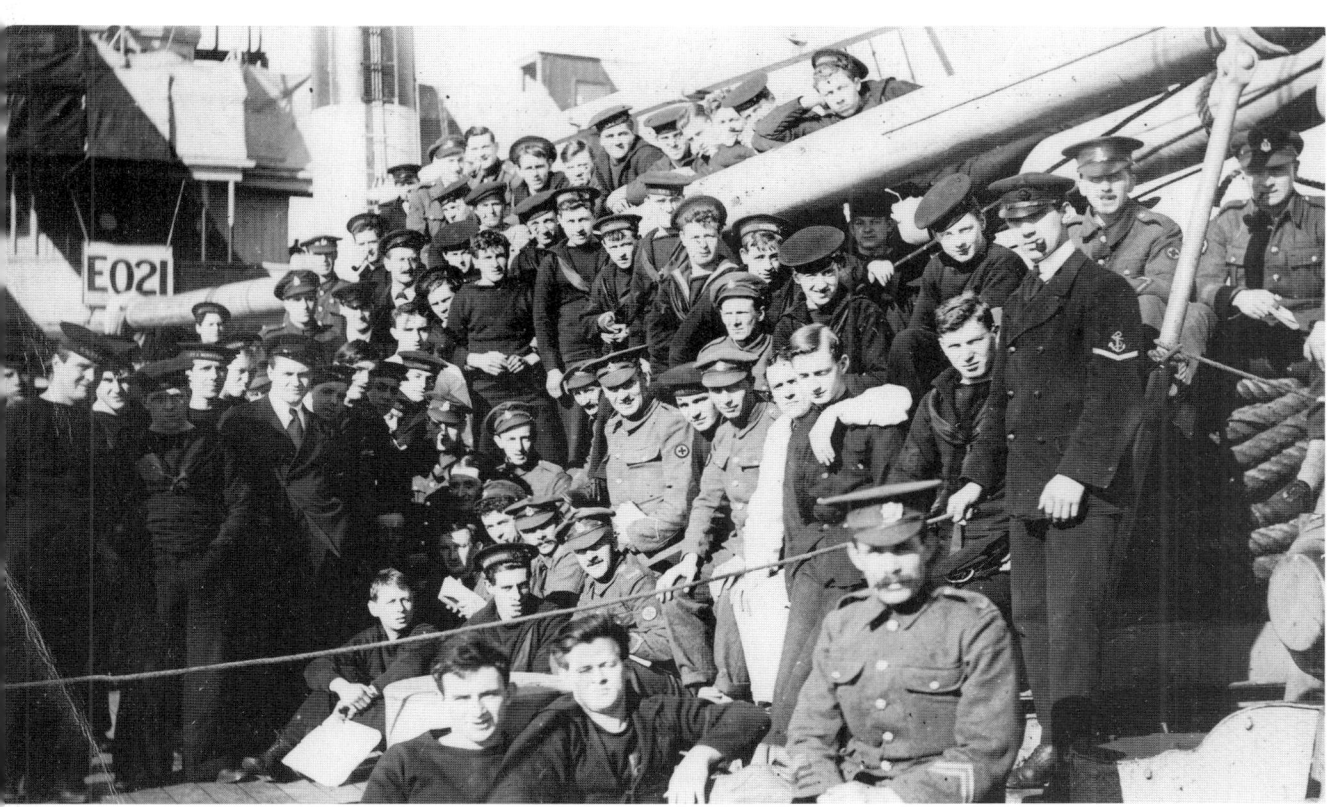
RAMC personnel and Royal Navy crew on the deck of HM Hospital Ship *Carisbrook Castle*.

Chapter 5

After the Conflict

Following the end of the First World War RAMC units continued to provide medical support around the globe, including as part of the Allied Occupation forces in Germany. Many who served with the corps were demobilised. However, some personnel continued to serve with regular RAMC units and also with the Territorial Army. Some were still serving with the RAMC at the outbreak of the Second World War.

During the First World War 6,873 personnel died serving in the RAMC; of these casualties an estimated 470 officers and 3,669 other ranks were either killed in action or died of wounds. Many more were wounded, injured or contracted diseases whilst on active service.

Old comrades associations were formed by veterans of RAMC units to remember their service together and commemorate members of their unit who died during the conflict. The associations met regularly and sometimes arranged to visit the battlefields where they served.

Photographs remain as tribute to the service and sacrifices made by members of the RAMC and medical services during the First World War.

(**Opposite, above**) 45th Field Ambulance, RAMC, 25th December 1918. A photograph of personnel who had served with the Unit throughout the conflict. *(Mr Andrew Read)*

(**Opposite, below**) The band of the 2nd Field Ambulance RAMC, Bonn, Germany, 1919. Three of the band members, including the sergeant (seated centre), wear the cap badge of the Royal Army Service Corps.

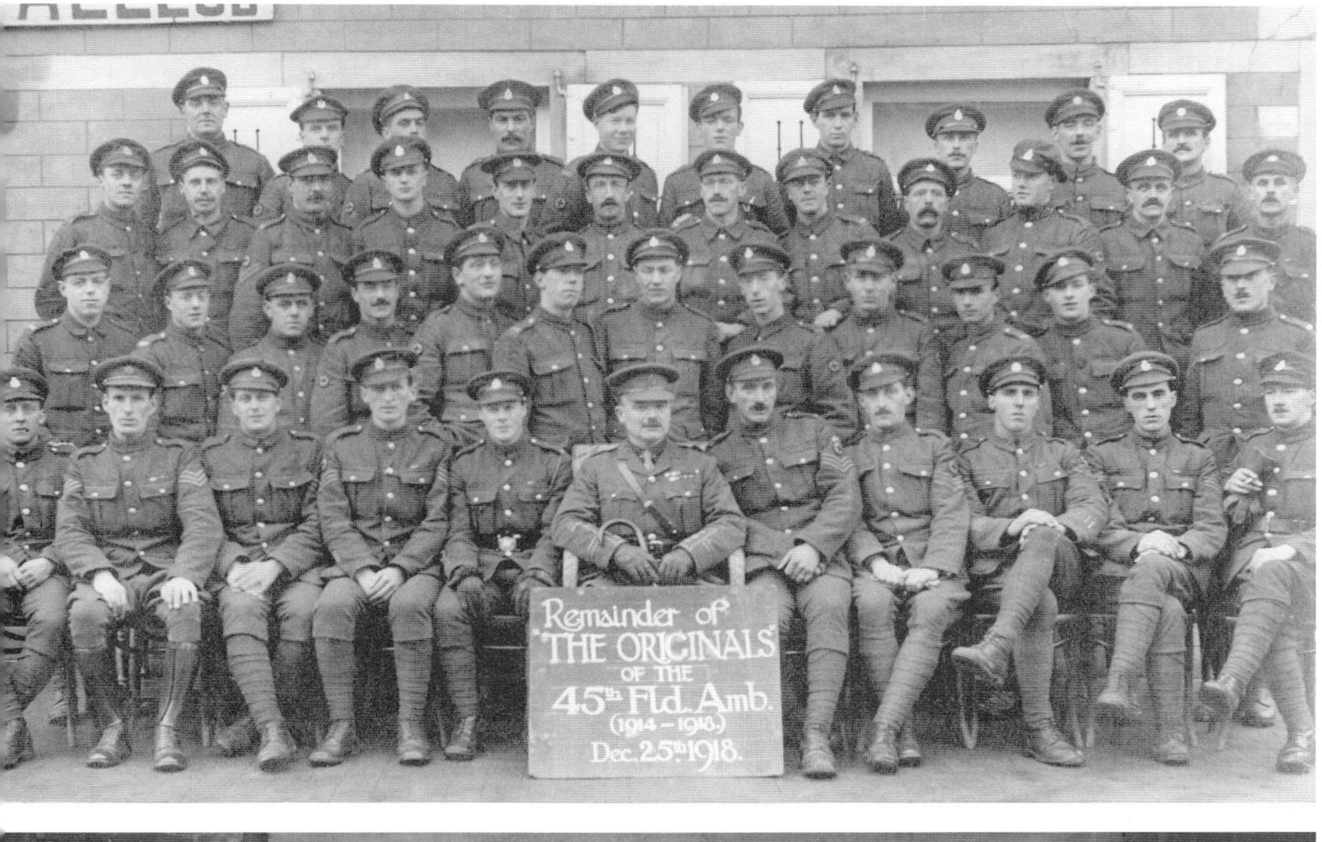

Remainder of THE ORIGINALS of the 45th Fld. Amb. (1914–1918) Dec. 25th 1918.

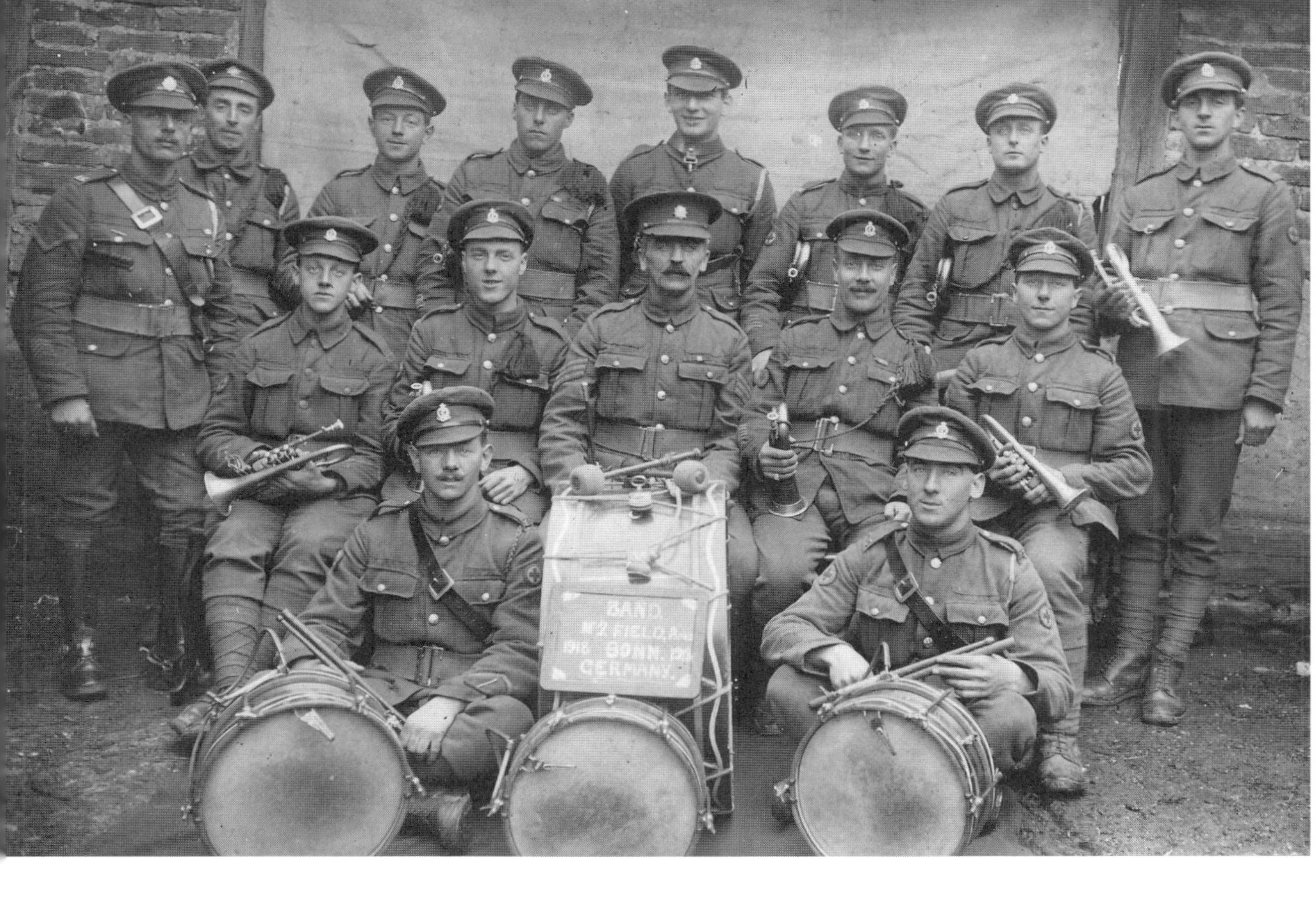

Band, No 2 Field Amb, Bonn, Germany

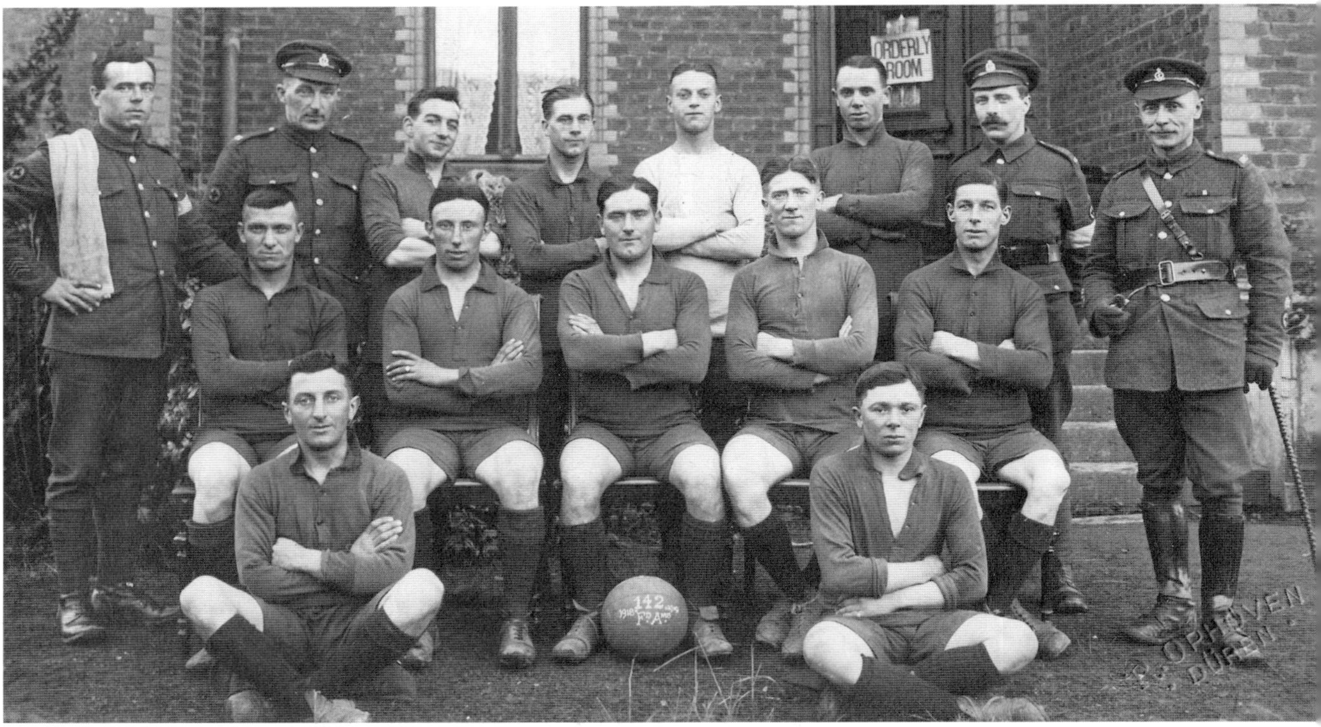

Football team of the 142nd Field Ambulance, RAMC, Düren, Germany, 1919.

A group of soldiers serving with the RAMC in Germany, part of the British Army of the Rhine. Three servicemen wear 9th (Scottish) Division Thistle patches and two (standing) wear the ribbon of the Military Medal (MM). The private, seated right, wears a wound stripe on his left cuff.

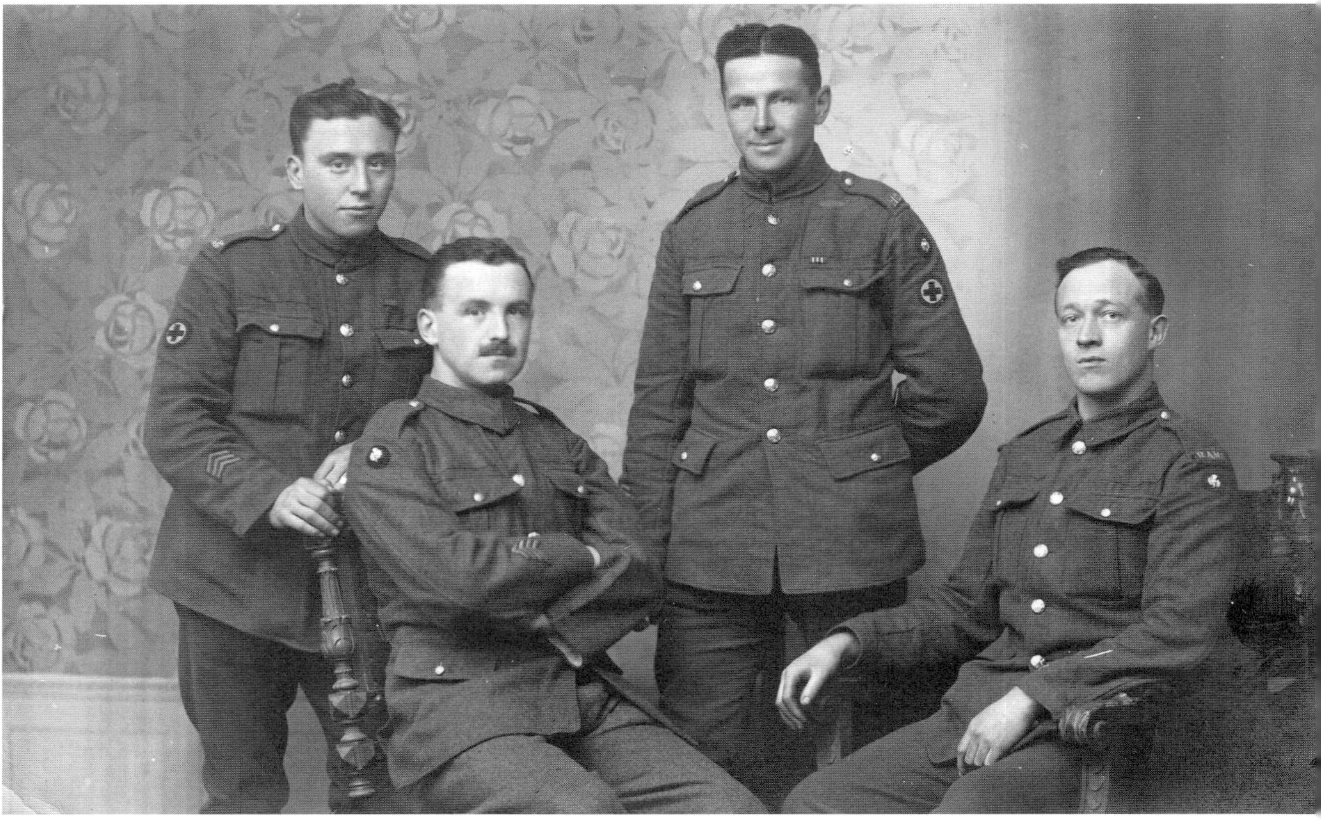

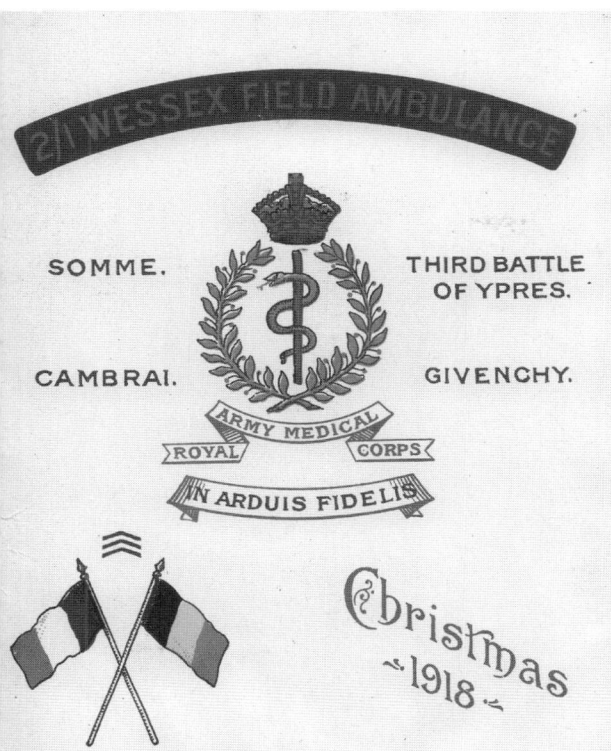

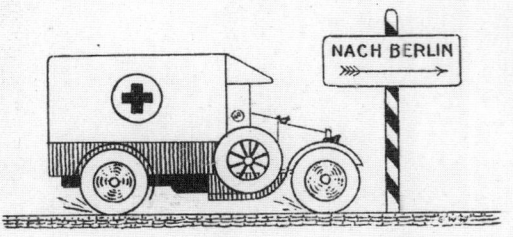

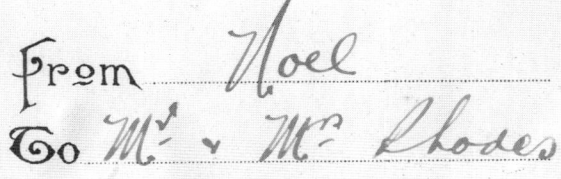

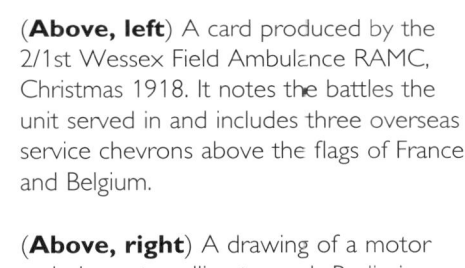

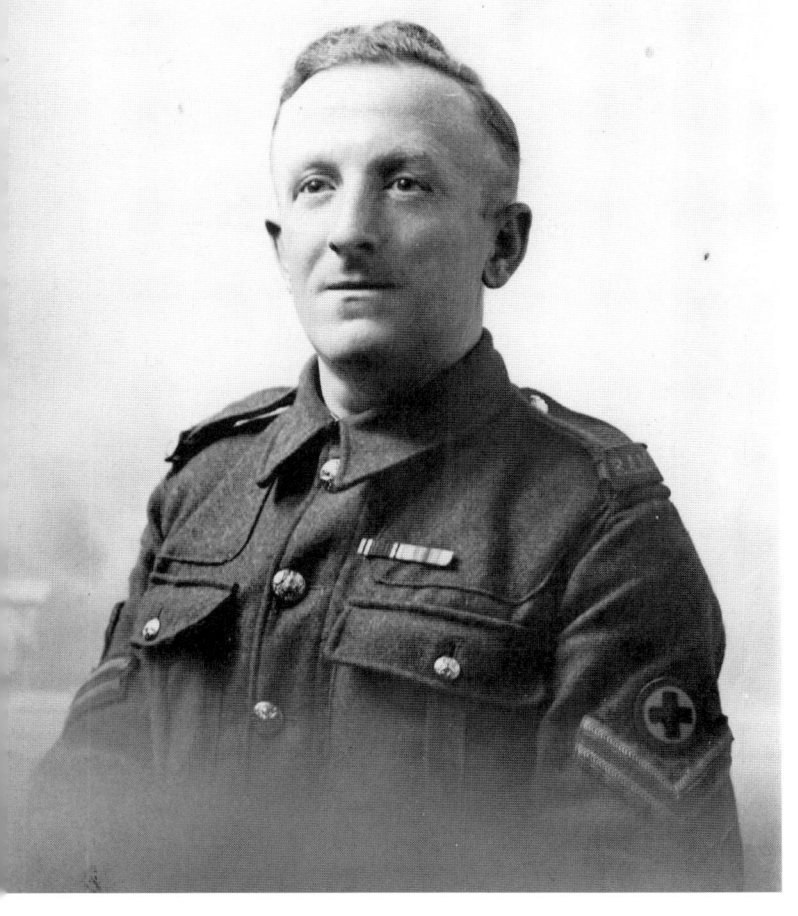

(**Above, left**) A card produced by the 2/1st Wessex Field Ambulance RAMC, Christmas 1918. It notes the battles the unit served in and includes three overseas service chevrons above the flags of France and Belgium.

(**Above, right**) A drawing of a motor ambulance travelling towards Berlin is featured inside the 2/1st Wessex Field Ambulance Christmas card.

(**Left**) A RAMC corporal wearing the medal ribbons of the British War Medal and Victory Medal.

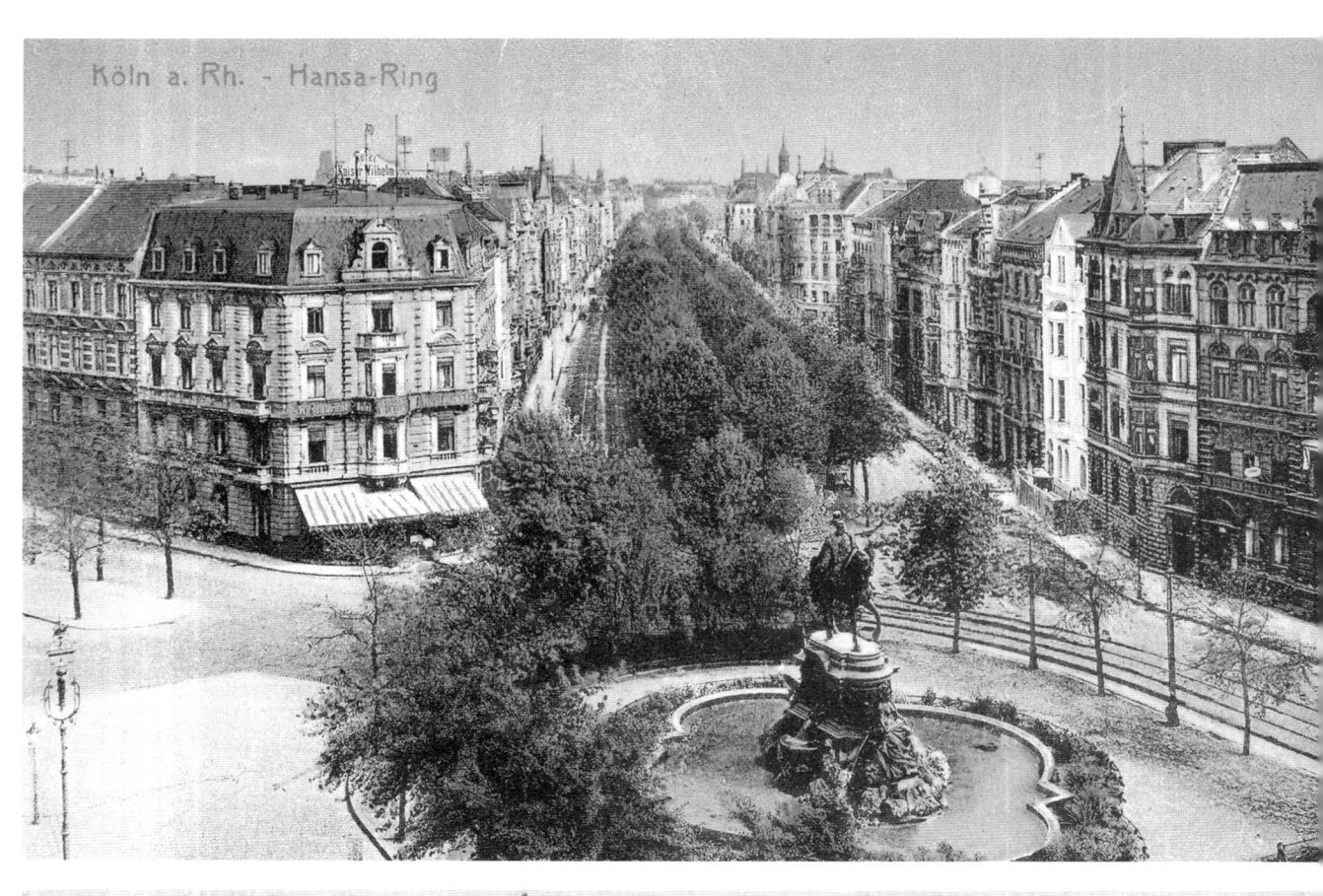

Köln a. Rh. - Hansa-Ring

C. L. K.   47912

Dear M.

Wednesday

Just off to No 3 General Hospital. Am only will likely be as soon as possible when arriving there. By Bye Lovie

R.H.B.

Miss M. Stuttle
30 Salisbury Ave
Colchester
Essex
England

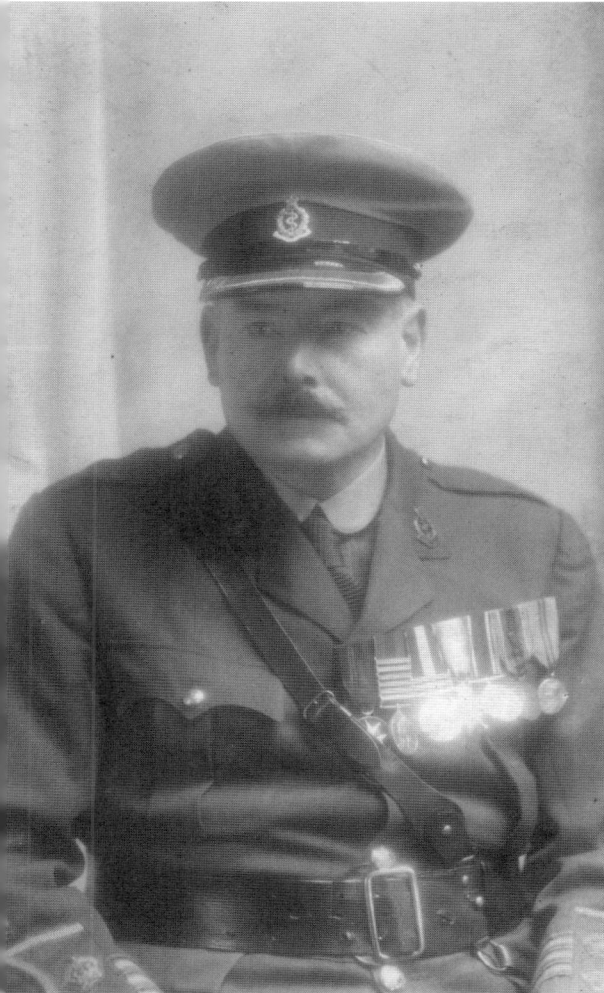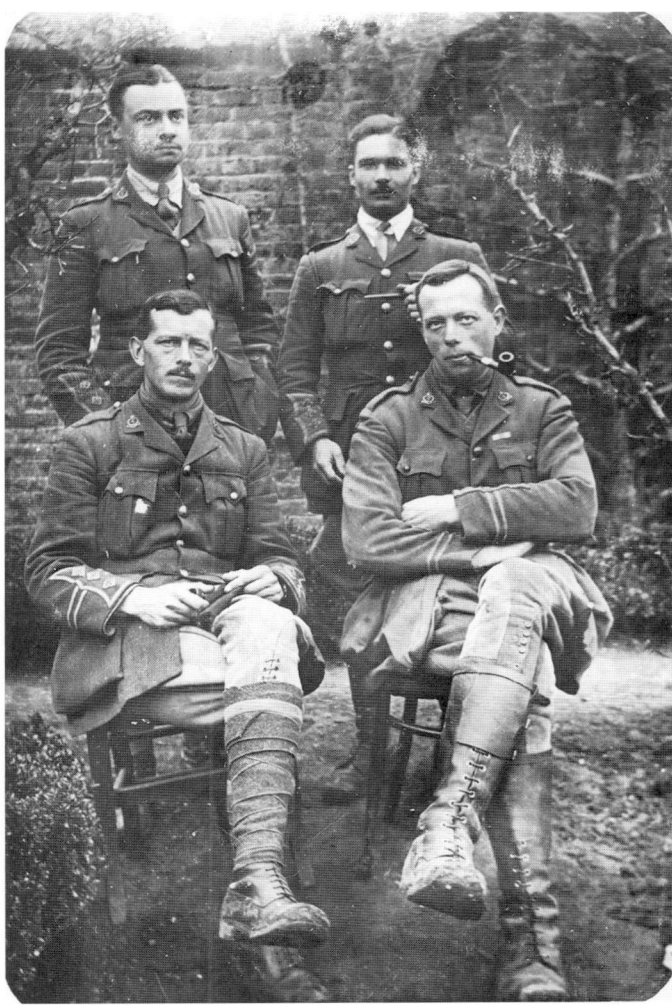

(**Opposite**) Postcard of Cologne posted by Private A. Hunter RAMC, 19 November 1919. In the message Private Hunter describes going on duty at No. 3 General Hospital.

(**Above, left**) A lieutenant colonel serving with the RAMC after the First World War. He wears First World War campaign medals in addition to the Order of St John, South African War campaign medals and the King George V Coronation Medal.

(**Above, right**) Dr George Bent Buckley (front right) and fellow RAMC officers, on the Western Front. Dr Buckley was born in Saddleworth. In 1912, at Manchester University, he qualified as a Member of the Royal College of Surgeons and as a Licentiate of the Royal College of Practitioners. He was awarded the Military Cross during the Battle of the Somme, at Flers, on 15 September 1916. The citation, published in the London Gazette, read: 'For conspicuous gallantry and devotion to duty. He tended and dressed the wounded under very heavy fire, displaying great courage and determination. He was wounded.' On 21 March 1918, whilst attached as medical officer to the 8th King's Royal Rifle Corps, he was taken prisoner of war. He was repatriated in January 1919. (*University of Manchester*)

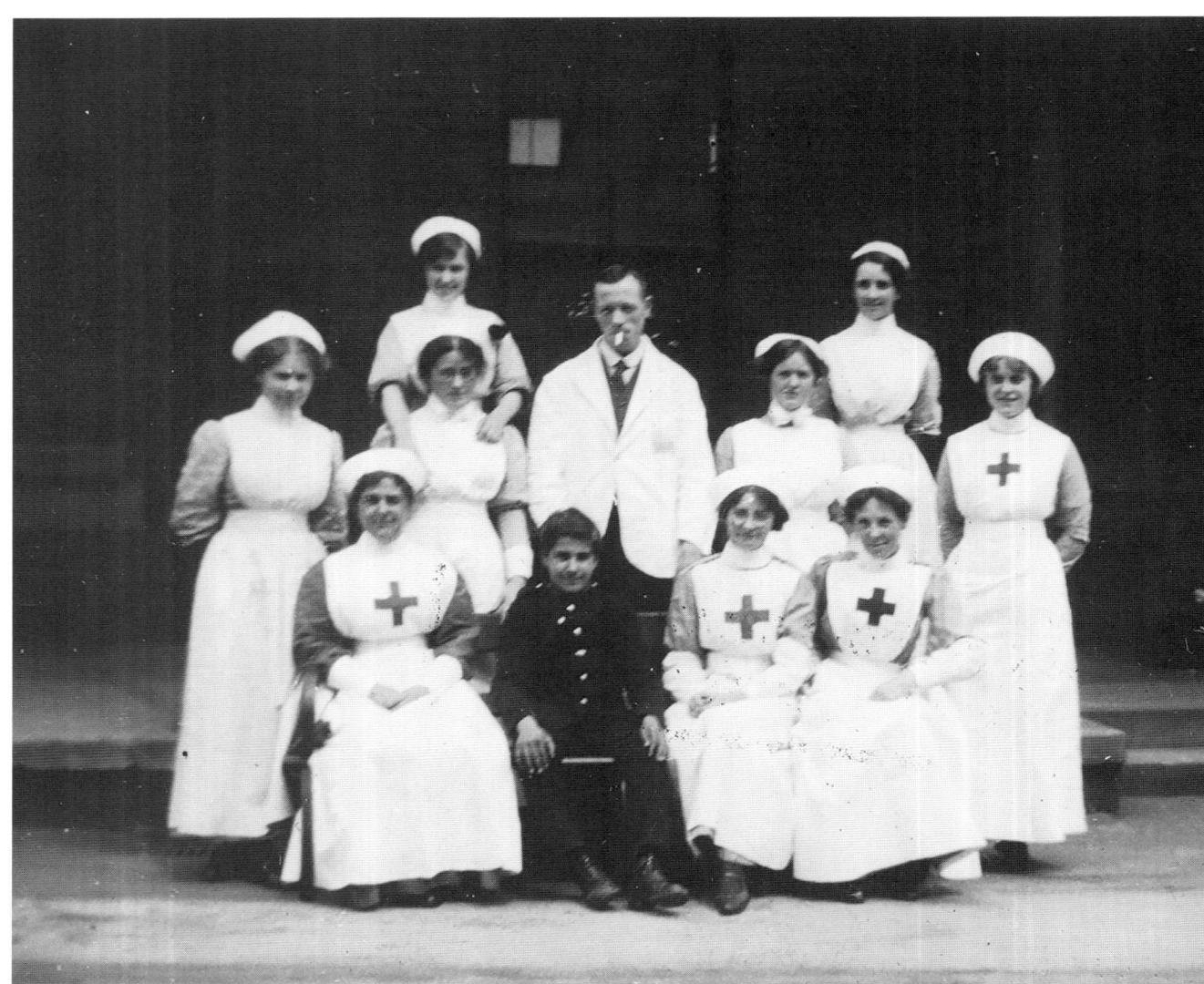

(**Above**) Dr George Bent Buckley (standing centre) with nursing staff. Prior to the First World War Dr Buckley worked at Manchester Royal Infirmary as an Accident Room House Surgeon and Senior House Surgeon. He was also a member of the Manchester Medical Society. In 1920 he was living in Greenfield and in 1921 in Weston-super-Mare. After he retired Dr Buckley became a celebrated cricket historian and an expert on the early history of the game. He died aged 77, on 26 April 1962 in Weston-super-Mare. *(University of Manchester)*

(**Opposite**) Following the First World War, veteran associations were formed by those who had served in RAMC units during the conflict. One such association was formed by veterans of the 4th London Field Ambulance, RAMC which held annual reunion dinners in the London area. This copy of the menu for the 4th London Field Ambulance RAMC reunion dinner of 1926 was signed by veterans of the unit. The back page of the menu included a brief summary of the service of the 4th London Field Ambulance RAMC on the Western Front.

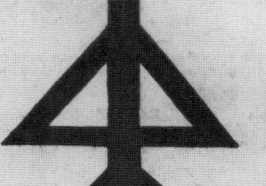

Fourth London — **4** — **Field Ambulance**

OLD COMRADES' ASSOCIATION

"Friendship Unfeigned but not Constraining."

EIGHTH

RE-UNION DINNER

TEMPLE BAR RESTAURANT,

Saturday, 20th March, 1926.

Major A. E. IRONSIDE, M.C., will preside
and will receive Members at 6.30 p.m.

ENGLAND.—August, 1914, to March 16th, 1915.
  Woolwich, Garston, Chelsea, Watford, Southampton.
FRANCE.—March 17th, 1915, to October 19th, 1916.
  Trek to the Front.—17.3.15 to 15.5.15.—Havre, Arques, St. Omer, Aires, Gauchy-à-la-Tour, Auchel, Rimbert, La Beuvrière (1st A.D.S. Essars, 7.5.15).
  Festubert.—15.5.15 to 31.5.15.
    Annezin-les-Bethune, Iodine House (Bearers in trenches collecting wounded for first time).
  Back at rest.—1.6.15 to 26.8.15.
    Drouvin, Alouagne, La Beuvrière (Divisional Sports).
  Loos Sector.—27.8.15 to 14.5.16.
    Noeux-les-Mines, Maroc, Les Brebis, Mazingarbe, Lone Tree, La Rutoire, Philosoph, Sailly Labourse (Xmas), Vermelles, Half-way House, Stansfield Road, The Hairpin.
    Lillers, Busnay.
  Vimy Ridge Sector.—15.3.16 to 26.7.16.
    Gauchin-le-Gal, Villers-au-Bois, Mont St. Eloi, Bethune Road, Death Valley, Quatre Vents, Sains-les-Mines, Bully Grenay, Estrée-Gauchy.
  Trek to the Somme.—26.7.16 to 14.9.16.
    Houdain, Grossart, Héricourt, Boffles, Conteville, Drucat, Bouchon, Naours, Beaucourt, Esbart, Franvillers (Rest Station).
  The Somme.—15.9.16 to 12.10.16.
    Fricourt, Bottom Wood, Flat-Iron Copse, Bazentin, High Wood Post, Cough Drop, Flers, Baucourt L'Abbaye, Butte de Warlencourt.
  Trek to Belgium.—13.10.16 to 20.10.16.
    Albert, Longprés, Bouchon, Caestre, Abeele, Boescheppe, Ouderdom.
BELGIUM.—(Ypres).—20.10.16 to 22.9.17.
  Brandhoek, Busseboom, Poperinghe, Reninghelst, Vlamertinghe, Voormezeele, Woodcote Farm, Bedford House, Bluff, Sunken Road, La Clytte, Westoutre, White Chateau, Cord Lane, Dickebush, Menin Road, Hell-fire Corner, Birr Cross Roads, Simon's Post, Bellewaarde Ridge.
FRANCE.—23.9.17 to the end (except for Tournai, etc., in Belgium).
  Arras Sector.—21.9.17 to 21.11.17.
    Maroeuil, Mont St. Eloi, Oppy.
  Trek, original destination Italy, but deflected to Cambrai (across desolate Somme country), 22.11.17 to 29.11.17.
    Montenescourt, Wanquetin, Courcelles, Beaulencourt, Doignies, Trescault.
  Cambrai Sector.—30.11.17 to 21.3.18.
    Havrincourt, Bourlon Wood, Hindenburg Line, Gun Pits Aid Post, Brick Kilns, The Retirement, Senlis (Xmas.), Heilly, Maricourt, Ytres, Lechelle.
  The Great Retreat.—22.3.18 to 29.3.18.
    Le Mesnil, Rocquigny, Les Boeufs, Le Transloy, Albert, Millencourt, Henencourt, Senlis, Bouzincourt, Louvencourt, Toutencourt, Raincheval, Warloy, Herrisart.
  The Stand at Aveluy Wood.—29.3.18 to 7.4.18.
    Englebelmer, Martinsart, Railway Dugout.
  The Long Wait.—8.4.18 to 30.8.18.
    Herrisart, St. Hilaire, Canchy, Warloy (Divisional Sports), Beaucourt, Mollens-au-Bois, Montigny, Saissemont, Querrieu, Méaulte.
  The Second Somme Attack.—30.8.18 to 7.9.18.
    Maricourt, Maurepas, Needle Wood (Division withdrawn early for Lille).
  Lille.—8.9.18 to 26.11.18.
    Heilly, Chocques, La Beuvrière, Belval, Listrem, Merville, Laventie, St. Venant, Rombly, Lomme, Fismes, Tressin, Kain, Tournai, Harbourdain.
  The Last Days.—From 27.11.18.
    The Long March, Harbourdin to Fonquières viâ La Bassee, 27.11.18.
    Auchel 28.11.18 to 20.3.19.
    Unit reduced to Cadre and transferred to Pernes, 20.3.19.
ENGLAND.—
  Southampton, 13.5.19; Lowestoft, 14.5.19.
  Last three men demobilised, 30.6.19.

THE TOASTMASTER WILL ASK THE COMPANY
TO STAND DURING THE SINGING OF GRACE.

Words by BURNS   "Grace"   Music—WALTER W. HEDGCOCK
    (FOR SOLO VOICE)
    MR. WILFRID PLATT

MENU

SOUP.

Consommé Julienne

Tomato

FISH.

Boiled Turbot   Lobster Sauce

JOINT.

Roast Lamb   Mint Sauce

VEGETABLES.

Boiled and Baked Potatoes   Cauliflower

SWEETS.

Compôte of Fruit

Ices

Cheese   Coffee

THE COMPANY WILL KINDLY REFRAIN FROM SMOKING
UNTIL AFTER THE FIRST TOAST—"THE KING"—IS GIVEN.

PROGRAMME.

Toast Master - Mr. O. PENNY

Accompanist - Mr. E. HAYWOOD

I. The KING - The President
    ("God Save the King")

II. Our GUESTS - The President

III. Our FALLEN COMRADES   Mr. R. H. Ridges
    "How sleep the Brave"   Mr. Wilfrid Platt
    (SAMUEL LIDDLE)

IV. Recollections of the War
    No. 3 A Plain Unvarnished Tale   Mr. J. W. WOOD
                                                 D.C.M.

V. Report by the Secretary

VI. The Toastmaster will endeavour to restrain us

VII. Auld Lang Syne

Au Revoir 19th March, 1927.

REGISTRATION. Please complete enclosed Form and send to the Hon. Secretary and Treasurer with a Booking Fee of 10/- per person. The whole cost may be paid at time of Registration if desired. If an acknowledgement is not received within 7 days, address inquiry to:—

Mr. W. N. DENOON,
84, Earlshall Road, Eltham, S.E.9

Please Register as early as possible, but in any event not later than 23rd FEBRUARY.

BALANCE OF FARE. May be paid by instalments of not less than 10/- but in order to allow adequate time for final detailed arrangements, the last payment must be made by March 7th, when lists will be closed.

PASSPORTS. No Passports, Photographs, or other means of identification are necessary.

LUGGAGE. Members are strongly advised to limit their luggage to an amount which can be handled at all points by themselves.

PROVINCIAL MEMBERS. For provincial members return tickets to London, tickets at reduced fares (fare and a half) will be available if required. Tickets or Vouchers will be supplied direct by:—

Messrs. THOS. COOK & SON, Ltd.
81, Cheapside, London, E.C.2.

To whom application together with covering payment for Railway Ticket should be made.

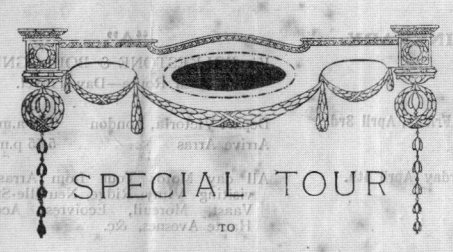

SPECIAL TOUR
to
ARRAS AND DISTRICT

EASTER 1931.

FOR MEMBERS OF THE

2/4th LONDON FIELD AMBULANCE

and R.A.S.C. Transport Section,

Their WIVES RELATIVES AND FRIENDS.

Under the direction of
Messrs. Thos COOK & SON, Ltd.
81, Cheapside, London, E.C 2

ITINERARY. "A"
Via FOLKESTONE & BOULOGNE.
Short Sea Route—Day Travel.

Good Friday, April 3rd.	Depart Victoria, London 9.0 a.m. Arrive Arras ... 5.55 p.m.
Saturday April 4th.	All day Motor Tour from Arras, visiting Vimy Ridge, Neuville-St-Vaast, Moreuil, Ecoivres, Acq, Haute Avesnes, &c.
Sunday, April 5th.	Day left free for members to spend as they wish.
Monday, April 6th.	Leave Arras ... 7.0 a.m. Arrive Victoria, London 3.30 p.m.

TRAVEL. Third Class England., Second Class Boat and France.

HOTEL ACCOMMODATION. Dinner on arrival at Arras, April 3rd. (Members should bring a packed luncheon for consumption on the outward journey)
Breakfast, Table d' Hote or packed Luncheon, Dinner and Bedroom on April 4th. and 5th.
Packed Lunch for Return Journey April 6th.

NOTE.—Will male members of the party please assist by filling in details respecting sleeping accommodation at foot of Registration Form. Endeavour will be made to give each lady a separate room, but similar details would be useful in the case of lady members of the party.
Married couples will be billeted together.

COST OF TOUR "A" £4-15-0 per person.
This covers all Rail and Boat Fares, Motor Excursion, Hotel Accommodation as shown, Service and Gratuities and all Expenses except those of a personal nature.

ITINERARY. "B"
Via TILBURY & DUNKIRK.
Long Sea Route—Night Travel.

Thursday April 2nd,	Depart St. Pancras, London 10.30 p.m
Good Friday, April 3rd.	Arrive Arras ... ... 9.15 a.m. Day left free for members to spend as they wish.
Saturday April 4th.	All day Motor Tour from Arras, Visiting Vimy Ridge, Neuville-St-Vaast, Moreuil, Ecoivres, Acq, Haute Avesnes, &c.
Sunday, April 5th.	Day left free for members to spend as they wish. Depart Arras 9.30 p.m.
Monday, April 6th	Arrive St. Pancras, London. 8.9 a.m.

TRAVEL Third Class England and Boat. Second Class France.

HOTEL ACCOMMODATION. Breakfast, Table d' Hote or packed Luncheon, Dinner and Bedroom on April 3rd, 4th and 5th.
(Members should make their own arrangements as to food on the night journeys, both outward and return.)

NOTE.—Will male members of the party please assist by filling in details respecting sleeping accommodation at foot of Registration Form. Endeavour will be made to give each lady a separate room, but similar details would be useful in the case of lady members of the party
Married couples will be billeted together.

COST OF TOUR "B" £3-14-6 per person.
This covers all Rail and Boat Fares, Motor Excursion, Hotel Accommodation as shown, Service and Gratuities and all expenses except those of a personal nature.

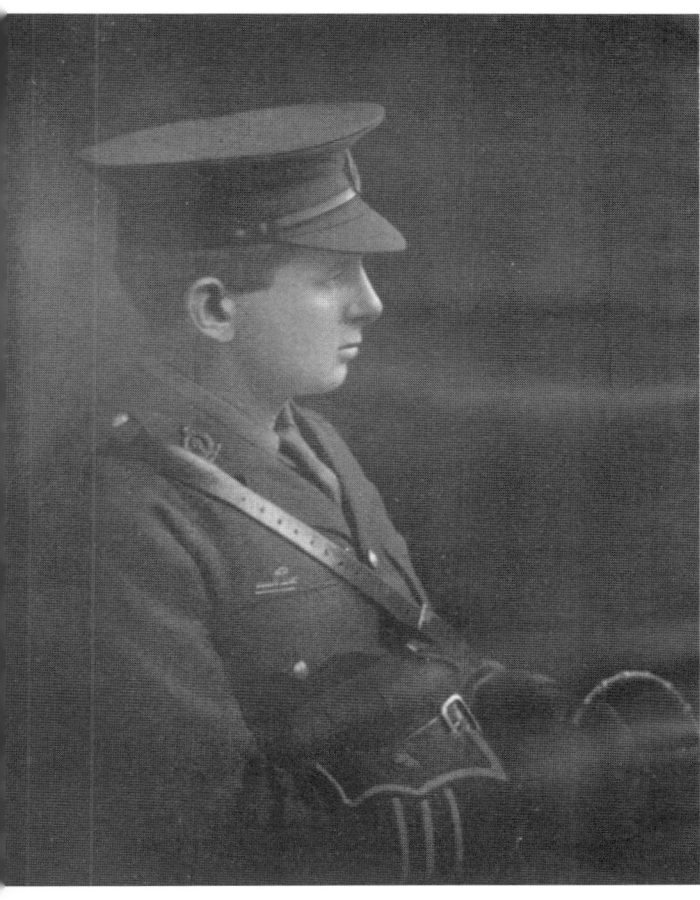

Lieutenant Colonel Thomas Bramley Layton, 2/4th London Field Ambulance, RAMC. Thomas Bramley Layton was born on 8 June 1882 and was educated at Bradfield College and Guy's Hospital Medical School, where he graduated in 1906 with honours. He became a Fellow of the Royal College of Surgeons in 1909. He was made surgical registrar at Guy's in 1908, specialising in otolaryngology (diseases of the ear and throat). In 1909 he married Miss Edney Eleanor Sampson, a nurse at Guy's and in 1912 travelled to study in Vienna and Berlin. Lieutenant Colonel Layton joined the Officers' Training Corps of London University, and was mobilized on the outbreak of war serving with the Territorial Force. He was on the Western Front from 22 June 1916, as the commanding officer of the 2/4th London Field Ambulance RAMC. He later commanded the unit in Salonika and the Middle East. In recognition of his services he was awarded the Distinguished Service Order and twice Mentioned in Despatches. He returned to Guy's soon after the end of the war as a throat and ear surgeon and was also appointed a consultant otologist to the London County Council, a post which he held until 1944. He was the first medical chairman of the London Insurance Committee. During the Second World War Lieutenant Colonel Layton became Director of Medical Services (DMS) in Sicily. Subsequently he served as Medical Superintendent of the hospital established by the United Nations Relief and Rehabilitation Administration (UNRRA) at Belsen Concentration Camp. He retired from Guy's in 1947 on reaching the age of 65. In recognition of the leading position that Dr Layton held in his specialty he was made Hunterian Professor of the Royal College of Surgeons in 1919; was awarded the John Hunter bronze medal and triennial prize for 1928–31 and delivered the Erasmus Wilson lecture in 1935. He had also been elected president of the laryngological section of the Royal Society of Medicine in 1939–41 and master of the Society of Apothecaries in 1940–41. His short book, *An Industry of Health* (1944), expressed his thoughts on how best to provide a comprehensive health service for the nation. Dr Layton died on 17 January 1964.

(**Opposite**) In the years following the First World War veterans also arranged to visit the battle areas where they served. In 1931 veterans of the 2/4th London Field Ambulance RAMC arranged a tour to visit the Arras area, where they had been during 1916. The itinerary of the 1931 tour arranged for veterans of the 2/4th London Field Ambulance RAMC, provides details of the travel arrangements and the areas which would be visited.

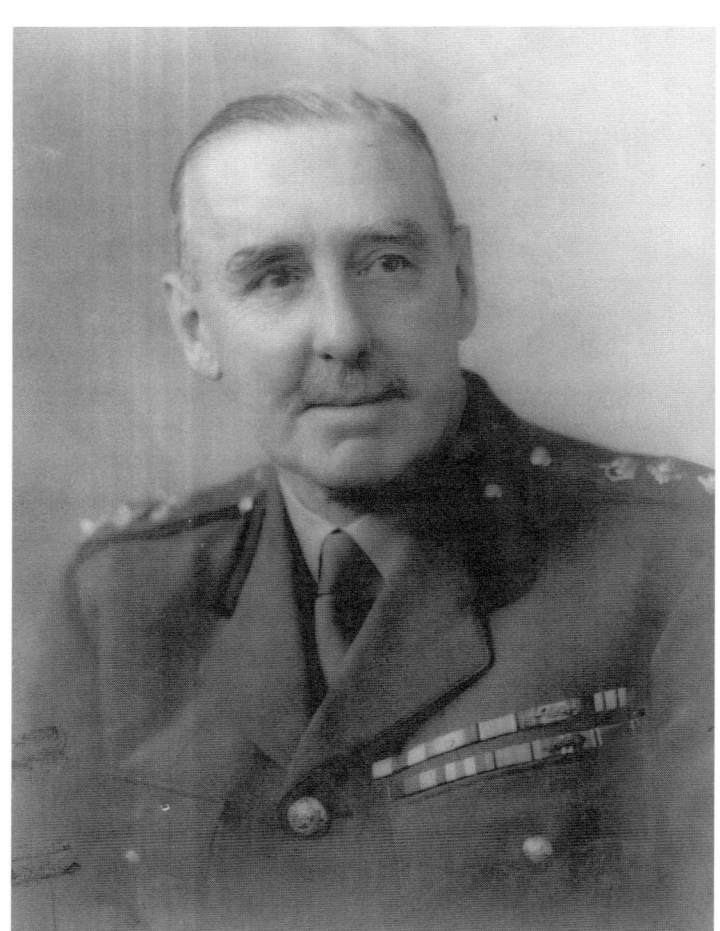 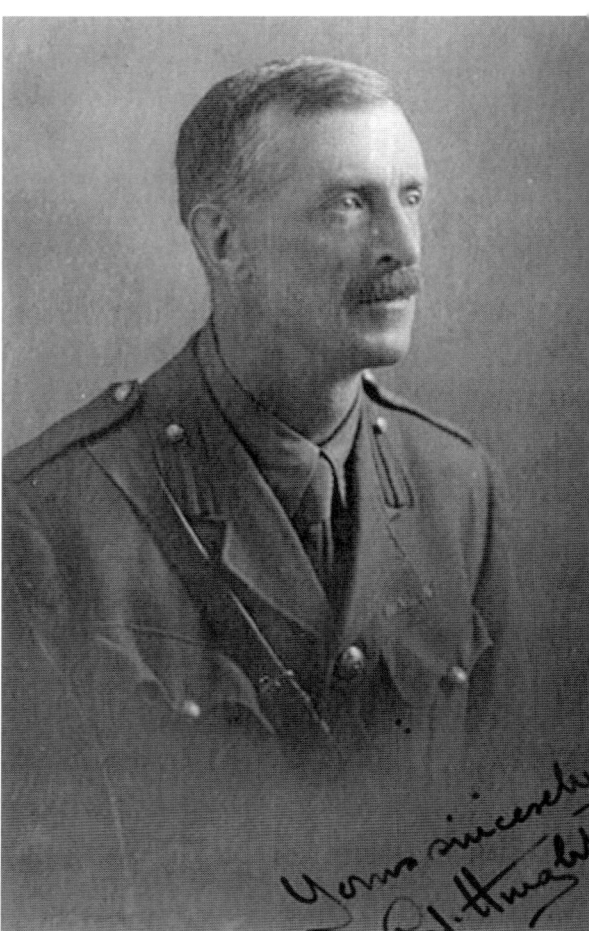

(**Above, left**) Charles Dudley Maybury Buckley was born at Glengeary, Ireland in December 1890 and qualified in medicine in Dublin. Commissioned as a second lieutenant in the Royal Army Medical Corps in August 1914, he embarked for France that October and remained on the Western Front until 1917, when he transferred to the Italian Front in the acting rank of major. For services during the First World War he was awarded the Military Cross and Mentioned in Despatches. Seconded to the Colonial Office in 1919, Major Buckley embarked for East Africa and served in the Somaliland operations of 1920, prior to taking up a post as a specialist in pathology in India, where he was promoted to substantive major in August 1926. Latterly employed there as Deputy Assistant Director of Pathology in Baluchistan District 1928–30, and at the Enteric Laboratory in Kasauli, he returned home in 1933, to take up appointment as Pathological Specialist at the Royal Victoria Hospital, Netley. Having then served again in India – as a lieutenant colonel and Deputy Assistant Director of Pathology in Madras 1936–38 – he was appointed Assistant Director of Pathology in Southern Command in 1938. On the outbreak of the Second World War he was serving as Assistant Director of Hygiene and Pathology at GHQ. In 1941 Dr Buckley re-embarked for India, where he served in the rank of colonel as commanding officer of the British Military Hospital at Bangalore, following which, in 1944, he returned to the UK to take up an appointment as commanding officer of the military hospital at Shenley. In 1945 he was appointed Commanding Officer of 111 General Hospital in North-West Europe. In recognition of his service in North-West Europe he was awarded the Belgian Order of Leopold I and Mentioned in Despatches. An award recommendation noted: 'Colonel Buckley has been responsible for running one of the most important British General Hospitals in BLA since 29 January 1945. This 1200 bedded hospital has handled a very large number of cases of an extremely complex variety of types. These include specialist departments for the treatment of prisoners of war, Belgian Type A forces and cases of venereal disease. The high standard of administrative arrangements in the hospital and the keenness and enthusiasm of the staff are directly attributable to the example in zeal and energy set by the Commanding Officer. This officer's consistent devotion to duty has thus been a material contribution to the acknowledged successful treatment of many hundreds of hospital cases.' Colonel Buckley was placed on the Retired List in February 1947, having ended his career as commanding officer of Cambridge Military Hospital at Aldershot. He died in London in June 1961.

(**Opposite, right**) Colonel George John Houghton was born at Rathmines, Dublin in September 1873. After studying medicine, he was commissioned as a lieutenant in the RAMC in April 1900. He served in South Africa, during operations in the Transvaal and the Orange River Colony. Promoted to captain in April 1903 and to major in January 1912, during this time he served in India and West Africa. Colonel Houghton served on the Western Front from May 1915, where he commanded the 112th Field Ambulance from December 1915 until May 1918. Whilst in command of 112th Field Ambulance he recorded the movements and services of the Field Ambulance in the unit War Diary. The 112th Field Ambulance was with the 16th (Irish) Division on the Western Front. The War Diary records services of the unit when the 112th Field Ambulance was out of the front line area, including medical support for local civilians and refugees, work to treat scabies, the training of other units and the building of dressing stations. On 9 April 1916, representing a typical day whilst the unit was stationed at Noeux-les-Mines supporting the 16th Division in the front line, Colonel Houghton noted: 'Admitted 1 officer wounded; Admitted 24 other ranks wounded; Admitted 15 other ranks sick. Two high explosive shells exploded in garden beside Ambulance Headquarters. Urinals damaged by earth shower – no casualties.' The War Diary also details the medical support the 112th Field Ambulance provided during major operations including during the gas attack at Hulluch in April 1915; during the Battle of the Somme at Guillemont and Ginchy in September 1916; at Messines in June 1917; at Langemarck during August 1917 and during the German Spring Offensive of 1918. During each of these operations, and when the 16th Division was holding the front line, the field ambulance treated large numbers of casualties. An example of the challenges it faced was recorded on 7 June 1917, the first day of the Battle of Messines; the first cases arrived around 5.00am and by 11.30pm 445 casualties had been treated, including six German prisoners of war. On 16 August 1917, when the unit was providing support during the Battle of Langemarck, during the day around 1,400 casualties passed through the unit; 575 were from units serving with the 16th Division. During these battles Colonel Houghton treated casualties in main dressing stations and advanced dressing stations and he records visiting the front line trenches to ensure all casualties had been evacuated. From May 1918 Colonel Houghton served as Assistant Director of Medical Services in the 30th Division and was promoted to the acting rank of colonel. For his services during the First World War, he was awarded the Distinguished Service Order, the Belgian *Croix de Guerre* and was twice Mentioned in Despatches. He served in Iraq during 1919–20, where he commanded a Field Ambulance and was Mentioned in Despatches, then in India 1919–25, in the British Army of the Rhine 1925–26 and in Egypt 1926–28. He was placed on the Retired List, in the rank of colonel, in September 1928. Colonel Houghton died at Farnham Royal, Buckinghamshire in November 1946.

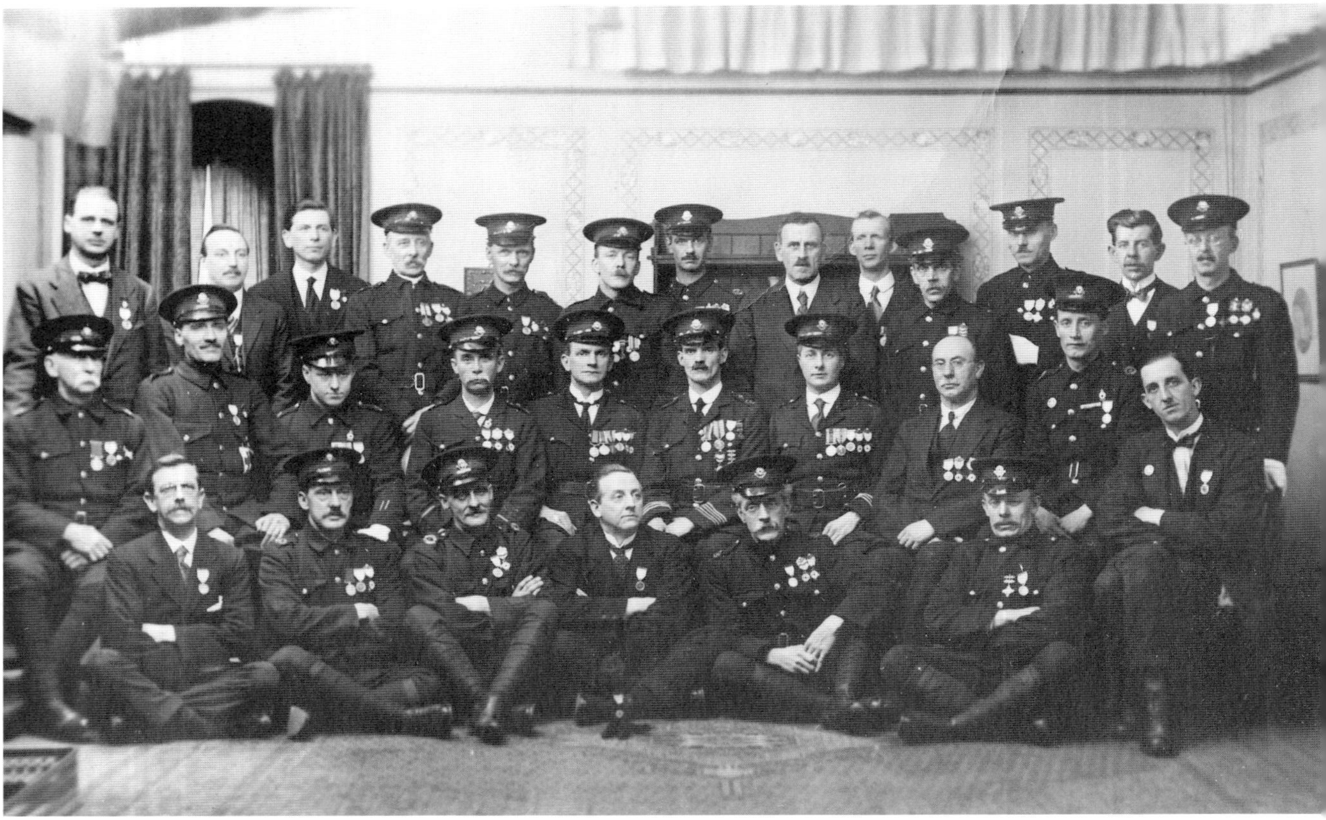

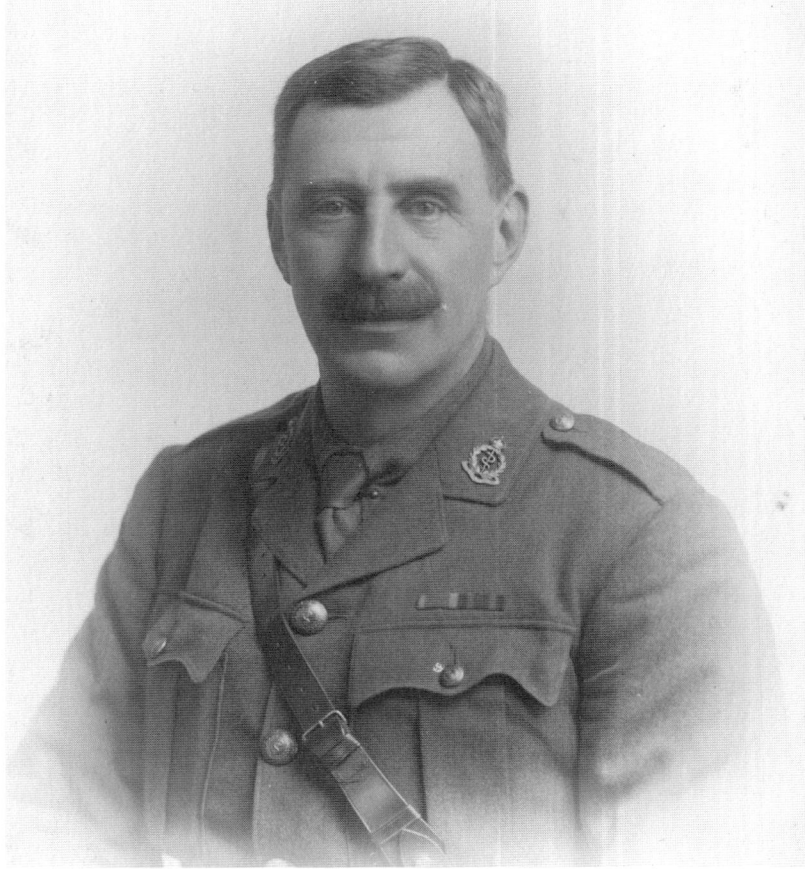

Red Cross volunteers photographed after the conflict wearing First World War service medals. During the war Red Cross volunteers served in the UK and overseas, supporting the RAMC and nursing services. Some also volunteered to serve with RAMC units.

Colonel George John Houghton, DSO, RAMC, on the Western Front, early 1918. He is wearing the medal ribbons of the Distinguished Service Order and the Queen's South Africa Medal.

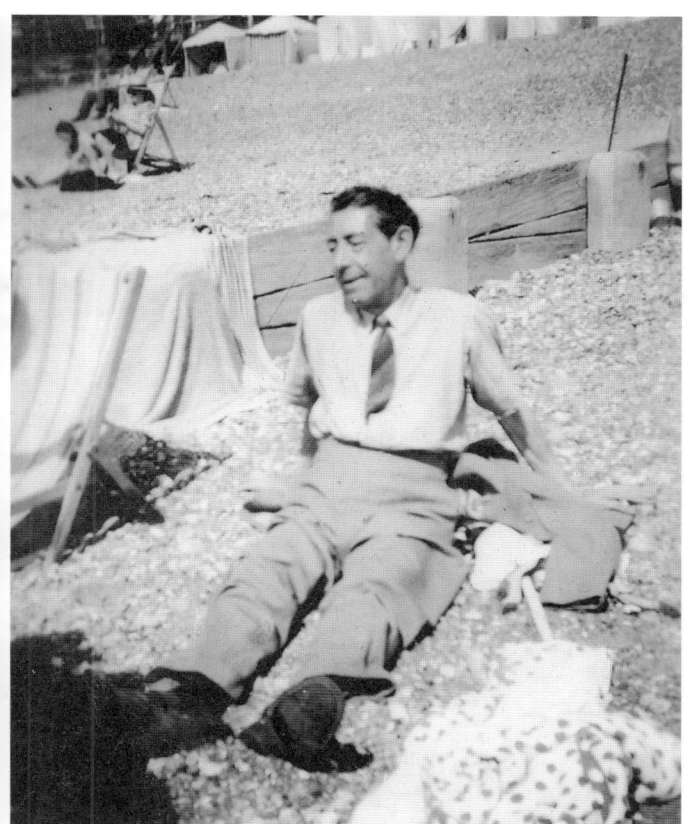 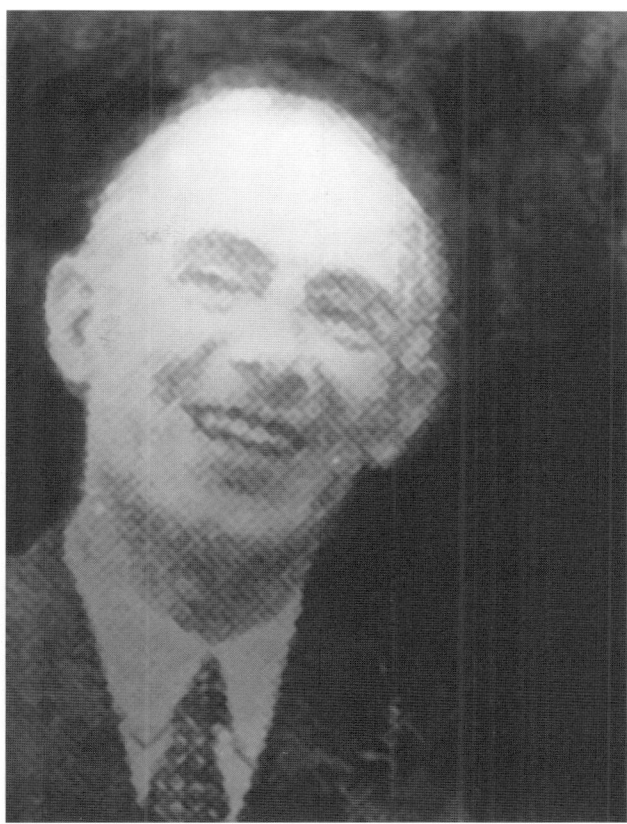

(**Left**) Norman Beyfus, photographed at Bexhill in 1949. Norman Beyfus was born on 29 March 1891. In 1911, aged 20, he was living with his uncle and aunts in London and working as a wool broker's assistant. During the First World War he served overseas with the 1st London Field Ambulance, RAMC (TF), enlisting on 3 August 1914, the day before the declaration of war. He was discharged on 26 March 1919, with a Silver War Badge, having suffered illness or wounds during his service with the RAMC. On 2 August 1923 he sailed for Montreal, from Southampton, on board the SS *Melita*, giving his occupation as a harvester and his address as Daisy Lodge, Holmwood, Surrey. On 18 November 1923 he returned on board the SS *Andania*, giving his occupation as a farmer. In 1926 he married Florence Barker in Chelsea. From the 1930s Norman Beyfus wrote a number of published poetry collections including *Sedlescombe and Other Verse* and *Through a Mist*. He died in Hastings in 1975.

(**Right**) Dr Andrew Fisher Calwell qualified as a Batchelor of Medicine and Surgery at Edinburgh University in 1912. During the early part of his career he worked as a Clinical Assistant at the Crichton Royal Institution, Dumfries and as a House Surgeon at York County Hospital. He also worked at the Thomas Hope Hospital in Langholm, Dumfriesshire. In 1915, he was living at 8 Charles Street New, Langholm. Prior to his service in the RAMC, early in the First World War, Dr Calwell was medical Officer at Langholm Red Cross Auxiliary Hospital; joint medical officer at the Eskdale Fever Hospital and joint medical officer for examining military recruits from the Langholm area. These responsibilities were in addition to his role as a General Practitioner in Langholm. Whilst serving with the RAMC on the Western Front, attached to the 13th Battalion of the King's Royal Rifle Corps, Lieutenant Calwell was awarded the Military Cross for treating wounded soldiers. On 10 December 1919 the citation for his award was published in the *London Gazette*: 'For gallantry and devotion to duty during the attack on Louvignies on 4th November 1918. He attended to the wounded under very heavy shell fire and subsequently removed them to a place of safety. Later, he went through a barrage and remained dressing them in the open for two hours until all had been attended to'. Returning to Langholm after the First World War, he resumed his role as a General Practitioner, working in the area until 1939. (*Ms Brenda Morrison and the Langholm Archive Group*)

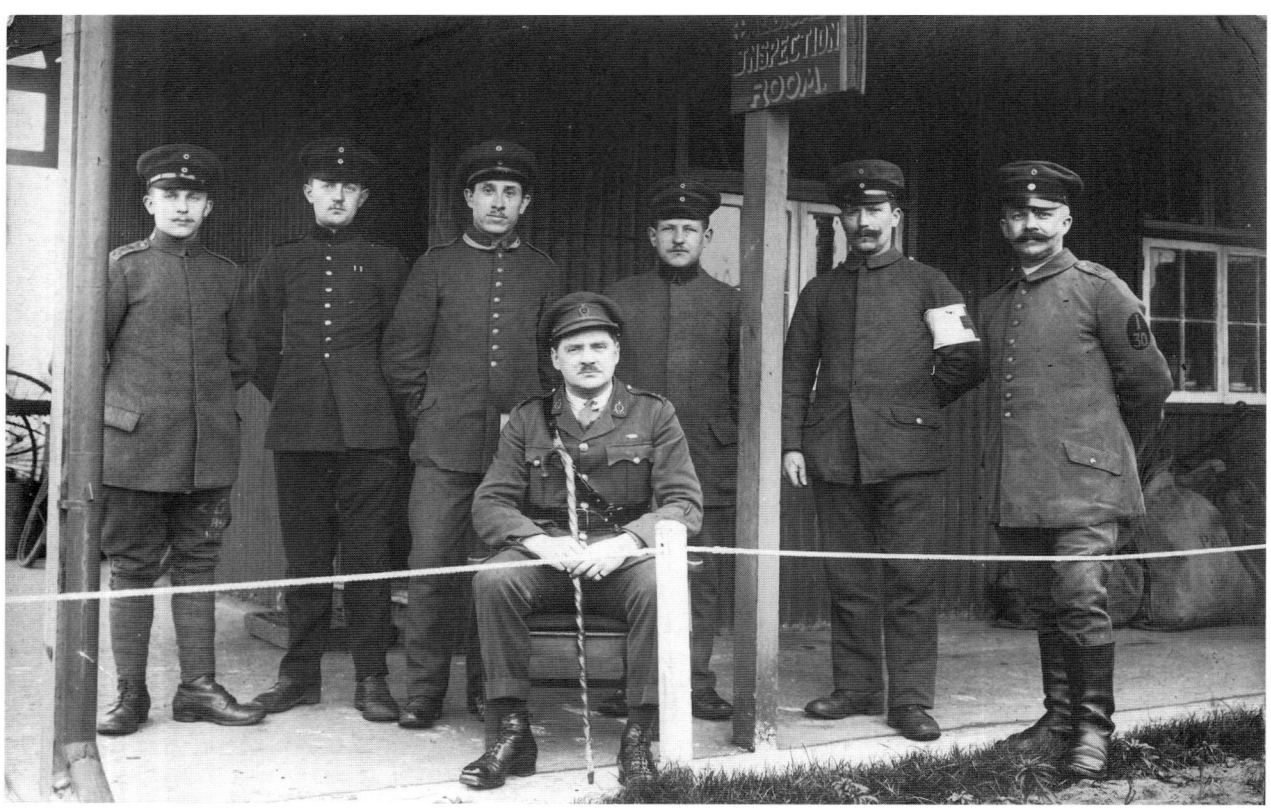

Captain Thomson, RAMC, and German Army Medical Staff, Le Havre, France, March 1919. They are photographed under a Medical Inspection Room sign. The German army medical personnel, taken prisoner on the Western Front, would have been providing medical support with the RAMC prior to their return to Germany.

Bibliography

Primary Sources
The Annandale Herald and Moffat News
The Annandale Observer
Dumfries and Galloway Courier and Herald
Dumfries & Galloway Standard & Advertiser
The Eskdale and Liddesdale Advertiser
The London Gazette
RAMC unit war diaries
Military records of service personnel
Census entries
Medical Directory entries

Secondary Sources
Chappell, Mike and Westlake, Ray, *British Territorial Units 1914–18* (Oxford: Osprey Publishing Ltd., 1991).

Macpherson, Major General Sir W.G., *Medical Services General History – Official Medical History of the War, Volumes I–IV* (Uckfield: The Naval & Military Press in association with the Army Medical Services Museum, facsimile edition, 2015).

Mitchell, Major T.J. and Smith, Miss G.M., *Casualties and Medical Statistics of the Great War* (Uckfield: The Naval & Military Press in association with the Imperial War Museum, facsimile edition, 2010).

Penny, Anne, *Ambulance Flotilla* (Blurb Inc., 2014).

Westlake, Ray, *Kitchener's Army* (Tunbridge Wells: The Nutshell Publishing Co. Ltd., 1989).

Websites
RAMC in the Great War – www.ramc-ww1.com
The American Hospital of Paris – www.american-hospital.org
The Commonwealth War Graves Commission – www.cwgc.org
The Queen Alexandra's Royal Army Nursing Corps – www.qaranc.co.uk